Information Management

IN

nursing
and
health care

Mary Etta C. Mills, ScD, RN, CNAA
Chair, Department of Education, Administration, Health Policy and Informatics
School of Nursing
University of Maryland at Baltimore

Carol A. Romano, PhD, RN, FAAN
Director, Clinical Systems and Quality Improvement
Clinical Center
National Institutes of Health

Barbara R. Heller, EdD, RN, FAAN
Dean and Professor
School of Nursing
University of Maryland at Baltimore

Springhouse Corporation
Springhouse, Pennsylvania

Senior Publisher
Minnie B. Rose, RN, BSN, MEd

Clinical Consultants
Patricia Dwyer Schull, RN, MSN; Franklin A. Shaffer, RN, EdD, DSc

Art Director
John Hubbard

Senior Associate Art Director
Stephanie Peters

Designer
Cindy Marczuk

Copy Editor
Janet Hodgson

Associate Acquisitions Editor
Betsy K. Snyder

Editorial Assistant
Stephanie Franchetti

Manufacturing
Deborah Meiris (director), T.A. Landis

Printed in the United States of America. For information, write Springhouse Corporation, 1111 Bethlehem
Pike, P.O. Box 908, Springhouse, PA 19477-0908.

IMNHC-020296

A member of the Reed Elsevier plc group

**Library of Congress Cataloging-in-
Publication Data**

Mills, Mary Etta.
    Information management in nursing and
health care/Mary Etta Mills, Carol A. Romano,
Barbara R. Heller.
    p. cm.
    Includes index.
    1. Nursing informatics. 2. Medical
informatics. I. Romano, Carol Ann. II. Heller,
Barbara R. (Barbara Roxanne), 1940- . III.
Title.
    [DNLM: 1. Information Systems—
organization & administration. 2. Nursing Care.
3. Nursing. WY 26.5 M657i 1996]
RT50.5.M555 1996
610.73'0285—dc20
DNLM/DLC
ISBN 0-87434-835-8
                                    95-21318
                                    CIP

Contents

Contributors vi

I. Introduction

A Conceptual Basis for Information Management in Nursing and Health Care 2
Carol A. Romano, PhD, RN, FAAN; Mary Etta C. Mills, ScD, RN, CNAA;
Barbara R. Heller, EdD, RN, FAAN

II. Establishing a Data Base for Decisions

√A Model for Defining Nursing Information System Requirements 7
Carole A. Gassert, PhD, RN

√Standardizing Nursing Language for Computerization 16
Joanne Comi McCloskey, PhD, RN, FAAN

√ One Nursing Minimum Data Set: A Key to Nursing's Future 28
Rhonda Anderson, MPA, RN, CNAA, FAAN

√ Significance of the Nursing Minimum Data Set for Decision Support in Acute Care 32
Connie Delaney, PhD, RN

The Omaha System: A Data Base for Ambulatory and Home Care 39
Karen A. Martin, MSN, RN, FAAN

√Decision-Support Systems for Nurse Managers 45
Nancy K. Meehan, PhD, RN

III. Strategies for Managing Information Systems

Information Systems: Use in Strategic Planning and in a Managed Competitive
Environment 56
Mary Etta C. Mills, ScD, RN, CNAA; Barbara R. Heller, EdD, RN, FAAN;
Carol A. Romano, PhD, RN, FAAN

Joint Commission on Accreditation of Healthcare Organizations: Standards for
Information Systems 64
Carole H. Patterson, MN, RN

Applying Technology Assessment to Information Systems 74
Barbara A. Happ, PhD, RN

Organizational Impact of Information Systems 83
Carol A. Romano, PhD, RN, FAAN

Choices of Nursing Systems 92
  Shirley Hughes, RN

Benefits Management 99
  Barbara J. Hoehn, MBA, RN

Systems Design and Implementation: Team Building Between Nurse Executive and
Vendor 108
  Linda Edmunds, MS, RN

The Nursing Manager's Role in Successful System Implementation 116
  Patricia A. Abbott, MS, RN

Training Issues in System Implementation 128
  Rita D. Zielstorff, MS, RN, FAAN, FACMI

IV. Strategies and Support for Managing Clinical Information

The Computer-Based Patient Record 138
  D. Kathy Milholland, PhD, RN; Barbara R. Heller, EdD, RN, FAAN

Technology and Case Management 144
  Roy L. Simpson, RN,C; Carol Falk, MS, RN

Information Systems to Measure the Cost/Quality of Patient-Centered Outcomes 153
  Alexis A. Wilson, MPH, RN

Using the Computer to Measure Outcomes of Nursing Care 167
  Mary S. Tilbury, EdD, RN, CNAA

Electronic Networking for Nurses 174
  Susan M. Sparks, PhD, RN, FAAN

New Electronic Health Care Community: The Denver Free-Net 181
  Diane J. Skiba, PhD, RN; Drew T. Mirque, BA

Quality Improvement via Clinical Information Systems 193
  Carol A. Romano, PhD, RN, FAAN

V. Strategies and Support for Managing Administrative Information

Integration of Managed Care with Information Systems 200
  Bonita Ann Pilon, DSN, RN, CNNA; Maria Hill, MS, RN

Maximizing Technology for Cost-Effective Staff Education and Training 216
  Susan K. Newbold, MS, RN

The Value of Bedside Computer Systems in Restructuring Nursing Care 222
  Karen E. Dennis, PhD, RN

Communication Technologies for Nurse Executives 230
  LTC(P) Nancy T. Staggers, PhD, RN (Army Nurse Corps)

Nurse-Designed Voice-Activated Computer Systems for Nursing Documentation 239
  Joan Trofino, EdD, RN, FAAN

Automated Systems for Staffing, Scheduling and Resource Management 245
  P.J. Maddox, EdD, RN, CNAA

VI. Professional Perspectives on Information Issues

Ethical Issues in the Management of Patient Data: Maintaining Confidentiality in a
Reformed Health Care System 257
  Sara T. Fry, PhD, RN, FAAN; Gail Ann DeLuca Havens, MS, RN, CNA

Confidentiality: Computer Security and Data Protection 264
  Patricia C. McMullen, MS, JD, RNC; Nayna C. Philipsen, PhD, JD, RN

The Role of the Professional Association in Policy Development Related to
Information Standards 272
  D. Kathy Milholland, PhD, RN

Standards of Practice and Preparation for Certification 280
  Teresa L. Panniers, PhD, RN, CRNP; Carole A. Gassert, PhD, RN

Nursing Informatics: Education for a New Specialty and Career 288
  Barbara R. Heller, EdD, RN, FAAN; Mary Etta C. Mills, ScD, RN, CNAA;
  Carol A. Romano, PhD, RN, FAAN

Research Focus Areas in Informatics 295
  Carol A. Romano, PhD, RN, FAAN; Barbara R. Heller, EdD, RN, FAAN;
  Mary Etta C. Mills, ScD, RN, CNNA

A Global Perspective on the Future of Informatics 303
  Marion J. Ball, EdD

Index 309

Contributors

Patricia A. Abbott, MS, RN
Clinical Specialist for Information
Systems
Geriatric Research Education Clinical
Center (GRECC)
Baltimore Veterans Administration
Medical Center
Baltimore, Maryland

**Rhonda Anderson, MPA, RN, CNAA,
FAAN**
Vice-President of Patient Operations
Hartford Hospital
Hartford, Connecticut

Marion J. Ball, EdD
Vice President for Information Services
University of Maryland at Baltimore
Baltimore, Maryland

Connie W. Delaney, PhD, RN
Associate Professor
College of Nursing
The University of Iowa
Iowa City, Iowa

Karen E. Dennis, PhD, RN
Chief for Nursing Research, Nursing Service
Baltimore Department of Veterans Affairs
Medical Center
Associate Professor, School of Nursing
University of Maryland at Baltimore
Baltimore, Maryland

Linda Edmunds, MS, RN
Director of Design
Highland Reserves, Inc.
Atlanta, Georgia

Carol Falk, MS, RN
Professional Nurse Case Management/Patient
Care Services
Carondelet St. Mary's Hospital and Health Center
Tucson, Arizona

Sara T. Fry, PhD, RN, FAAN
Henry R. Luce Professor of Ethics
School of Nursing
Boston College
Boston, Massachusetts

Carole A. Gassert, PhD, RN
Assistant Professor
Department of Education, Administration,
Health Policy and Informatics
School of Nursing
University of Maryland at Baltimore
Baltimore, Maryland

Barbara A. Happ, PhD, RN
Senior Consultant in Healthcare Information
Services
Hamilton/KSA
Fairfax, Virginia

Gail Ann DeLuca Havens, MS, RN, CNA
Doctoral Candidate, Nursing Ethics
School of Nursing
University of Maryland at Baltimore
Baltimore, Maryland

Barbara R. Heller, EdD, RN, FAAN
Professor and Dean
School of Nursing
University of Maryland at Baltimore
Baltimore, Maryland

Maria Hill, MS, RN
Senior Consultant
The Center for Case Management
South Natick, Massachusetts

Barbara J. Hoehn, MBA, RN
Senior Manager
KPMG Peat Marwick
New York, New York

Shirley Hughes, RN
Principal
SJ Hughes Consulting
Chandler, Arizona

P.J. Maddox, EdD, RN, CNAA
Associate Professor
College of Nursing and Health Sciences
George Mason University
Fairfax, Virginia

Karen A. Martin, MSN, RN, FAAN
Health Care Consultant
Omaha, Nebraska

Joanne Comi McCloskey, PhD, RN, FAAN
Distinguished Professor of Nursing
College of Nursing
Adjunct Associate Director
University of Iowa Hospitals and Clinics
The University of Iowa
Iowa City, Iowa

Patricia C. McMullen, MS, JD, RNC
Uniform Services University
Washington, D.C.

Nancy K. Meehan, PhD, RN
Assistant Professor
Department of Nursing Science
Clemson University
Clemson, South Carolina

D. Kathy Milholland, PhD, RN
Senior Policy Fellow, Research and Databases
Department of Practice, Economics and Policy
American Nurses Association
Washington, D.C.

Mary Etta C. Mills, ScD, RN, CNAA
Associate Professor and Chair
Department of Nursing Education,
Administration, Health Policy and Informatics
School of Nursing
University of Maryland at Baltimore
Baltimore, Maryland

Drew T. Mirque, BA
Project Administrator
University of Colorado Health Sciences Center
Denver, Colorado

Susan K. Newbold, MS, RN
Doctoral Student, Nursing Informatics
University of Maryland at Baltimore
Baltimore, Maryland

Teresa L. Panniers, PhD, RN, CRNP
Assistant Professor
Department of Nursing Education,
Administration, Health Policy and Informatics
School of Nursing
University of Maryland at Baltimore
Baltimore, Maryland

Carole H. Patterson, MN, RN
Associate Director, Standards Development
Department of Performance Measures
Development
Joint Commission for Accreditation of Healthcare
Organizations
Oakbrook Terrace, Illinois

Nayna C. Philipsen, PhD, RN, JD
Compliance Analyst
Board of Physicians
Quality Assurance
Baltimore, Maryland

Bonita Ann Pilon, DSN, RN, CNNA
Assistant Professor
Director, Nursing Administration Program
School of Nursing
Vanderbilt University
Nashville, Tennessee

Carol A. Romano, PhD, RN, FAAN
Director, Clinical Systems and Quality
Improvement
Clinical Center
National Institutes of Health
Bethesda, Maryland

Roy L. Simpson, RN,C
Executive Director, Nursing Affairs
HBO and Company
Atlanta, Georgia

Diane J. Skiba, PhD, RN
Associate Professor and Director of Informatics
Center for Nursing Research
University of Colorado Health Sciences Center
Denver, Colorado

Susan M. Sparks, PhD, RN, FAAN
Research Education Specialist
Educational Technology Branch
National Library of Medicine
Lister Hill Center
Bethesda, Maryland

LTC(P) Nancy T. Staggers, PhD, RN
Deputy Director for Clinical Policy Support
Health Affairs, Health Services Operations
Office of the Assistant Secretary of Defense
Washington, D.C.

Mary S. Tilbury, EdD, RN, CNAA
Assistant Professor
Department of Nursing Education,
Administration, Health Policy and Informatics
School of Nursing
University of Maryland at Baltimore
Baltimore, Maryland

Joan Trofino, EdD, RN, FAAN
Vice President, Patient Care Services
Riverview Medical Center
Red Bank, New Jersey

Alexis A. Wilson, MPH, RN
President, Wilson & Associates
Outcome Concept Systems
Gig Harbor, Washington

Rita D. Zielstorff, MS, RN, FAAN, FACMI
Assistant Director, Laboratory of Computer
Science
Associate Computer Scientist, Department of
Medicine
Staff Specialist, Department of Nursing
Massachusetts General Hospital
Boston, Massachusetts

Introduction

A Conceptual Basis for Information Management in Nursing and
Health Care 2

A Conceptual Basis for Information Management in Nursing and Health Care

Carol A. Romano, PhD, RN, FAAN
Director, Clinical System and Quality Improvement
National Institutes of Health Clinical Center

Mary Etta C. Mills, ScD, RN, CNAA
Chair and Associate Professor
Department of Education, Administration, Health Policy and Informatics
School of Nursing
University of Maryland at Baltimore

Barbara R. Heller, EdD, RN, FAAN
Dean and Professor
School of Nursing
University of Maryland at Baltimore

Introduction

The delivery of health care services is a complex endeavor that depends extensively on information. Information is needed about the science of care, the patient, the provider, the outcomes, and the processes and systems for the delivery of health care. Because health services are provided by many individuals, disciplines, and specialists, the information related to these services must be integrated, coordinated and managed. The management of information is a central component of the ongoing operations and strategic decisions made within organizations and agencies that focus on delivering health care; it plays a significant role in the rapidly changing and evolving delivery systems of the future (National Center for Nursing Research, 1993).

Information Management

Information management is a function that focuses on meeting an individual's or organization's need for meaningful data or information. This function includes a set of processes and activities directed to acquire needed information, to transmit, to store, to represent, to assimilate and to use information in an economical, efficient and productive way (Joint Commission for Accreditation of Healthcare Organizations, 1994). Information as a concept consists of three aspects—data, information, and knowledge. Information in this generic sense is considered a critical phenomenon of study for information based disciplines such as nursing (Graves and Corcoran, 1989).

From this perspective, data is defined as discrete entities objectively described, without interpretation or context. Data that are interpreted, organized, structured and given meaning are referred to as information. Information that has been synthesized in such a way so as to create formalized, identifiable relationships is referred to as knowledge. Knowledge is used both in making decisions as well as in making new discoveries and can be thought of as data and information transformed into decision and discoveries. This transformation of data or information from one form to another is referred to by Graves and Corcoran (1989) as processing. Information, in the generic sense, then, needs to be managed (aggregated, organized, transmitted, etc.) so that it can be transferred or processed to support appropriate decision making.

It is noted that information is conceptualized as data that are structured so as to create meaning. It is the meaningfulness of the data, not its structure alone, that allows for the support of decision making. The "informated" health care provider, or the "informated" work environment, then, is the person or area through which information circulates for the purpose of the expansion of knowledge—knowledge in terms of what it means to be productive in delivering or managed health care and or services (Zuboff, 1984). The goal of information management, then, is to improve the effectiveness of the data assimilation, interpretation, and representation so that informed decisions are made.

Framework

The paradigm of fueling the transformation of data into information to create the expansion of knowledge forms the conceptual framework for information management in nursing and health care. The content of the information reflects the clinical or administrative aspects required in the delivery of health care or the management of delivery systems. The extent to which information is successfully managed is measured by the extent to which appropriate decisions are made and knowledge and learning occur.

A study of information management in nursing and/or health care encompasses a study of five dimensions—1) the data base required, 2) the strategy to manage the transformation of data, and the systems/processes that channel it, 3) the clinical content of data, and the core purposes for which data is collected, 4) the administrative systems which support the core purpose, and 5) the context,—the social, political, legal, and professional environments—in which the other processes occur.

Data Bases

The study of information management includes issues related to the development and use of a consistent language that represents the domain of the health care professional. This data base is needed for several purposes. A common, uniform, comprehensive approach to the representation of nursing and medical information is needed to express the details of observation, diagnosis, and patient management (Evans, Cimino, Hersh, Huff, and Bell, 1994). It is also used to index, sort, retrieve, and classify nursing data in clinical records, health information systems, medical and nursing literature and in research.

The development of a data base needs to reflect consistency in language to address the needs of different settings and perspectives. That is, the data base needs to reflect the information requirements for acute care, ambulatory care and long term care. In addition, it needs to support the decision-making requirements for clinical and administration decisions.

Information Systems

The second perspective of information management addresses strategies for managing the transformation of data through well defined, manual and automated information systems. This dimension encompasses the review of existing models for defining information requirements, the planning, organizing, directing and evaluating of information systems and their impact, the relationship of information systems to strategic planning, and the regulatory standards that affect information management requirements.

Managing information systems includes a critical focus on anticipated and actual benefits of information systems, the vendor and nursing role expectations, and the complex issues of orchestrating change in light of the evolution of new information practices and technologies.

Clinical Information

The third dimension of information management focuses on clinical information content and the processes and technologies needed to support clinical decision making. This dimension encompasses a review of the trend toward the computerized patient record and the impact of new electronic communication technologies for patient care and delivery systems. The relationship between information technology and quality outcomes frame the context of this dimension from the perspective of improving clinical care through improved information management.

Administrative Information

The fourth dimension of information management addresses the administrative data required to direct health care organizations and the new technologies that support the processing of this type of data. Administrative activities related to the management of manpower resources, the establishment and monitoring of the competency of care providers, facilitation of organizational communications, and the restructuring of care delivery systems all require informed decisions. In addition, these activities need to be supported with innovative information technology strategies that enhance the clinical outcomes of the health care system while creating more efficient administrative methods to handle information requirements.

Environmental Context

The fifth dimension of information management addresses the social, political, legal and ethical context in which health information is processed and managed. The environmental context also includes the role of professional associations and the establishment of standards of practice for the processing and management of clinical and administrative information. It also includes the educational institution's perspective on preparing nurses and health care professionals to function in a changing environment in which information technology continues to proliferate. Finally the global context of health care delivery and the scientific context of knowledge development through research in this area need to be addressed. These contexts provide an integrated whole in which multiple perspectives intermingle to create the "informated" health environment of the future.

Information Management in the Coming Age

A paradigm shift from sick care and profit centers to well care and cost centers is occurring throughout the health care delivery system. This shift will bring increasing diversity to patient care through shorter lengths of stay in acute care settings, an emphasis on community based care, and a growing emphasis on the development of health care networks and managed care. New approaches to reduce the costs of care and to increase continuity will emphasize illness prevention and health promotion, global pricing of services, a capitated system of reimbursement, and competitive bidding by providers.

Health Care Networks

In an effort to remain competitive in a managed care environment, health care providers will place an increasing emphasis on offering care across a continuum of client needs. This will lead to expanded health care network development in which there is a corporate relationship between patient care services designed to meet health care needs across the life span continuum. These services will include features such as primary care, community based services, acute care, mental health, rehabilitation, long term care, and home health care. The need to coordinate information within and across these services will significantly increase the importance of electronic networks and computer based patient records.

Standards for health care networks were published by the Joint Commission for Accreditation of Healthcare Organizations in July, 1994. These standards emphasize the ability of multiple delivery sites to work as a system to track a client through the entire process of care—for example, from admitting through rehabilitation—with no duplication of effort and consistent information across all providers and areas of care. To reach this goal, information management systems will need to be developed which provide for the integration and coordination of services, management of professional staff, safeguards of patients rights and confidentiality, measurement of quality, facilitation of education and communication, and support of decision making at every level of the network.

The development of health care service networks must be supported by baseline data on the health status of specific communities and careful strategic planning of services. This will lead to further development of Comprehensive Community Health Information Networks [C-CHIN]. These networks will need to provide "rigorous patient identification; cross-referencing; data sharing and transaction services; basic patient data; links to providers, reference laboratories and billing systems; data formatting and interfacing; and network management and services plus basic network functions, including e-mail, imaging support, forms processing, scheduling and library services" (Wenzlick, 1994, p.23).

The objective of taking a "broad view" of comprehensive information systems development is to support continuous and integrated care, where services are matched to need, duplication and concomitant costs are reduced and provider accountability is enhanced. This type of system can only be developed through the careful determination of clinical and administrative information needed to support patient care and patient care organizations, and the planning, design and implementation of responsive information systems.

Summary

Health care leadership needs to carefully consider the key dimensions of information management in order to effectively plan and support the development of electronic systems facilitative of data driven decisions. These dimensions include data base requirements, the strategy and systems to transform and process data, the clinical content of data, the administrative systems which support decision making, and the context in which care delivery processes occur. Systems must be built in consideration of the information content required to underpin excellent patient care and the environmental context in which care will be organized and delivered.

References

Evans, D., Cimino, J., Hersh, W., Huff, S., and Bell, D. (1994). Toward a medical-concept representation language. *Journal of the American Medical Informatics Association*, (3), 207-217.

Graves, J.R. and Corcoran, S. (1989). The study of nursing informatics. *Image: Journal of Nursing Scholarship, 21*, 227-231.

Joint Commission on Accreditation of Healthcare Organizations. (1993). Joint Commission Indicators for the Indicator Monitoring System. In *Accreditation Manual for Hospitals 1994 edition. Vol. 1 Standards*. Oakbrook Terrace, IL: Author.

National Center for Nursing Research. (1993, May). *Nursing Informatics: Enhancing Patient Care—National Nursing Research Agenda*. (NIH Publication No. 93-2419).

Wenzlick, P. (1994, September). Extending the utility of community health information networks. *InfoCare*, 20-24.

Zuboff, S. (1984). *In the Age of the Smart Machine*. New York: Basic Books, Inc.

Establishing a Data Base for Decisions

A Model for Defining Nursing Information System
Requirements 7
Standardizing Nursing Language for Computerization 16
One Nursing Minimum Data Set: A Key to Nursing's Future 28
Significance of the Nursing Minimum Data Set for Decision
Support in Acute Care 32
The Omaha System: A Data Base for Ambulatory and
Home Care 39
Decision-Support Systems for Nurse Managers 45

A Model for Defining Nursing Information System Requirements

Carole A. Gassert, PhD, RN
Assistant Professor
Department of Education, Administration, Health Policy and Informatics
University of Maryland at Baltimore
School of Nursing

Introduction

The emergence of health care as an information-intensive industry has been well- documented. More recently, there has been a shift to emphasize the importance of using information technology to make decisions that are data driven. As an example, in the Institute of Medicine report on medical records (Dick & Steen, 1991), Detmer indicates that computer-based patient records will serve as the infrastructure for supporting information management needs of health care professionals, including nurses. Zielstorff, Hudgings, and Grobe (1993) support this paradigm shift by referring to the need for atomic-level data that can be transformed and presented using information systems, into information for making nursing decisions.

A frequent prediction for health care in the future is that influences such as health care reform and more limited financial and personnel resources will push health care agencies even more to select or develop and install comprehensive information systems (IS) within the next few years. Hard (1993) further suggests that although many health care investments are currently on hold, it is prudent to invest in information technology. If information technology (IT) is to support data driven decisions, the software must be responsive to health care providers' information needs. This author believes that in order to match information system functionality and information management needs to obtain the most effective systems, requirements must be carefully defined *before* information systems are purchased. The suggestion that end users, including nurses, be involved in the processes of defining requirements for information system selection is repeatedly heard.

Historically, nurses have been excluded from the process of selecting IS that impact their practice (Berg, 1983), resulting in the installation of systems that have not adequately processed nursing information (Rieder & Norton, 1984). During the 1980s, the need for nurse involvement to ensure appropriate system purchase was stressed (Cook, 1983; Rieder & Norton, 1984). Nurse participation in system selection has increased, but despite the recognized importance of including nurses in this process, Dunbar reports that less than half of more than 200 nurse executives surveyed were included in purchase decisions for an IS that would be used extensively by nurses (Dunbar, 1992). Informal discussions with nurses at informatics conferences support these findings. Oral histories of their experiences indicate that small groups of individuals often make decisions about an information system purchase with little or no input from nurses.

Some may argue that nurses are unprepared to participate in the information systems selection process. Although formal nursing informatics education programs specifically designed to prepare nurses for IS design and development, selection, implementation, and evaluation have been available only since 1988 (Gassert, 1991a; Heller, Romano, Moray, & Gassert, 1989), nurses have entered into roles that focus on these job functions since the late 1970s. Several articles, written by nurses practicing in informatics, appeared in earlier literature and presented guidelines for the selection process (Ball & Hannah, 1984; Berg, 1983; Cook, 1982; Drazen, 1983; Hoffman, 1985; Powell, 1982; McAlindon, Danz, & Theodoroff, 1987; McCarthy, 1985; Rieder & Norton, 1984; Romano, McCormick, & McNeely, 1982; Romano & McNeely, 1985; Weaver & Johnson, 1984; Zielstorff, 1975).

Ten years after the initial interest in system selection in health care environments, nurses continue to seek information about selecting IS. Their interest is demonstrated by the oversubscription of a professional development summer institute that focused on system selection, implementation, and evaluation (Gassert, 1994) and the continued appearance of literature about system selection (Behrenbeck, Davitt, Ironside, Mangan, O'Shaughnessy, & Steele, 1990; Korth & Morris, 1993).

Selection of information systems is a lengthy process that generally takes 18 months to complete. If included in the selection process, nurses are asked to identify their system requirements, which are then woven into the request for proposal (RFP) issued by the agency to software vendors. Some vendors and health care agencies have advocated that traditional methods of selection be abandoned to shorten the process (Casper, 1993).

An alternative to eliminating a thorough analysis of information management needs is to expedite the process. Therefore, the Model for Defining Nursing Information System Requirements (MDNISR) was developed as a graphic model to depict the process of identifying nursing information system requirements and to facilitate decisions about the adequacy of information systems for nursing (Gassert, 1988, 1989, 1990, 1991b). This model could be used by nurses to describe the way an information system is expected to perform. It could be used in selecting, evaluating, enhancing, or developing information systems that support nursing. The MDNISR model is the focus of this chapter.

Model Description

A descriptive research study was conducted to develop and test the model (Gassert, 1988). Techniques for development included structured analysis and content validation. The Model for Defining Nursing Information System Requirements has a pentagonal shape and five elements that are linked together in sequential order (see Figure 1). Within each model, element data are received as inputs, undergo specific processing, are considered in relation to identified influences, and result in unique information or outputs for that element. Collectively, the five-model element outputs, nursing information functions, nursing information processing requirements, nursing system outputs, nursing data requirements, and nursing system benefits, specify an agency's requirements for a nursing information system (NIS).

Definitions

Definitions for each of the model elements and sub-elements within them are given here, along with some examples of each sub-element.

Nurse Users Element

This element is defined by the processes of relating nursing functions, practice responsibilities, and information handling needs to identify nursing information functions.

Nursing functions. Nursing functions are defined as all activities performed by nurses in particular roles; as clinicians—in diagnosing and treating human response to actual or potential health problems, or in assisting clients to perform health maintenance behaviors; as administrators—in managing care and resources; as researchers—in

Figure 1
Model for defining nursing information system requirements.

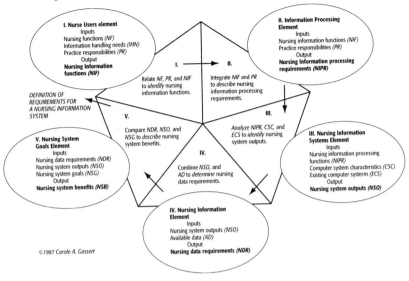

©1987 Carole A. Gassert

studying nursing; as educators—in providing educational experiences for learners; and as informatics nurse specialists—in applying information technology to nursing.

Information handling needs. Information handling needs include those documents containing data that must be read, recorded, or used for reporting by nurses while performing their defined nursing functions. Examples are as follows: obtain assessment data about a patient and his/her needs, gather information about patient's status of care and acuity.

Practice responsibilities. Practice responsibilities are the nursing roles of clinicians, administrators, researchers, educators, or informatics nurse specialists that describe the categories of activities performed by nurse users.

Nursing information functions. The outputs of the first model element are nursing information functions and are defined as those activities requiring information handling that are associated with nurses' roles. For example, documenting care, coordinating discharge information, making decisions about managing nursing resources, conducting studies related to nursing care, and conducting studies related to the teaching of nursing procedures are information functions.

Information Processing Element
This element is defined by the processes of integrating nursing information functions and practice responsibilities to describe nursing information processing requirements.

Nursing information processing requirements. Nursing information processing requirements are the functional processes that users feel a computer must perform as it manipulates data into information for nurses. Manipulative tasks that are required of the computer are dependent upon users' specific practice responsibilities. Examples of nursing information processing requirements are: generate a written plan of care or critical pathway from input received, provide a reminder of deficiencies in recorded data, determine staffing variances, generate monthly unit schedules, and determine educational needs from personnel records.

Nursing Information Systems Element

This element is defined by the processes of analyzing nursing information processing requirements, computer system characteristics, and existing computer systems to identify nursing system outputs.

Computer system characteristics. Computer system characteristics are the descriptive traits of a computer system that are expressed in computer language terms. These characteristics reflect the state of current information technology and its capabilities. Rapid response time, ease of use, graphical user interface, point of care data capture, and real-time data processing are examples of computer system characteristics.

Existing computer system(s). A computerized system that has already been installed in a facility or that is planned for installation is an existing computer system. Economy and efficiency of information handling dictate that IS be linked together to allow transfer of data across these systems.

Nursing system outputs. Nursing system outputs are the statements describing outputs, i.e., computer screens or printouts, obtained from processing nursing information with a nursing information system. Examples of nursing system outputs include: a report with notations of missing data categories, a flow sheet for documenting treatments, a digital image of a surgical wound on a previous visit, and the recorded nursing history from a previous admission.

Nursing Information Element

This element is defined by the processes of combining nursing system outputs and available data to determine nursing data requirements.

Available data. Available data is defined as computerized patient data that is available from other automated sources for storage, processing, or retrieval by a nursing information system. Examples of available data are a nursing history from a previous admission, social and demographic data from outpatient records, a census report from a previous month, and unit staffing patterns.

Nursing data requirements. Nursing data requirements are categories of data or characteristics of data that must be included on the computer for nurses to perform and document their nursing information functions or to aggregate data for later decision making. Examples of nursing data requirements include nursing diagnoses, nursing interventions, nursing outcomes, standards for staffing practices, and intensity of nursing care.

Nursing System Goals Element

This element is defined by the processes of comparing nursing data requirements, nursing system outputs, and nursing system goals to describe nursing system benefits.

Nursing system goals. Statements describing the desired end-points of information handling to which a nursing information system is directed are the nursing system goals. System goals might be (1) to reduce the cost of information processing, (2) to increase documentation of patient outcomes, and (3) to improve the readability of patient records.

Nursing system benefits. Nursing system benefits are statements identifying the effects or outcomes of using an automated system to process nursing information. Some examples of nursing system benefits include the ability to determine which nursing interventions are used successfully with identified problems or nursing diagnoses, improved clinical decision making, use of longitudinal data in making economic decisions affecting health care delivery, and reduction of overtime payments for charting purposes.

Model Development

Four major steps were used to develop the Model for Defining Nursing Information System Requirements. As a first step, Schwirian's model for nursing informatics research was used as a mind-set to guide an extensive review of nursing informatics literature. Schwirian describes a pyramid-shaped model with the three elements of information, nurse and computer systems forming a triangular base of nursing informatics activity that reaches toward a fourth element, the goal (Schwirian, 1986). The literature review included information systems, information processes, needs and problems, and guidelines for developing or selecting systems.

The four elements suggested by Schwirian were analyzed and sub-elements were identified. Several analyses or decompensations were needed to logically explain the processes needed to decide about information systems. The resulting sub-elements supported the addition of a fifth element, information processing element, to the model.

In the second step of model development, a structured analysis approach (Gassert, 1990) was used to conceptually decompose or breakdown each of the five model elements. Structured analysis (SA) was initially suggested by Ross and Schoman (1977) as a means of describing a computer system and later by Borich and Jamelka (1982) as a vehicle for program evaluation. Structured analysis is an organized and patterned approach for graphically documenting what someone thinks about a topic. A topic of interest is conceptually broken down into subtopics and represented graphically as a series of diagrams. The set of diagrams is arranged in levels demonstrating the properties of modular configuration, hierarchical structure, and means-end continuum (Ross & Schoman, 1977; Borich & Jamelka, 1982), thus establishing sequential relationships among the processes described. The first diagram presents an overview of the topic being analyzed (see Figure 2). Each lower diagram shows a smaller portion of information, greater detail, and further defines the topic (Ross & Schoman, 1977). A topic may be decomposed to any level of depth the analyst feels necessary for understanding.

Specific SA language symbols are used to label diagrams within the set (Ross, 1977). At each level the diagram is composed of boxes, arrows, natural language names, and symbolic notations. A box indicates that a transaction has occurred and an arrow indicates relationships between various parts of the whole. A transaction may be an activity, a process or an event. Inputs or objects a transaction uses, enter the box from the left. Outputs or objects produced by or resulting from the transactions exit the box from the right. Constraints, positive or negative influences that modify a transaction, push down on the transaction box from above. Mechanisms or means of activating a transaction press upward on the box. Using a box and arrow syntax, a graphic model can demonstrate the following: structure and process, linkage between activities and outcomes, relationship of values to outcomes, and relationship between a topic and its environment (Borich & Jamelka, 1982).

Figure 3 depicts application of SA techniques and language symbols. In this example the transaction is "Judge compatibility of information system and health care agency." Inputs or information the transaction uses enter the box from the left and are "Adequacy of IS for allied health services; Adequacy of IS for pharmacy services, etc." Constraints or influences that modify the judgment of compatibility are "computer technology innovation, health care agency aims, accrediting standards, etc." In this example there are no mechanisms pressing upward on the transaction. The transaction result or output in this example is the "Decision about proposed information system."

Using SA the MDNISR was decomposed as the fourth level of the topic "Judging the compatibility of an information system and a health care agency" (see Figure 4). SA tech-

Figure 2.

Decomposition of topic: Judging the compatibility of an information system and a health care agency.

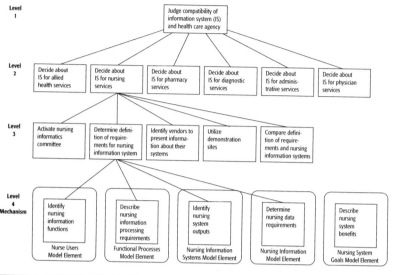

Figure 3.

Decomposition of level 1 transaction, judge compatibility of an information system and a health care agency.

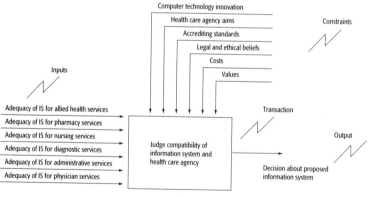

niques identified sub-elements within each element and produced a graphic model of the inputs, outputs, processes, and constraints for each element. The graphic model also showed the relationships or linkages of elements and sub-elements.

The third step of model development content establishes validity of the model's sub-elements. A matrix was used to compare the sub-elements with published guidelines. Thirteen publications that discussed guidelines for system selection were used in the matrix (Ball & Hannah, 1984; Berg, 1983; Cook, 1982; Drazen, 1983; Hoffman, 1985; Powell, 1982; McAlindon, Danz, & Theodoroff, 1987; McCarthy, 1985; Rieder & Norton, 1984; Romano, McCormick, & McNeely, 1982; Romano & McNeely, 1985; Weaver & Johnson, 1984; Zielstorff, 1975). Labels for the sub-elements either appeared

Figure 4.
Decomposition of level 4: Model for defining nursing information system requirements.

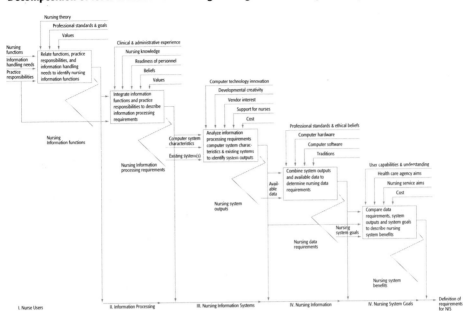

directly in the literature or were synthesized from information presented. Twelve of the 13 sets of guidelines reviewed included sub-elements from each of the five model elements. The remaining set included sub-elements from four of the five elements, thereby establishing content validity. Once the graphic model demonstrating the mechanism for defining requirements for a nursing information system was developed, it became necessary to extract a portion of the model and present it to users in a shortened and less detailed version. To add to the content validity of the model, experts in nursing informatics judged the extracted model and offered suggestions regarding the naming of sub-elements and the ordering of events. Figure 1 depicts the graphic model deduced from the fully decomposed version known as the MDNISR.

Model Testing

At the time of its development the MDNISR was tested with a purposive sample of 75 registered nurses from throughout the United States who had participated in planning, designing, selecting, enhancing, or evaluating NISs. A self-administered questionnaire, emanating from the model's content, was used to test the clarity, completeness and usefulness of the model. Although model testing is an important part of development, this article only briefly summarizes the results of testing. A more complete discussion is available in the literature (Gassert, 1988, 1989). Clarity of model element outputs was tested and supported by asking study participants to develop examples of their own that demonstrated the model's sub-elements. Subjects were able to use the definitions provided to generate examples that were correct more than 66% of the time.

Completeness of the MDNISR was also upheld during testing. To determine completeness, three different analyses were used. First, subjects were asked to indicate data items they had considered in deciding about NISs that had not been included in the model. Only two items that had not been part of the larger model were named. Both of these items were constraints. No new model elements were suggested. Second, subjects were asked whether anything was missing from the model; no suggestions were given for adding data to the model. And finally, subjects' mean scores on the questionnaire indicated that all of the model element outputs listed are essential to include in the model.

MDNISR's usefulness was likewise defended. To determine the characteristic of usefulness subjects were asked to indicate the extent to which they had actually considered the model element output when deciding about the information systems in their agencies. Again, subjects' mean scores on the questionnaire showed they had actually used the information listed in the model. Initial testing, therefore, supported clarity, completeness and usefulness of the MDNISR in deciding about information systems for nursing.

Future Application

Needless to say, it was very exciting to learn that the model was supported during its initial testing. The real, and probably most important, test of the MDNISR, however, will come with determining its utility in defining requirements of information systems for nursing in specific health care environments. Current work is being done by the author to operationalize each of the model element transactions.

(The author wishes to acknowledge that the research to develop and test the model was done as part of the requirements for completing the doctoral degree at the University of Texas at Austin. The author also wishes to thank the following students for their comments regarding MDNISR: J. Byrne, A. Creech, K. Davis, B. Harris, and C. Wark.)

References

Ball, M. J., & Hannah, K. J. (1984). *Using Computers in Nursing.* Reston, VA: Reston Publishers.

Behrenbeck, J. G., Davitt, P., Ironside, P., Mangan, D. B., O'Shaughnessy, D., & Steele, S. (1990). Strategic planning for a nursing information system (NIS) in the hospital setting. *Computers in Nursing, 8*(6), 236-242.

Berg, C. M. (1983). The importance of nurses' input for the selection of computerized systems. In M. Scholes, Y. Bryant & B. Barber (Eds.), *The Impact of Computers on Nursing* (pp. 42-58). Amsterdam: Elsevier Science Publishers B. V.

Borich, G. D., & Jamelka, R. P. (1982). *Programs and Systems: An Evaluation Perspective.* New York: Academic Press.

Casper, M. (1993). A non-traditional request-for-proposals. *Healthcare Informatics, 10*(1), 22, 24.

Cook, M. (1982). Selecting the right computer system. *Nursing Management, 13*(8), 26-28.

Cook, M. (1983). Using computers to enhance professional practice. In M. Scholes, Y. Bryant & B. Barber (Eds.), *The Impact of Computers on Nursing* (pp. 84-90). Amsterdam: Elsevier Science Publishers B. V.

Dick, R. S., & Steen, E. B. (Eds.). (1991). *The Computer-Based Patient Record: An Essential Technology for Health Care.* Washington, DC: National Academy Press.

Drazen, E. L. (1983). Planning for purchase and implementation of an automated hospital information system: A nursing perspective. *Journal of Nursing Administration, 13*(9), 9-12.

Dunbar, C. (1992, March) Nurses want I/S selection power, but do they have it? *Computers in Healthcare,* 20-22, 24.

Gassert, C. A. (1988). *Development of a nursing informatics model: A description of nursing elements needed to obtain essential data for deciding about nursing information systems.* Unpublished doctoral dissertation, University of Texas at Austin.

Gassert, C. A. (1989). Defining nursing information system requirements: A linked model. In L.C. Kingsland (Ed.), *Proceedings of the Thirteenth Annual Symposium on Computer Applications in Medical Care*, (pp. 779-783). Los Angeles: Computer Society Press.

Gassert, C. A. (1990). Structured analysis: A methodology for developing a model for defining nursing information system requirements. *Advances in Nursing Science, 13*(2), 53-62.

Gassert, C. A. (1991a). Preparing for a career in nursing informatics. In P. B. Marr, R. L. Axford & S. K. Newbold (Eds.), *Nursing Informatics '91: Proceedings of the Post Conference on Health Care Information Technology: Implications for Change* (pp. 163-166). New York: Springer-Verlag.

Gassert, C. A. (1991b). Validating a model for defining nursing information system requirements. In E. J. S. Hovenga, K. A. McCormick, K. J. Hannah, & J. S. Ronald (Eds.), *Proceedings of Nursing Informatics '91* (pp. 215-219). New York: Springer-Verlag.

Gassert, C. A. (1994). Summer Institute: Providing continued learning in nursing informatics. In S. Grobe & E. S. Pluyter-Wenting (Eds). *Nursing Informatics: An International Overview for Nursing in a Technological Era*. Amsterdam: Elsevier, pp. 536-539.

Hard, B. (1993, September). Multisite Lutheran General uses information systems to create care continuum. *Computers in Healthcare*, 16-18, 20.

Heller, B. R., Romano, C. A., Moray, L. R., & Gassert, C. A. (1989). Special follow-up report: The implementation of the first graduate program in nursing informatics. *Computers in Nursing, 7*(5), 209-213.

Hoffman, F. M. (1985). Evaluating and selecting a computer software package. *Journal of Nursing Administration, 15*(11), 33-35.

Korth, S. K., & Morris, M. (1993). Selecting an information system. *Nursing Management, 24*(4), 62-64, 66.

McAlindon, M. N., Danz, S. M. & Theodoroff, R. A. (1987). Choosing the hospital information system: A nursing perspective. *Journal of Nursing Administration, 17*(10), 11-15.

McCarthy, L. J. (1985). Taking charge of computerization. *Nursing Management, 16*(7), 35-40.

Powell, N. M. (1982). Designing and developing a computerized hospital information system. *Nursing Management, 13*(8), 40-45.

Rieder, K. A., & Norton, D. A. (1984). An integrated nursing information system—A planning model. *Computers in Nursing, 2*(3), 73–79.

Romano, C. A., & McNeely. L. (1985). Nursing applications of a computerized information system: Development, implementation, utilization. In K. J. Hannah, E. J. Guillemin, & D. N. Conklin (Eds.), *Nursing Uses of Computers and Information Science* (pp. 43-49). Amsterdam: Elsevier Science Publishers B. V.

Romano, C., McCormick, K. A., & McNeely, L. D. (1982). Nursing documentation: A model for a computerized data base. *Advances in Nursing Science, 4*(2), 43-56.

Ross, D. (1977). Structured analysis (SA): A language for communicating ideas. *IEEE Transactions on software Engineering, SE-3*(1), 16-34.

Ross, D. T., & Schoman, K. E. (1977). Structured analysis for requirements definition. *IEEE Transactions on Software Engineering, SE-3*(1), 6-15.

Schwirian, P. M. (1986). The NI pyramid—A model for research in nursing informatics. *Computers in Nursing, 4*(3), 134-136.

Weaver, C. G., & Johnson, J. E. (1984). Nursing participation in computer vendor selection. *Computers in Nursing, 2*(2), 31-34.

Zielstorff, R. D. (1975). The planning and evaluation of automated systems: A nurses' point of view. *Journal of Nursing Administration, 5*, 22-25.

Zielstorff, R. D., Hudgings, C. I., Grobe, S. J., & NCNIP. (1993). *Next-Generation Nursing Information Systems: Essential Characteristics for Professional Practice*. Washington, DC: American Nurses Publishing.

Standardizing Nursing Language for Computerization

Joanne Comi McCloskey, PhD, RN, FAAN
Distinguished Professor in Nursing
College of Nursing and Adjunct Associate Director of Nursing
University of Iowa Hospitals and Clinics
The University of Iowa

This chapter is based on a presentation given at the Summer Institute in Nursing Informatics '93 held in Baltimore, Maryland, July 18, 1993. The author wishes to thank the other members of the Implementation Team who are working to include the Nursing Interventions Classification (NIC) in the computer systems of five health care agencies. They are, from the University of Iowa College of Nursing: Gloria Bulechek, Tom Kruckeberg, Sue Moorhead, Bill Donahue, and Joan Carter; from the University of Iowa Hospitals and Clinics: Colleen Prophet, Marita Titler, and Vicki Kraus; from Oaknoll Retirement Residence in Iowa City: Jeanette Daly and Sue Bush; from Mercy Hospital in Davenport, Iowa: Peg Mehmert, Mary Clark and colleagues; from Dartmouth-Hitchcock Memorial Hospital in Hanover, N.H.: Pat Button and Priscilla Hall; and from Loyola University Medical Center's Mulcahy Outpatient Center in Chicago, Illinois: Ida Androwich, Cheryl Russow and colleagues. Support for the research comes from a grant from the National Institute of Nursing Research, NIH (2RO1NR02079-04), J. McCloskey and G. Bulechek, Co-PIs.

Introduction

The planning and documentation of nursing care is being increasingly automated. In the past, no standardized system for describing the treatments that nurses perform existed. Each health care agency developed a unique set of nursing orders or actions, copying ideas from one another either by using lists of orders that have been generated from care plans used at the institution or modifying a list supplied by a vendor. If an agency could agree on a standardized list of interventions for all units, it was unlikely that this list was the same as another agency's list. This resulted in the inability to collect data that are comparable from one institution to another, or even from one unit to another. In 1983, a study group, at a conference on nursing information systems, pointed out that even though nurses spend much of their time documenting their care, this documentation has not been systematically organized or used to advance nursing knowledge, to develop nursing practice, or to improve patient care (Study Group on Nursing Information Systems, 1983). In 1984, Zielstorff asserted that the major impediment to the development of computerized nursing information systems is the deficiencies in nursing's knowledge base:

> Those who work in the design and development of nursing information systems constantly bemoan the fact that there are so few clinical problems in nursing for which the etiology, symptoms, treatments, and expected outcomes are known. There are no known probability estimates for prevalence or incidence of common nursing problems; or for relating symptoms to diagnosis, or treatment to outcome. Indeed, there is neither a standard terminology nor a widely accepted format for data gather-

ing. It is impossible to derive hard and fast rules for computer assistance in decision making with such an ill-defined data base (p. 9).

At a January 1988 Conference on Research Priorities in Nursing Science, the National Center for Nursing Research identified as a high priority the development of nursing information systems (National Center for Nursing Research, 1988). With the coming of the Computer-based Patient Record (CPR), nursing needs to agree upon standardized classifications of nursing knowledge in order to communicate with one another and to be able to construct research data bases that can be used to evaluate the effectiveness of nursing care. Simpson (1991) has outlined 12 requisites that a computerized record must possess. Requisite Number 10 is "The CPR supports structured data collection in a manner which adequately supports practitioners' direct entry and stores that information according to a defined vocabulary" (p. 28).

A goal that the profession is working toward is the implementation of the Nursing Minimum Data Set (NMDS), or the uniform collection of essential nursing information (Werley and Lang, 1988). The purpose of the NMDS is to foster comparability of nursing data across patient populations, with the ultimate goal of improving health care. Sixteen data elements are included in the proposed NMDS, including four nursing care elements: diagnoses, interventions, outcomes, and intensity of nursing care. While the proposal for a NMDS has been widely acclaimed by the professional community, implementation has proved difficult largely because of the lack of a comprehensive classification in the area of nursing interventions. With the development of the NIC, this roadblock has been removed. Now nurses can communicate their treatments in a common language which will further facilitate communication and research. The NIC, in conjunction with classifications of nursing diagnoses and patient outcomes, will provide the nursing profession with the data elements for an automated patient record.

Background

The need for a classification of nursing interventions has been motivated by developments both within and outside of the profession. Within nursing, before the development of the NIC (Iowa Intervention Project, 1992), nursing interventions were viewed as discrete actions, e.g., "Position the limb with sandbags"; "Raise the head of the bed 30 degrees"; or "Explore the need for attention with the patient." There was little conceptualization of how these discrete actions would fit together. Nursing textbooks, care planning guides, and nursing information systems have typically addressed nursing interventions at the most discrete level. Long lists of nursing actions are given for each type of patient; the list in one source is not the same as the list in another even though the same patient condition is being discussed. For example, if we compare the suggested nursing interventions for the nursing diagnosis of Activity Intolerance in several books, we find major differences. For treatment of Activity Intolerance, Moorhouse, Geissler, and Doenges (1987) list six independent interventions (e.g., "Check vital signs before and immediately after activity") and one collaborative intervention ("Follow graded cardiac rehabilitation and activity program"); McFarland and McFarlane (1989) list three goals with 24 interventions (e.g., "Assess the patient's past and present activity pattern"); and Carpenito (1989) lists eight major categories of interventions and 46 discrete activities (e.g., "Instruct person to practice controlled coughing four times a day").

At the opposite extreme of the long lists of discrete nursing actions are classification schemes for nursing interventions composed of large categories. Examples of these include: Henderson's (1961) components of basic nursing; Benner's (1984) seven domains of nursing; the National Council of State Board Study's categories of nurse activities

(Kane, Kingsbury, Colton, and Estes, 1986); the Visiting Nurse Association of Omaha's classification scheme for community health interventions (Martin and Scheet, 1992; Visiting Nurse Association of Omaha, 1986); Verran's taxonomy of ambulatory care nursing (Cohen, Arnold, Brown, and Brooten, 1991; Verran, 1981); the Joel classification (1988) adapted from the New Jersey Department of Health; Bulechek and McCloskey's (1987) beginning taxonomy of nursing interventions; the minimum data set intervention lists (Werley and Lang, 1988); Sigma Theta Tau's (1987) International Classification of Nursing Knowledge; and Saba and colleagues' (1991) intervention taxonomy for home health care. Most of these schemes contain only broad categories which are not clinically useful.

The review of existing intervention terminology and classifications (see McCloskey and Bulechek, 1993) demonstrates that we have thousands of discrete action statements and a number of large conceptual categories, but little descriptive language in between these two extremes. The identified need was the development of clinically useful intervention concept labels that are more abstract than the very discrete action statements, but less abstract and more useful than the large categories.

Within nursing, the most important work has been the effort by the North American Nursing Diagnosis Association (NANDA) to define a standardized list of nursing diagnoses to describe patient conditions that nurses diagnose. The widespread use of NANDA's nursing diagnosis language has increased an awareness of the need for similar standardized classifications in the areas of interventions and outcomes.

Several developments outside of nursing have also motivated the development of a standardized language for nursing interventions. The push for guideline development by the Agency for Health Care Policy and Research (Agency, 1990) has clarified the need. Guidelines are needed to help practitioners determine which of several courses of action are best given a particular set of circumstances: that is, based on research, what interventions are most effective for patients with a particular diagnosis or set of diagnoses. While medicine has used standardized data bases to guide the evaluation of medical care, nursing's use of large data bases and our knowledge about the effectiveness of nursing care is limited.

The federal government, insurance companies, and the medical community have been collecting standardized health information for a number of years for purposes of reimbursement and research. To facilitate the data collection, several Uniform Minimum Health Data Sets have been developed; for example: Uniform Hospital Discharge Data Set, Ambulatory Medical Care Minimum Data Set, and the Long-term Health Care Minimum Data Set (Pearce, 1988). Once variables are defined, there needs to be a classification system for each variable. The major systems for classification are the *International Classification of Diseases, The Current Procedural Terminology,* the *Diagnostic and Statistical Manual of Mental Disorders,* the *Systematized Nomenclature of Pathology,* and the *Systematized Nomenclature of Medicine* (Gebbie, 1989). None of these coding classifications or the data sets of which they are a part represent nursing practice (Zielstorff, 1992). If nursing variables are to be included in health care data sets, we need standardized classifications of nursing knowledge. Since a major portion of the work of nursing is the treatments that nurses perform, a classification of nursing interventions is essential.

Development of Nursing Interventions Classification

The Nursing Interventions Classification was published in May 1992. This document contains a standardized list of 336 direct care nursing interventions, each with a definition, a set of activities that a nurse does to carry out the intervention, and a short list of background readings. Five chapters delineate the ongoing research effort to develop and expand the Classification. The Classification is the work of a large research team at the University of Iowa. Two grants from the National Institute of Nursing Research, NIH (RO1-NR02079 and 2RO1-NR02079), as well as other support from the Rockefeller Foundation and the University of Iowa have facilitated the effort. The development work completed in five steps includes:

1. Identification and resolution of the conceptual and methodological issues
2. Generation of an initial list of interventions
3. Refinement of the intervention labels and defining activities
4. Arrangement of the interventions in a taxonomic structure
5. Validation of the interventions and taxonomic structure.

Step 1: Identification and resolution of the conceptual and methodological issues

During the first step of the research a number of methodological and conceptual issues were resolved. For example, a major conceptual issue was the question of what sorts of nursing activities should be included in an intervention taxonomy. Nursing interventions, by definition, represent nurse actions or behaviors. This differs from nursing diagnoses and nursing outcomes, which represent the patient's actions or behaviors.

Nurses, in fact, perform many activities to benefit the client. Seven groups of nursing activities were identified (Bulechek and McCloskey, 1989):

1. Assessment activities to make a nursing diagnosis
2. Assessment activities to gather information for a physician to make a medical diagnosis
3. Nurse-initiated treatments, in response to nursing diagnoses
4. Physician-initiated treatments in response to medical diagnoses
5. Daily essential function activities that may not relate to either medical or nursing diagnoses but are done by the nurse for clients who cannot do these for themselves
6. Activities to evaluate the effects of nursing and medical treatments. These are also assessment activities but they are done for purposes of evaluation, not diagnosis
7. Administrative and indirect care activities that support the delivery of nursing care.

After discussion of these groups of activities, it was decided that the intervention taxonomy should include all direct care treatment activities (both physician-prescribed and nurse-prescribed) that nurses do on behalf of patients and the activities in areas 4, 5 and 6 above were targeted for inclusion.

Step 2: Generation of an initial list of interventions

We began with the idea that nurses have documented their treatments for decades, but at a very concrete level of action. Nursing textbooks, published care planning guides, and nursing information systems contain innumerable concrete nursing activities. These rich sources of data were an excellent starting point for organizing, categorizing and labelling the activities at higher levels of abstraction. We reviewed and rated more than 30 possible data sources. We choose 14 of the highest rated sources for use in eight content analysis exercises to create an initial list of intervention labels. Each content analysis procedure was done as follows: (1) approximately 250 concrete nursing activities from two related sources were randomly selected and entered into a computer file; (2) each activity was printed on a separate slip of paper and the slips distributed to all members of the research team; and (3) each team member independently categorized the activities and gave each category an intervention label. In the beginning, each label had to be generated by team members based upon their knowledge and experience. As the list of labels grew, members selected a label already identified or added a new label if an appropriate one was not on the list. After eight exercises, the number of new labels being generated was small, and the team felt it was time to go on to the next step: further development from the literature and validated through expert opinion.

Step 3: Refinement of the intervention list and defining activities

Following the literature-based exercises, we had a list of approximately 350 intervention labels, each associated with from one to several hundred activities. Many of these activities were redundant as different sources proposed the same activity with different wording. The task was the refinement of the labels and activities to begin to establish face and content validity. Two methods were used: expert survey and focus group.

The expert survey process used a two-round Delphi questionnaire given to certified master's prepared nurses in particular specialty areas. Groups of related intervention labels were selected, lists of their accompanying activities generated by the computer, and, after some cleaning for face validity, each activity was rated as to the extent it is characteristic of the label. Each survey used a Delphi technique with an adaptation of the Fehring method (1986; 1987) for establishing content validity. Between June 1989 and March 1991, we validated 138 interventions in 14 surveys of 483 nurse experts. Twelve of the surveys were published in the June 1992 issue of *Nursing Clinics of North America* (Bulechek and McCloskey, 1992).

The second method, using a focus group, was instituted when it became apparent that the survey process was too time-consuming and not appropriate for all labels. The focus group methodology consisted of repeated discussions of successive drafts of an intervention. First, a team member prepared a draft of the intervention's label, definition, and activities for initial review by a small group of six core team members. After group discussion, the intervention was revised and then reviewed again. This was repeated until the core group was satisfied, and then the intervention was sent for a similar review by the entire research team, which included more than 20 people. Each intervention underwent usually 3 to 5 reviews, with each review leading to further refinement of the label, definition, and activities. Through the focus group method, 198 interventions were prepared in 12 months. At this point in the research, we submitted the manuscript to NIC, which was then published in May of 1992. While the work was by no means finished, we believed that it was necessary to introduce this research into the literature so the project would be known and others could use the interventions and provide feedback. Since then, we have continued to work to identify and standardize interventions and to organize them into a taxonomy.

Step 4: Arrangement of the intervention list in a taxonomic structure

Once we had the interventions defined we needed to identify an organizing structure that is easy to use and clinically meaningful. We used similarity ratings and hierarchical clustering techniques to guide the development of a system of classification, or *taxonomy* of nursing interventions. Hierarchical cluster analysis groups interventions into clusters of related interventions. These interventions can, in turn, be combined into "super-clusters" of similar groups (Everitt, 1974; Sokal, 1974).

At this time, we have identified an initial 26 groups of interventions, which we are calling "classes," and we have six super-groups, which we are calling "domains." A manuscript describing the methodology for developing the taxonomy was published in *Image* in the fall of 1993 (Iowa Intervention Project, 1993). The top level of the taxonomy comprises the six domains, which are entitled Physiological: Basic, Physiological: Complex, Behavioral, Family, Health System, and Safety. At the middle level are the classes; for example, Activity and Exercise Enhancement, Medication Management, Cognitive

Therapy, Family Care, Health System Management, and Crisis Management. At the third level are the 336 interventions published in NIC, plus 21 more developed since the publication of NIC.

Step 5: Validation of the interventions and taxonomy

If the classification is to be used, it needs validation from nurses in practice. To this end, we have taken several actions. In the summer of 1992 we distributed a questionnaire asking for feedback from the 32 clinical specialty nursing organizations participating in the American Nurses' Association Committee on Nursing Practice Standards and Guidelines. A similar questionnaire was distributed in December 1992 to a national sample of approximately 300 nurses in clinical practice in order to gain the practicing nurse perspective. Also, we have included a review form in the book, *Nursing Interventions Classification,* and we have recently developed a review process to evaluate and incorporate the feedback we receive. In addition, a questionnaire to assess the meaningfulness of the classes and domains was distributed in May of 1993 to a sample of nurses who were expert in theory development and analysis. Based upon this survey, some modifications in the taxonomy have been made.

In summary, then, NIC is intended to include all interventions that nurses perform on behalf of patients, including both independent and collaborative interventions. From the validation surveys we have learned that all of the interventions in NIC are used in practice by nurses from at least two specialty groups. We also know that we have some additional interventions that should be developed further and then added to NIC. From the surveys, we have gathered suggestions for approximately 50 additional interventions; most of these are specialized. We have placed these suggestions on an "under consideration" list and will be developing them in the future.

The NIC is useful to nurses in all specialties and in all settings. While an individual nurse will have expertise in only a limited number of interventions, the entire classification captures the expertise of all nurses. The interventions have been placed in a 3-level taxonomic structure that facilitates selection of an intervention and use of the Classification on a computer. NIC has been endorsed by the American Nurses Association as one of the nursing classifications that should be part of a unified nursing language, and in January 1993, it was one of the first two nursing languages to be included in the National Library of Medicine's *Methathesaurus for the Unified Medical Language System.*

Development and refinement work on nursing classification is continuing. Current efforts of the research team center on the development of indirect care interventions (interventions done away from the patient's bedside but on behalf of a patient or group of patients); coding of the classification for ease in computerization; articulation with other classifications for use in reimbursement; and on field testing the classification in five clinical sites.

Implications for Computerization

Implications for computerization will be discussed in two areas: (a) improving tomorrow's patient care and (b) facilitating today's patient care.

The key to improving patient care in the future is nursing research. Simplistically, let's divide the methods for nursing research into two groups. In the first group we can list the research steps as follows: define a purpose, state the research questions or hypotheses, choose a study design, get a sample and collect data, and analyze the data. This approach, in which data are collected proactively for each study, is one that nurses have typically used with a good deal of success. The resulting samples are small, however, and it is difficult to compare studies on the same topic. By contrast, a different research approach uses data already generated: define a purpose, state the research questions or hypotheses, find a large data set with variables that will answer the questions, and conduct the analysis. This approach is more common in other disciplines than in nursing. We need to add it to our repertoire of research skills but to do so means that we first must construct the data bases with the desired variables. To achieve this, nursing information systems need to include standard classifications of diagnoses, interventions, and outcomes. When nurses systematically use a common standardized language to document the diagnoses of their patients, the treatments they performed, and the resulting patient outcomes, then we will be able to determine which nursing interventions work best for a given population. Several lines of research are possible with large data bases that are not possible or are difficult without them; for example, the following three:

1. Identifying interventions that typically occur together

When we systematically collect information about the treatments we perform, we will be able to identify clusters of interventions that typically occur together for certain types of patients. For example, in caring for a burn patient, we would expect to see interventions used from the NIC classes on Electrolyte and Fluid Management, Physical Comfort Promotion, Psychological Comfort Promotion, Nutrition Support, Coping Assistance, Risk Management and perhaps others depending on the location of the burn. We need to begin to identify interventions that are frequently used together for certain types of patients so that we can study their interactive effects. This information will also be useful in the construction of critical paths, in determining costs of services, and in planning for resource allocation.

2. Identifying the use rate of particular interventions

Large standardized data bases allow us to study and compare the use rate of particular interventions by type of unit and facility. We do not expect any particular group of nurses to use all 336 interventions. We do not know, however, which interventions are associated with specific nursing specialties. Determining the interventions used most frequently on a particular type of unit or in a specific agency will help to determine which interventions should be on that unit's nursing information system. It will also help in the selection of personnel to staff that unit and in the structuring of the continuing education provided to the personnel on these units. Since the practice of nursing is based so heavily on tradition, we would expect to find "area variations" in the selection of interventions from facility to facility.

Since the early 1970s, John Wennberg and his colleagues have been studying the variations in procedures performed by physicians (Wennberg and Gittelsohn, 1973). Even when these studies were performed within small and comparable communities and used controls for differences in age, race, and demographics, major differences in the medical care received were found (Salive, Mayfield, and Weissman, 1990; Wennberg, Freeman, and Culp, 1987). The documentation of the variations in medical care played a leading role in the move to outcomes evaluation. The Patient Outcomes Research Teams, funded by AHCPR, evolved from the studies on area variations.

Nursing has not produced similar studies comparing the use of nursing interventions by different providers, or even by type of unit. This has been difficult for a number of reasons. The development and implementation of a standardized list of nursing treatments makes it possible now to compare interventions used in one setting versus those used in another.

3. Identifying core nursing diagnoses and outcomes for specific interventions

Large data bases should make it easier to determine what nursing diagnoses, DRG categories, and patient outcomes are associated with particular interventions. At this point, the linkages to patient outcomes are most difficult to determine as the language in this area has not yet been standardized. The construction and use of retrievable clinical data bases would allow nursing to build a body of science based upon the study of actual patient care. Documentation of care with standardized classifications allows for the integration of research and practice. Researchers can use the data collected by practitioners in different settings to address more complex research questions.

Before we can achieve these kinds of studies, however, we need to bring NIC into computerized nursing information systems that are used by nurses in practice to facilitate patient care of today. Several challenges lie ahead related to implementation and use. Some of these can be illustrated by a brief account of the issues that we have encountered in just a few months of working with our field sites. Part of our second grant, which began funding in June 1993, provided for implementation of NIC in five field sites. The participating sites and a brief description of their computer system follows:

Mercy Hospital in Davenport, Iowa, is a 265-bed community hospital with 12 inpatient departments, four outpatient departments, and a nursing staff of 600. Since 1982, nursing diagnosis has served as the focus for planning patient care. Since 1984, a mainframe Spectra 2000 computerized nursing information system based on the NANDA list of diagnoses has been used to generate and document patient care plans.

The University of Iowa Hospitals and Clinics in Iowa City, Iowa, is an 820-bed teaching hospital and a regional tertiary care center with a staff of 1,500 Registered Nurses. The hospital has been computerized since the early 1970s with an IBM mainframe system, which includes a locally distributed network of 1,100 cathode ray terminals and 200 terminal printers. The nursing information system called INFORMM was designed in-house and implemented for care planning in 1988. Online documentation is at the pilot stage.

Oaknoll Retirement Residence is an independent living complex and long-term care facility also located in Iowa City. It has 133 apartments for elderly persons able to live alone with minimal assistance and a 48-bed, long-term care facility (32 skilled and 16 intermediate). The nursing department employs 16 Registered Nurses. A nursing information system has recently been implemented and the staff are still being trained. The information system is on an IBM compatible personal computer and uses a MED-COM medical records software program.

Dartmouth-Hitchcock Medical Center is a 435-bed teaching hospital and tertiary care center with a staff of more than 450 nurses located in Lebanon, New Hampshire. The hospital is working with the Cerner Corporation of Kansas City to develop its nursing information system. The Cerner applications run on Digital hardware and represent a strongly integrated system based on a relational data base.

Loyola University Medical Center's Mulcahy Outpatient Center in Chicago, Illinois, is a multispecialty ambulatory care facility. The Community Nursing Service provides approximately 1,000 nursing visits monthly. A Hospice program began providing services in 1993. A faculty-run Nurse Managed Center, initiated in 1981, provides approximately 1,000 visits a year for prenatal, maternal and child, and elder care. The medical center hospital uses a Technicon (TDS) medical information system called LUCI. The system is installed in the Outpatient Center but the care planning and documentation functions are not yet on-line.

While the challenges related to computerization of NIC differ by type of facility, by

Table 1.
Reasons Nurses Document

1. To communicate to others what they know about the patient in order to facilitate care planning and delivery

2. To identify individual patterns or norms so that deviation from these is noted as soon as possible

3. To communicate to other caregivers what still needs to be done; to have a mechanism whereby nursing "orders" to others are noted

4. To illustrate how the general plan of care (interventions) has been tailored to the individual, so that outcomes of care can be more closely evaluated

5. To protect themselves and their employers from threats of malpractice claims

6. To provide a record that can serve as a basis for patient billing of care delivered

7. To provide evidence that assists in the determination of patient acuity which can be used to determine staffing requirements

8. To help build and provide a retrievable institutional data base which can serve to study linkages between interventions and other variables and be used to help improve care

9. To adhere to the mandates of the Joint Commission on Accreditation of Healthcare Organizations, or other regulatory bodies

whether or not they already have a nursing information system, and by sophistication of the staff, several issues are common to all. Issues identified to date include the following:

1. How to use NIC for both care planning and documentation of care delivered; specifically, whether activities in NIC as well as intervention labels should be charted, and if so, whether all activities should be charted

2. Whether NIC activities can or should be modified to better meet the needs and practices of the facility

3. Space considerations and the fact that all of the systems restrict the number of characters, making it difficult to list the activities as they are stated in NIC

4. Articulation with vendors and need for licensing agreements

5. Articulation with the agency's current care planning and documentation system

6. Articulation with the agency's policies and procedures related to some NIC interventions

7. Best ways to introduce NIC to staff members and gain their support

8. Whether to establish linkages with diagnoses and outcomes and priorities or just let nurses search and choose from lists

9. How to ensure that the documentation is electronically retrievable in order to minimize manual data extraction and to provide for comparative studies across multiple sites.

We all know that nurses spend a good deal of time documenting what they do and that they complain about how much time this takes. One of the major challenges of implementation of NIC is to sort out the area of documentation. We have begun to do this by listing the reasons why nurses document (see Table 1) and what they document (see Table 2). Documentation in this context is defined as "anything written and relied upon to record or prove something" (Webster's *Dictionary*).

NIC can help with documentation of plans of care, care provided, and discharge status. The area of "care provided" is the most complex of the six listed in Table 2, as it is complicated by the issue of how to ensure that the care gets provided (nursing orders) as well as recording what care was provided.

Working out the relationship between using NIC to build a research data base and using NIC to document care will not be easy. Turley (1992) would call the former, the "nursing knowledge model" and the second, "the transaction record." In his article, he challenged nursing to reevaluate the current mode of record keeping, saying "any frame-

Table 2.
What Nurses Document

     Nurses document:

     1. assessments

     2. diagnoses or needs

     3. plans of care

     4. care provided

     5. outcomes of care

     6. discharge status

work that maps and organizes professional knowledge cannot have an exact link to the transaction record." Future nursing information systems "must accommodate both the needs of the transactional model and the needs of the nursing knowledge model." Reporting only detailed transactions "gives the appearance that nurses' responsibilities are solely task fulfillment and masks the elements of professional nursing." Conversely, "a model driven solely by nursing knowledge will create problems for legal or ethical monitoring and reimbursement" (p. 177-181).

Clearly, nurses should be taught to use standardized language in the areas of diagnoses, interventions, and eventually, when we have the language, outcomes. This approach to knowledge development and care delivery admittedly has limitations. These include the need to keep the language clinically useful and understandable and the effort that will be needed to keep the classifications current. Use of the classifications in clinical practice should not be rigid. For example, nurses should not be expected to know the exact NIC term in order to locate it on a computer. A thesaurus of terms (NIC has one) can be put on the computer and "behind the screens" can assist nurses to find the appropriate NIC term when they type in a related word or idea. Also, there should always be a place for writing in new interventions that may not yet be a part of NIC.

The burden on nurses to learn the new language has led some researchers in both nursing and in informatics to develop another approach. For example, Susan Grobe (1993) believes that computers themselves should be used to standardize nursing language, rather than expecting nurses to learn and use standardized terminology. Grobe advocates the development of automated systems that will accept all nursing statements and then classify the statements.

Grobe's approach has three disadvantages. First, the necessary equipment and expertise to do this is currently available only in linguistics laboratories. Nurses need nursing information systems *now* to deal with the increasing complexity of patient care. Current systems require standardized language and nursing needs to provide this language so that we are using the available technology. Second, not every practicing nurse and health care institution has access to a computer. Standardized language can be used by all providers whether they document care through a manual system, a personal computer, or a mainframe. The computer technology is important but will vary greatly across location and time; the constant anchor for an individual's practice will always be the standardized language. Third, nurses don't want things decided for them behind computer screens. The representation of nursing knowledge should be up front and visible and very much a part of how we think and communicate with each other. Language is a part of life and a part of culture; nurses who share a common language will reap many benefits.

Grobe correctly accesses the benefits of narrative charting. Many of the reports about the use of new charting systems demonstrate that nurses like to write and that they resist moving to another system. The reason may be that they were taught narrative charting in school so this is what they know best. Another reason, however, is that the best way to communicate the details of care that are unique to one individual is through narrative writing. It seems probable that the best computerized nursing information system of the future will combine standardized documentation with narrative charting.

Summary

The Nursing Interventions Classification is the first comprehensive classification of nursing treatments, and as such, it represents an important milestone in the development of nursing science. The Classification names the treatment concepts for nursing's practice discipline. The systematic naming and classifying of our interventions makes possible new types of studies and demonstrates areas of needed research. The profession of nursing can now more fully participate in the growing world of computerized data bases. Linkages among diagnoses, interventions, and outcomes can now be studied using actual clinical data. The computerization of nursing care through the use of NIC makes possible the determination of both the effectiveness and the cost of the nursing care. The language has been standardized; now it is the responsibility of the nursing community to use this language to improve nursing care.

References

Agency for Health Care Policy and Research. (1990, August). *AHCPR Program Note*. Rockville, MD: DHHSPHS.

Benner, P. (1984). *From Novice to Expert*. Menlo Park, CA: Addison-Wesley Publishing Co.

Bulechek, G. M., and McCloskey, J. C. (1987). Nursing interventions: What they are and how to choose them. *Holistic Nursing Practice, 1*(3), 38.

Bulechek, G., and McCloskey, J. C. (1989). Nursing interventions: Treatments for potential diagnoses. In E. M. Carroll-Johnson (Ed.), *Proceedings of the Eighth Conference, NANDA* (pp. 23-30). Philadelphia: J. B. Lippincott Co.

Bulechek, G. M., and McCloskey, J. C. (Eds.). (1992, June). Symposium on nursing interventions. *Nursing Clinics of North America*. Philadelphia: W. B. Saunders Co.

Carpenito, L. J. (1989). *Nursing Diagnoses: Application to Clinical Practice* (3rd ed.). Philadelphia: J. B. Lippincott Co.

Cohen, S. M., Arnold, L., Brown, L., and Brooten, D. (1991). Taxonomic classification of transitional follow-up care nursing interventions with low birthweight infants. *Clinical Nurse Specialist, 5*(1), 31-36.

Everitt, B. (1974). *Cluster Analysis*. London: Heinemann.

Fehring, R. J. (1986). Validating diagnostic labels: Standardized methodology. In M. E. Hurley, (Ed.), *Classification of Nursing Diagnoses: Proceedings of the Sixth Conference*. St. Louis: C. V. Mosby Co.

Fehring, R. J. (1987). Methods to validate nursing diagnoses. *Heart and Lung, 16*(6), 625-629.

Gebbie, K. M. (1989). Major classification systems in health care and their use. In *Classification Systems for Describing Nursing Practice: Working Papers*. Kansas City, MO: American Nurses Association.

Grobe, S. J. (1993). Response to J. C. McCloskey's and G. M. Bulechek's paper on nursing intervention schemes. In *Canadian Nurses Association: Papers from the Nursing Minimum Data Set Conference*. Canada: The Association.

Henderson, V. (1961). *Basic Principles of Nursing Care*. London: ICN House.

Iowa Intervention Project. (1992). J. McCloskey and G. Bulechek (Eds.), *Nursing Interventions Classification (NIC)*. St. Louis: C. V. Mosby Co.

Iowa Intervention Project. (1993). The NIC taxonomy structure. *Image, 25*(3), 187-192.

Joel, L. (1988). Data requirements for clinical practice. In H. H. Werley and N. M. Lang (Eds.), *Identification of the Nursing Minimum Data Set* (p. 149). New York: Springer Publishing Co.

Kane, M., Kingsbury, C., Colton, D. and Estes, C. (1986). *A Study of Nursing Practice and Role Delineation and Job Analysis of Entry-level Performance of Registered Nurses.* Chicago: National Council of State Boards of Nursing, Inc.

Martin, K. S., and Scheet, N. J. (1992). *The Omaha System: A Pocket Guide for Community Health Nursing.* Philadelphia: W. B. Saunders Co.

McCloskey, J. C., and Bulechek, G. M. (1993). Defining and classifying nursing interventions. In P. Moritz, (Ed.), *Patient Outcomes Research: Examining the Effectiveness of Nursing: Proceedings of the State of the Science Conference.* Sponsored by the National Center for Nursing Research, September 11-13, 1991. Washington, DC: USDHHS, DHS NIH Pub. No. 93-3411.

McFarland, G. K., and McFarlane, E. A. (1989). *Nursing Diagnosis and Intervention.* St. Louis: C. V. Mosby Co.

Moorhouse, M. F., Geissler, A. C., and Doenges, M. E. (1987). *Critical Care Plans: Guidelines for Patient Care.* Philadelphia: F. A. Davis Co.

National Center for Nursing Research. (1988). *Report on the National Nursing Research Agenda for the Participants in the Conference on Research Priorities Nursing Science.* Washington, DC: NCNR, NIH.

Pearce, N. D. (1988). Uniform minimum health data sets: Concept, development, testing, recognition for federal health use, and current status. In H. H. Werley and N. M. Lang. (Eds.), *Identification of the Nursing Minimum Data Set* (pp. 122-133). New York: Springer Publishing Co.

Saba, V. K., O'Hare, A., Zuckerman, A. E., Boondas, J., Levine, E. and Oatway, D. M. (1991). A nursing intervention taxonomy for home health care. *Nursing and Health Care, 12*(6), 296-299.

Salive, M. E., Mayfield, J. A., and Weissman, N. W. (1990). Patient outcomes research teams and the Agency for Health Care Policy and Research. *Health Services Research, 25*(5), 697-708.

Sigma Theta Tau International Honor Society of Nursing. (1987). *Introduction to the International Classification of Nursing Knowledge.* Indianapolis: Sigma Theta Tau.

✓ Simpson, R. L. (1991). Computer-based patient records. Part II. IOM's 12 requisites, *Nursing Management, 22*(11), 26-28.

Sokal, R. R. (1974). Classification: Purposes, principles, progress, prospects. *Science, 185,* 1115-1123.

Study Group on Nursing Information Systems. (1983). Computerized nursing information systems: An urgent need. *Research in Nursing and Health, 6*(2), 101-105.

Turley, J. P. (1992). A framework for the transition from nursing records to a nursing information system. *Nursing Outlook, 40*(4), 177-181.

Verran, J. (1981). Delineation of ambulatory care nursing practice. *Journal of Ambulatory Case Management, 4,* 1-13.

Visiting Nurse Association of Omaha. (1986). *Client Management Information System for Community Health Nursing Agencies.* (Pub. No. HRP-0907023) U.S. Washington, DC: Department of Health and Human Services.

Wennberg, J. E., Freeman, J. L., and Culp, W. J. (1987). Are hospital services rationed in New Haven or over-utilized in Boston? *Lancet, 1*(8543), 1185-1189.

Wennberg, J., and Gittelsohn, A. (1973). Small area variations in health care delivery. *Science, 182,* 1102-1108.

Werley, H. H., and Lang, N. M. (Eds.) (1988). *Identification of the Nursing Minimum Data Sets.* New York: Springer Publishing Co.

Zielstorff, R. D. (1984). Why aren't there more significant automated nursing information systems? *Journal of Nursing Administration, 14*(1), 7-10.

Zielstorff, R. D. (April 1992). *National Databases: Nursing's Challenges.* Presented at 10th Conference on Classification of Nursing Diagnosis, San Diego, CA.

One Nursing Minimum Data Set: A Key to Nursing's Future

Rhonda Anderson, MPA, RN, CNAA, FAAN*
Vice President of Patient Operations
Hartford Hospital, Hartford, Connecticut.
President, American Organization of Nurse Executives—1993–1994.
* Assisted by Debra Stock, AONE Staff Member.

Introduction

Who will be the significant players in health care reform in the 1990s and the coming decade? Will there be winners and losers? How will success in a reformed health care system be measured? Such questions are of vital concern to the health care industry today. Every professional, hospital, home health agency and system, or a representative of these groups, is scrambling for a position as health care reform evolves, each hoping to be the winner or, at least, a significant player. Because such reform principles are directed toward a healthier population, universal coverage, and convenient access to a cost-effective, quality-oriented health care system, outcome data will be essential. These accrued data will be used to negotiate the capitated dollars that will flow to the accountable health plans.

Historically, the ability to quantify the contributions that nursing practice makes to the outcomes of patient care has been a struggle. Now, as health care reform generates new opportunities for nursing, it is even more important that data about nursing practice and nursing management practice be systematically and uniformly gathered across the continuum of care. Such data can be used for creative decision making as well as shared within the new health care networks and with public policy makers. Accordingly, the American Organization of Nurse Executives (AONE), the nation's professional organization for nursing leadership, has set as a top priority the establishment, acceptance, and implementation of one uniform data set for the practice of nursing management.

The Importance of Data to Nursing Practice

From the beginning of the nursing profession, starting with Florence Nightingale, the gathering of patient-related data has been recognized as critical to evaluate and advance the nursing profession, as well as to enhance patient care. Florence Nightingale was an early (and a futuristic) proponent of the importance of documenting and analyzing patient data. In her writings, Nightingale discussed the need to statistically compare outcome data by treatments, interventions, and by hospitals. In addition, she was an early advocate of the use of comparative data to evaluate the quality of medical care, and to examine the cost-effectiveness of care through a cost-benefit analysis (Ulrich, 1992, p. 30).

Since Nightingale's efforts during the last century, nursing itself has come to recognize that standardized data is essential if the profession is to exert influence on public health care policy. The capability of documenting nursing's contributions to patient care outcomes places the profession in a strong position to influence national health policy and to advance the nursing health agenda. Possession of such hard data gives the nursing profession leverage as a political player (Huber, Delaney and Crossley, 1992). In the past, however, the profession of nursing has failed to consistently and comprehensively identify the core data needed, to systematically collect the information, and to utilize it for either management or public policy purposes. To date, the obstacle has been the lack of one accepted minimum data set for nursing practice and nursing management practice across the continuum of care. Principal information gathered in the past has focused on comparative productivity data not linked to outcomes. Thus, while nurse executives contend that because there are great differences among patient populations, severity of illness, practice patterns, delivery systems, levels of productivity, and skill mix of workers, the information that has been collected until now has not allowed nursing to prove those suppositions by making effective, outcome-based comparative analyses across settings.

In today's high tech health care environment, such contentions are no longer acceptable. Why do we want a data set? MaryAnn Fralic, Vice President for Nursing, Johns Hopkins Hospital, asks the provocative question, "Is the development of a data set intended to support our own position or to test our biases?" To use excuses to justify why a certain skill mix is necessary is an old paradigm. The "bottom line" expectation by those distributing the monies in the reformed health care system will be to show the outcome data correlated to the cost information. Under the terms of health care reform, a more cost-effective mix of providers leading to the same or better outcomes will be the winning delivery system. This is not a new thought, but what was "incentivized" between 1965 and 1982 was a "more is better" attitude. What is being re-emphasized and will be incentivized in 1995 is the low-cost, reasonable quality phenomenon.

In 1860, Florence Nightingale emphasized the cost-effective delivery of care and the use of data to prove this to the public.

> These statistics would show subscribers how their money was being spent, what amount of good was really being done with it, or whether the money was doing mischief rather than good. . . . They would enable us to ascertain the mortality in different hospitals, as well as from different diseases and injuries at the same and different ages, the relative frequency of different diseases and injuries among the classes which enter hospitals in different countries, and in different districts of the same country. They could enable us to ascertain how much of each year of life is wasted by illness (Ulrich, 1992, p. 30).

What Florence Nightingale emphasized is the following:

1. Clinicians have a responsibility to spend their customers' money wisely.
2. Clinicians are accountable to the consumer for their practice and should share their outcomes with the customer or payor.
3. Data should be used to determine appropriate "cuts."
4. Clinicians should be able to measure the improved level of health in the community due to their interventions.

Why hasn't nursing followed through on the wisdom of Ms. Nightingale's admonition to develop a data set to monitor, compare, and bench mark over the years?

The Impact of Health Care Reform

Health care reform will create a dramatically new paradigm for health care delivery. These changes include the establishment of integrated provider networks linking multiple service delivery points, a holistic, patient-driven system with an emphasis on prevention and health maintenance, fixed-financing, and an enlarged consumer role (Anderson, 1993).

Within a reformed care delivery environment, solid opportunities exist to maximize the traditional essence of the nursing profession's practice and to expand nursing roles. Nursing has always been the discipline to use a holistic approach in caring for patients. Nursing as a profession has also engaged patients in their own care and helped these patients reach realistic restorative outcomes based on the patient's response to illness. Creating the appropriate system and capitalizing on the principles of basic nursing practice, however, is contingent upon having consistent data to scientifically support and articulate the profession's contribution to patient outcomes in the redesign of hospital-based and other point-of-service care delivery redesign. It is of utmost importance to make the case for the cost-effectiveness and the quality of care impact which expanded nursing practice and new nursing roles will and can make within a developing health care network. Nursing must have a distinct voice in the deliberations of health care reform at the local, state, and national tables. As the discussions occur and policies develop around an integrated network to provide the continuum of health, illness, and restorative care, nursing, with good data, can influence the cure versus care debates.

Bench marking is another concept that will be key to management decision making under health care reform, and it is a concept which clearly relies on solid data. Bench marking is defined as "the process of comparing practices and results with the best organizations anywhere in the world and adapting the key features to your organization." Its outcomes are "accelerate(d) organizational learning, customer-driven quality, and continuous organizational learning, customer-driven quality, and continuous improvement" (O'Dell, 1993). In other words, best practices are used to learn from and continually improve how the organization functions. It is also important for members of an organization to create bench marks internally and continuously improve.

Bench marking "guards against jumping to quick conclusions or reaching for highly publicized results without understanding the driving forces behind those results" (Heidbreder, 1993). However, as the pace of change accelerates with health care reform, the ability to make rational, data-based decisions will be even more difficult but also more essential for managers and leaders. Now, it is essential to have one accepted, utilized nursing minimum data set which includes the management data necessary to benchmark effective new systems designs. Use of the data set will help direct who cares for patients and where and how care takes place in the new systems.

Nursing Minimum Data Set

The Nursing Minimum Data Set (NMDS) represents the nursing profession's initial attempt to standardize the collection, storage and retrieval of essential, comparable, core nursing data. Its creation was derived from the general concept of a Uniform Minimum Health Data Set, defined by the Health Information Policy Council (1993) as "a minimum set of items (or elements) of information with uniform definitions and categories, concerning a specific aspect or dimension of the health care system, which meets the essential needs of multiple users." As developed by Werley, the NMDS includes 16 elements that have been categorized into three broad groups: (1) nursing care, (2) client demographics, and (3) service (Leske and Werley, 1992). Since the evolution of Werley's NMDS, other minimum data sets have been developed, for example, in long-term care and home health care. Each of these models, however, renders information at the service-delivery level only, and they do not address management data in nursing.

A Nursing Management Minimum Data Set (NMMDS) is a group of core data elements that links management practice outcomes and patient outcomes. A NMMDS is useful to nursing leadership for management decision making and to compare effectiveness across institutions and delivery settings (Huber et al., 1992). According to the University of Iowa research team working on developing the nursing management minimum data set, the NMMDS would "support patient outcomes related to cost of patient care, patient satisfaction, and quality of care" (Simpson, 1994). It would mean, for example, that nurse executives could evaluate patient outcomes, levels of staffing, nursing productivity, nursing workload, length of stay per nursing unit or the specific patient population profile for a unit (Flarey, 1993). The challenge is to combine these disparate minimum data sets into one accepted tool for use by all of the profession across all settings and types of nursing practice and management practice. If appropriately developed and used, the data will drive how the management of the business of patient care is most cost effective.

AONE'S Commitment

AONE has made a commitment to the profession to take the leadership role in bringing together all of the existing nursing minimum data sets into one tool for all of nursing across the continuum of health care delivery. AONE's role in this process is to bring together the experts on the issue, and to urge consensus on one data set for the profession, rather than to maintain several disparate data sets, as currently exists (Lambertus, 1993).

An advisory board composed of nursing minimum data set experts and nurse executives has been established to develop consensus on one nursing management minimum data set for a reformed health care system. Not only is this timely, but the pace must increase so this group can complete its work.

Summary

While the need for nursing data has long been established, the current era of health care reform makes it a mandate. AONE is committed to working toward consensus, on behalf of the nursing profession, on the development of *one* nursing management minimum data set that will allow the profession to delineate effective care delivery systems as they relate to outcome data. The contribution these management data will make in shaping the effective health care system or network of the future, as well as the public policies that allow for the system to flourish, will be invaluable to the profession and to the public.

References

Anderson, R. (1993). Nursing leadership and health care reform—Part III: Nurse executive role in a reformed health care system. *Journal of Nursing Administration, 23*(12), 8–9.

Flarey, D. (1993). Quality improvement through data analysis. *Journal of Nursing Administration, 23*(12), 21–30.

Heidbreder, J. (1993). Looking for the light—Not the heat. *Healthcare Forum Journal, 36*(1), 26.

Huber, D., Delaney, C., and Crossley, J. (1992). A nursing minimum data set. *Journal of Nursing Administration, 22*(7/8), 35–40.

Lambertus, T. D. (1993). Understanding bench-marking. *Journal of Healthcare Material Management, 11*(9), 36–40.

Leske, J. S. and Werley, H. D. (1992). Use of the nursing minimum data set. *Computers in Nursing, 10*(6), 259–263.

O'Dell, C. (1993). Building on received wisdom. *Healthcare Forum Journal, 36*(1), 17.

Simpson, R. L. (1994). A nursing management minimum data set. *Nursing Management, 24*(4), 24–25.

Ulrich, B. T. (1992). *Leadership and Management According to Florence Nightingale.* Norwalk, CT: Appleton & Lange.

Significance of the Nursing Minimum Data Set for Decision Support in Acute Care

Connie Delaney, PhD, RN
Associate Professor
College of Nursing
The University of Iowa

Introduction

The Nursing Minimum Data Set (NMDS) addresses the core data needed to support decision making in clinical nursing. In addition to the demographic and service data elements found in other health care data sets, the NMDS includes nursing diagnoses/problems, interventions to treat the diagnoses/problems, outcomes of nursing treatments, and intensity, a measure of nursing resources. Ready access to such data can generate information regarding the diagnoses that nurses treat, which interventions contribute to quality outcomes in patient care, and which treatment plans are most effective and efficient. Such data is needed for implementation of the Computerized Patient Record (CPR).

Implementation of computerized information systems is essential for data-driven decision support in clinical practice. Adoption of these systems has led to the growing realization that information systems are not just a vehicle to maintain a data base. Rather they affect both the structure and function of the organization, the quality of patient care as well as the work life of the employees, and ultimately the cost and quality of patient care.

This chapter discusses the use of the NMDS for decision support in acute care. The discussion focuses on the status of the NMDS, implications for data systems architecture, and use of the data to answer questions posed in clinical practice.

Status of the Nursing Minimum Data Set

The Nursing Minimum Data Set, built on the concept of the Uniform Minimum Health Data Sets, was consensually derived through the efforts of a national group of experts. The Murnaghan and White (1970) and Health Information Policy Council Subcommittee on Data Comparability and Standards (1983) criteria for minimum data sets as well as the design and implementation issues identified by Murnaghan (1978) have guided the development of the NMDS. By definition, the NMDS includes the essential nursing data used on a regular basis by most nurses across all settings in the delivery of care.

The purposes of the NMDS are fourfold (Werley and Zorn, 1988):

1. Establish comparability of nursing data across populations, settings, geographic areas, and time;

2. Describe the nursing care of patients or clients and their families in a variety of settings, both institutional and noninstitutional;

3. Demonstrate or project trends regarding nursing care needs and allocation of nursing resources to patients or clients according to their health problems or nursing diagnoses;

4. Stimulate nursing research through links to the detailed data existing in nursing information systems and other health care information systems (p. 107).

To date, the elements and working definitions of the NMDS (see Table 1), including

Table 1.
Elements of Nursing Minimum Data Set

Nursing Care	Service
1. Nursing diagnosis	10. Unique facility/service agency number
2. Nursing intervention	11. Unique health record number of patient
3. Nursing outcome	12. Unique number of principal registered nurse provider
4. Intensity of nursing care	13. Episode admission or encounter date
Patient or Client Demographic	14. Discharge or termination date
5. Personal identification	15. Disposition of patient or client
6. Date of birth	16. Expected payer for most of bill
7. Sex	
8. Race and ethnicity	
9. Residence	

nursing care, demographic, and service elements, have been outlined (Werley and Lang, 1988). Nursing care elements include nursing diagnosis, intervention, outcome, and intensity of nursing care. Personal identification, date of birth, sex, race and ethnicity, and residence constitute the patient demographic category. And last, the service category includes the unique facility number, unique health record number of the patient, unique number of principal registered nurse provider, episode admission or encounter data, discharge or termination date, disposition of patient, and expected payer for most of the bill.

Although most elements are contained and have been collected within other health care minimum data sets, namely the UHDDS, several implementation issues exist. First, consensus has not been reached within health care and society on what information will be used for the personal identification. Numerous working groups at state and national levels are considering resolutions that will protect individual privacy and confidentiality and provide for tracking of individual health care records across sites and settings from birth to death. Second, unique numbers for principal registered nurse providers have not been designated. Perhaps the work of the National Council of State Boards of Nursing in issuing unique provider numbers at the national level will provide this much needed data. Third, taxonomies and classifications for nursing care elements of nursing diagnosis, intervention, and outcomes of the NMDS are still under development.

Following more than 15 years of pioneering efforts by the North American Nursing Diagnosis Association (NANDA), the Nursing Taxonomy I of diagnoses was approved in 1987. The taxonomy has since been endorsed by the American Nurses' Association. Currently, 112 diagnoses (with associated etiologies and defining characteristics) have been identified (Gordon, 1987; Gordon, 1989; North American Nursing Diagnosis Association, 1989a, 1990). This taxonomy, as well as the problem classification outlined in the Omaha Classification, provides a framework for documenting what nurses treat.

The Nursing Intervention Classification is in the process of clinical testing in numerous sites and settings (McCloskey et al., 1990). In addition, the Omaha System (Martin and Scheet, 1992) offers a framework for nursing interventions for community health and other settings while Saba and colleagues' (1991) Nursing Interventions for Home Health Care has been developed for use in home health nursing services. Although no classification of nursing outcomes is currently available, a major research effort is currently funded by the National Institute of Nursing Research (Johnson and Maas, 1994).

The existence of synonyms and antonyms in different classifications systems raises questions of definition and data equivalency, measurement, and underlying theoretical assumptions. The ability of the NMDS to support comparability of nursing data, however, is being enhanced by the Board of the International Council for Nurses' work on the International Classification of Nursing Practice, which includes nursing diagnosis, intervention, and outcome elements of the NMDS (Lang, 1991).

And last, much confusion exists concerning the NMDS element of nursing intensity, which is defined as hours of care and staff mix. Intensity has been associated with interventions, episode of care, utilization, and acuity (Ryan et al., 1994).

Despite these issues, multiple studies have been conducted or are in process that document the availability and retrievability of the NMDS in manual and computerized information systems across sites and settings (Ryan and Delaney, 1994). Such pioneering work is beginning to provide direction for systems architecture that will enhance documentation of care, continued development and refinement of nursing classification systems, linkage to existing health care information systems and to state and national health-related data bases, and comparability of nursing care across site, setting, and geographical area. This work will aid health policy planning and decision-making, and further advance nursing as a research-based discipline.

Implications for Data (Systems) Architecture

Computerized information systems must support both the management and processing of the data comprising the NMDS. That is, the system must have the functional capacity to collect, aggregate, organize, move, and present the data in a way that is accurate, economical, efficient, and useful to the practitioner. In addition, the system must support the processing of the data, including clinical decision making of the practitioner, discovering knowledge by the researcher, and/or development of theory by nursing theorists. To this end, input must be logical, adequate processing must be assured, ample data storage and retrieval must be guaranteed, and the system's output must be valid and reliable. Specific implications for system design for each of these criteria follow.

Logical Input

Clear and unambiguous definitions of all data elements should be available and, if possible, incorporated into the system and made available in data dictionaries. For example, if NANDA nursing diagnoses are used, the conceptual definition and, when available, operational definitions of the diagnosis, related factors and defining characteristics should be made available. Help screens may facilitate this. It is necessary that the system possess the flexibility to accommodate new data items, change existing definitions to accommodate expanded definitions, and delete data items no longer necessary. Each data item should be clearly coded, thus allowing every data element to be a key field for data retrieval. The system should be built upon an underlying conceptual framework. Provision for periodic reorganization and updating of each classification implemented in the information system must be made. Although these updates are quite frequent, such updating is necessary to reflect current practice. Point-of-care data entry will facilitate more accurate and complete documentation of the NMDS.

Adequate Processing

Linkages between data elements and sets must be made. This allows study of the effects of nursing care among nursing diagnoses, interventions, outcomes and resources used over time, activity and patient population. With the development and implementation of the CPR and Community Health Management Information Systems, it is essential that linkages to relational data bases outside the institution be considered. Processing must be monitored to ensure that degradation of accuracy from programming errors or mistakes in computer processing does not occur. Adequate response time, minimal downtime, and planned installation of system enhancements ensure efficient data processing.

Ample Storage and Retrieval

All care planning data included in the NMDS should be archived, maintained, and used for research and quality improvement activities. If the data has been appropriately collected, coded, and stored, then population-based, problem-oriented, or procedure specific data can be retrieved.

Valid and Reliable Output

Validity and reliability of the content is increased if it has been derived through literature searches, consultation with nurse experts in practice, education, research, and administration, expertise of practicing clinicians, and use of classifications developed through a research process. Incorporation of all operational definitions of data elements and availability of these definitions on-line may enhance the validity of the clinical data. Validity and reliability studies should be ongoing within the institution to determine the diagnostic reasoning of the clinicians, measure nursing interventions prescribed for treatment of nursing diagnoses, describe nursing outcomes based on these interventions, and ascertain the costs associated with nursing care. Multiple levels of security and numerous procedures for maintaining data confidentiality are essential to the validity and reliability of the data. Policies governing the use of standardized language, documentation, and procedures for responding to system failure are essential to ensure complete, accurate, and quality data. Regular audits of each patient's care plan will help ensure data quality.

The usefulness of the data requires that the data be free from errors. Developing computer programs to complete regular consistency checks and specific logical relationships between certain data items provide a useful means of ensuring some degree of data accuracy (Rush et al., 1987). For many items in a data base such as the NMDS, entry of certain values dictates a restricted selection of values for subsequently recorded related data elements. Consistency, or inter-item checking (the verification of a relationship between data values), requires that values for two or more items of data be available simultaneously for comparison. Evaluation for coding errors and deviations from the coding schema should be included. Calculation of the frequencies for all data elements and review for logical inconsistencies assist in determining data quality. These calculated frequencies of occurrence of all data elements can be compared with in-house statistical reports to determine consistency. Last, evaluating the data base for meaningless, missing, and duplicative data further ensures the validity and reliability of the data.

The value of the data in the computerized system is influenced by the degree to which users have been oriented to the various elements of the system: standardized language, computers, pathway content, standards of nursing care, protocols, and critical paths. Ongoing staff development is mandatory to disseminate classification updates and related research findings. Supervision and performance appraisals of the nurses consistent with the implementation of standardized language will enhance compliance, and consequently, the data quality. Also, integral to maintaining data quality is the use of Quality Assurance-Improvement programs, on indicators set at both the unit, division, and nursing department levels to examine the relationship between nursing interventions prescribed for diagnoses, nursing interventions delivered, and outcomes resulting from nursing actions.

Using the Data Base to Address Clinical Questions

McCloskey (1988) asserts that the minimum data set provides a way of collecting nursing knowledge that would lead to the development of not only improved nursing information systems but also to modification of what we collect to construct the NMDS. Standardized data sets such as the NMDS provide a means for determining rates of health care events through a variety of sampling frames while realizing cost and time savings in data retrieval (Allison-Cooke, Griffin, Schwartz, and Malbon, 1991; Paul, 1991). One of the best strategies for providing a viable framework for looking at the potential of the NMDS to address clinical issues is to use nursing informatics as the conceptual basis for study of nursing's essential data, coupled with the taxonomy for nursing research using computerized data bases proposed by McCormick (1991). The taxonomy is composed of three major categories of research focus: Nursing Science in Patient Care, Efficacy of Nursing Strategies in Solving Patient Problems, and Nursing Care Organization and Delivery. Within each area of focus, research activities are ordered into aggregate, utility, abstractions, correlations, linear profiles, comparisons, and quality. Selection of any major category or categories and focus area(s), coupled with one or more elements of the NMDS, can provide information related to clinical practice. For example, if one applies Nursing Science in Patient Care with an aggregate focus to the patient demographic elements of date of birth, sex, and race/ethnicity and the nursing care element of nursing diagnosis, a demographic profile for each diagnostic label can be derived.

Zielstorff (1984) noted:

Those who work in the design and development of nursing information systems constantly bemoan the fact that there are so few clinical problems in nursing for which the etiology, symptoms, treatment, and expected outcomes are known. There are no known probability estimates for prevalence or incidence of common nursing problems; or for relating symptoms to diagnosis, or treatment to outcome (p. 9).

Numerous studies have begun to address these concerns. Studies have validated the availability and retrievability of the NMDS from computerized information systems in acute care (Devine and Werley, 1988; Delaney and Mehmert, 1990; Rios-Iturrino, Delaney, Mehmert, Kruckeberg, and Chung, 1991; Mehmert and Delaney, 1991; Delaney and Mehmert, 1991; Delaney, Mehmert, Prophet, Bellinger, and Ellerbe, 1991; Delaney, 1991; Mehmert, Delaney, Prophet, and Crossley, 1992; Delaney, Mehmert, Prophet, Bellinger, S. Gardner, and Ellerbe, 1992; Ryan et al., 1994), as well as in nursing centers, ambulatory, home health care, and long term care. Such findings set the stage for comparisons across settings. These studies unequivocally identify the costs savings realized from computerized versus manual data records. Since not all systems have established linkages among the NMDS data elements, the ability to quantify diagnoses, treatments, outcomes, and costs of nursing and to determine their inter-relationships is compromised. These studies have begun to describe the demographic variables for the patients nurses treat, determine the nursing diagnoses, interventions, and outcomes prevalent in different clinical populations, and quantify direct nursing care costs per nursing diagnosis and DRG category. Moreover, as McCloskey (1988) asserted, such work has begun to suggest modifications and enhancements to collection of the NMDS. For example, Huber, Delaney, Crossley, Mehmert, and Ellerbe (1992) have identified a Nursing Management Minimum Data Set to complement the ability of the NMDS to meet the needs of nurse executives.

Nursing leaders have identified national and regional data bases as the key to measuring patient outcomes. McPhillips (1992) noted "the importance of valid, complete, and accurate data cannot be stressed enough in the pursuit of our goal of identifying and promoting health care interventions that are of consistently high quality, appropriate, and cost effective" (p. 197). Stevic (1992) identified the "severe limitations that exist in the lack of large, standardized tests of data, elements or tools, and their relative acceptance within nursing practice" (p. 201).

Summary

All major national health care, research, professional, and accrediting organizations have recognized the importance of the NMDS. Simpson (1991) asserts that "although nurses stand to benefit a great deal from electronic medical charting, the nursing profession's current polyglot language of communication presents one of the greatest obstacles for their swift development. To have an electronic charting system, there must be standardized coding, screen formats, problem lists and encounter forms" (p. 14). Without a minimum data set, such activities are not possible. Simpson further states, "Nurses will not only have to adopt a minimum data set with all deliberate speed, but also demand nursing representation" (p. 13). The leadership of nursing in this area will not only help to fulfill the purpose of the NMDS but will also facilitate the direction of health care reform and the improvement of patient care.

References

Allison-Cooke, S., Griffin, J., Schwartz, R. and Malbon, A. (1991). Building a multi-state data base for research purposes. *Abstracts of the Sixth Annual Meeting of the National Association of Health Data Organizations*. Falls Church, VA: National Association of Health Data Organizations.

Classification of nursing interventions. *Journal of Professional Nursing, 6*(3), 151-157.

Delaney, C., and Mehmert, P. (1990). Electronic transfer of clinical NMDS facilitates nursing diagnoses validation. [Paper] In *Proceedings of the Fourteenth Annual Symposium on Computer Applications in Medical Care (SCAMC)* (pp. 899-901). Washington, DC: IEEE Computer Society Press.

Delaney, C., and Mehmert, P. (1991). Utility of NMDS is validation of computerized nursing diagnoses. In R. Carroll-Johnson (Ed.), *Classification of Nursing Diagnoses: Proceedings of the Ninth Annual North American Nursing Diagnosis Association* (pp. 175-179). Philadelphia: J. B. Lippincott Co.

Delaney, C., Mehmert, P., Prophet, C., Bellinger, S., Huber, D., and Ellerbe, S. (1992). Standardized nursing language for healthcare information systems. *Journal of Medical Systems, 16*(4): 145-149.

Devine, E., and Werley, H. (1988). Testing of the nursing minimum data set: Availability of data and reliability. *Research in Nursing and Health, 11*(2), 97-104.

Gordon, M. (1987). *Nursing Diagnoses* (2nd ed). New York: McGraw-Hill Book Co.

Gordon, M. (1989, May). *Theoretical Basis for Nursing Diagnosis*. Paper presented at University of Ottawa Conference, Nursing Theory, Nursing Diagnosis, Nursing Intervention.

Health Information Policy Council. (1983). *Background Paper: Uniform Minimum Health Data Sets* (Unpublished). Washington, DC: U.S. Department of Health and Human Services.

Huber, D., Delaney, C., Crossley, J., Mehmert, M., and Ellerbe, S. (1992). A nursing management minimum data set. *Journal of Nursing Administration, 22*, 35-40.

Johnson, M., and Maas, M. (1994). Nursing-focused patient outcomes: Challenge for the nineties. In J. McCloskey and H. Grace (Eds.), *Current Issues in Nursing* (4th ed., pp. 136-142). St. Louis: C. V. Mosby Co.

Lang, N. (November 22, 1991). Personal communication, Letter to J. McCloskey, G. Bulechek.

Martin, K. and Scheet, N. (1992). *The Omaha System*. Philadelphia: W. B. Saunders Co.

McCloskey, J. (1988). The Nursing Minimum Data Set: Benefits and Implications for Nurse Educators. In H. Werley and N. Lang (Eds.), *Identification of the Nursing Minimum Data Set*. New York: Springer Publishing Co.

McCloskey, J., Bulechek, G., Cohen, M., Craft, M., Crossley, J., Denehy, J., Glick, O., Kruckeberg, T., Maas, M., Prophet, C., Tripp-Reimer, T. (1990). Classification of nursing interventions. *Journal of Professional Nursing, 6*(3), 151-157.

McCormick, K. (1991). Future data needs for quality of care monitoring, DRG considerations, reimbursement and outcome measurement. *Image, 23,* 29-32.

McPhillips, R. (1992). National and regional data bases: The big picture. In *Patient Outcomes Research: Examining the Effectiveness of Nursing Practice. Proceedings of the State of the Science Conference—NCNR.* DHHS Pub. No. (NIH 93-3411).

Mehmert, P. and Delaney, C. (1991). Validation of defining characteristics of immobility using the computerized NMDS. *Nursing Diagnosis, 2*(4), 143-154.

Mehmert, P. A., Delaney, C., Crossly, J. and Prophet, C. (1992). Validation of nursing diagnostic labels across clinical sites using the NMDS and computerized information systems. In R. Carroll-Johnson and M. Paquette (Eds.), *Nursing Diagnosis—New Directions into the 21st Century. Tenth Conference on Classification of Nursing Diagnosis* (pp. 304-306). San Diego: NANDA.

Murnaghan, H., and White, K. (Eds.) (1970). *Hospital Discharge Data: Report of the Conference on Hospital Discharge Abstract Systems.* Philadelphia: J. B. Lippincott Co.

Murnaghan, J. (1978). Uniform basic data sets for health statistical systems. *International Journal of Epidemiology, 7*(3), 263-269.

North American Nursing Diagnosis Association. (1989a). *Taxonomy I—Revised 1989: With Official Diagnostic Categories.* St. Louis: Author.

North American Nursing Diagnosis Association. (1989b). *Proceedings of the Invitational Conference on Research Methods for Validating Nursing Diagnosis.* St. Louis: Author.

North American Nursing Diagnosis Association. (1990). *Taxonomy I—Revised 1990: With Official Diagnostic Categories.* St. Louis: Author.

Paul, J. (1991). Use of large databases in outcomes research. *Abstracts of the Sixth Annual Meeting of the National Association of Health Data Organizations.* Falls Church, VA: National Association of Health Data Organizations.

Rios-Iturrino, H., Delaney, C., Mehmert, P., Kruckeberg, T., and Chung, Y. (1991). Validation of defining characteristics for nursing diagnoses using the nursing minimum data set extracted from a computerized nursing information system. *Journal of Professional Nursing, 7*(5), 293-299.

Rush, R., Barwick, J., Elsinger, J., Crum, D., Foulkes, M., and Chantry, K. (1987). Maximizing detection of data inconsistency: The development of a consistency check interpreter. In *Symposium on Computer Applications in Medical Care* (pp. 848-851).

Ryan, P., Coenen, A., Devine, E., Werley, H., Sutton, J., and Kelber, S. (1994). Prevalence and relationships among elements of the Nursing Minimum Data Set. In S. J. Grobe and E. S. Pluyter-Wenting, (Eds.). *Nursing Informatics: An International Overview for Nursing in a Technological Era* (pp. 174-178). Amsterdam: Elsevier.

Ryan, P. and Delaney, C. (1994). The Nursing Minimum Data Set. *Annual Review of Nursing, 13.*

Saba, V., O'Hare, P., Zuckerman, A., Boondas, J., Levine, E., and Oatway, D. (1991). A nursing intervention taxonomy for home health care. *Nursing and Health Care, 12,* 296-299.

Simpson, R. (1991). Electronic patient charts: Beware the hype. *Nursing Management, 22*(4), 13.

Stevic, M. (1992). Patient-linked data bases: Implications for a nursing outcomes research agenda. In *Patient outcomes research: Examining the effectiveness of nursing practice. Proceedings of the State of the Science Conference—NCNR* (p. 201). DHHS Pub. No. (NIH 93-3411).

Werley, H., and Lang, N. (Eds.) (1988). *Identification of the Nursing Minimum Data.* New York: Springer Publishing Co.

Werley, H., and Zorn, C. (1988). The Nursing Minimum Data Set: Benefits and implications. In H. Werley and N. Lang (Eds.), *Identification of the Nursing Minimum Data Set.* New York: Springer Publishing Co.

Zielstorff, R. (1984). Why aren't there more significant automated nursing information systems? *Journal of Nursing Administration, 14*(1), 7-10.

The Omaha System: A Data Base for Ambulatory and Home Care

Karen A. Martin, RN, MSN, FAAN
Health Care Consultant
Formerly: Director of Research, VNA of Omaha
Partially funded by National Center for Nursing Research, NIH, grant R01 NR02192.
Portions of this chapter are excerpted from Martin and Scheet's book, The Omaha System: Applications for Community Health Nursing. Philadelphia: W. B. Saunders Co., 1992.
Reprinted with permission.

Introduction

The practice of nursing is a pluralistic combination of art and science. Donahue's illustrated history (1985) provides an outstanding graphic example in its depiction of the important similarities and differences in the practice of nursing from a national and international perspective. Equally rich and varied are the data that current clinicians generate from service settings for inclusion in management information systems. Such systems should assist clinicians to transform diverse data into patterns of information and knowledge which should also be valuable for management personnel, third-party payers, accreditors, educators, and researchers.

With such diversity of possible users, how can the profession address the issues of global information management and setting-specific clinical data bases? Much has been written about the past, present, and future of information systems. The nursing literature clearly documents the struggles and lack of consensus as well as the phenomenal progress within the profession (Abraham, Nadzam, and Fitzpatrick, 1989; Grady and Schwartz, 1993; Canadian Nurses Association, 1993; National Center for Nursing Research [NCNR], 1993; Werley and Lang, 1988; Zielstorff, Hudgings, Grobe, and NCNIP, 1993).

The title of a recent publication, *Next-Generation Nursing Information Systems* (Zielstorff et al., 1993) attests to the profession's progress. The authors predict:

...the system must be rebuilt on a design different from that of most approaches used today; it must be a data-driven rather than a process-driven system. A dominant feature of the new system is its focus on the acquisition, management, processing, and presentation of "atomic-level" data that can be used across multiple settings for multiple purposes. The paradigm shift to a data-driven system represents a new generation of information technology... (p. 3).

Various forces are encouraging such developments in nursing information systems. Health care providers are increasing their demands for useful systems capable of transforming data into information, despite the lack of standardization involving content and form of client records across service settings. Within those settings, management personnel are becoming more concerned about the inaccessibility, incompleteness, and inaccuracies of client records. Managers are also concerned about the inefficiency and rising costs of their health care settings and becoming interested in the potential benefits of the principles of total quality management or continuous quality improvement, if used, throughout their setting. Furthermore, effectiveness of services can rarely be assessed and its absence is being challenged by third-party payers, accreditors, and researchers.

Progress is evident when nurses can describe features of the next-generation systems as noted in the earlier quotation, even though no such system or data base yet exists. In reality, a single system or data base may never exist capable of meeting the needs of all nurses, or even all nurses practicing in ambulatory and home care settings. Barriers frequently associated with existing systems, which must be addressed and will be difficult to eliminate, include control, cost, integration, uniform nursing language, user interface, and direct entry.

Data Needs

Ambulatory and home care nurses represent a significant and rapidly increasing force in professional practice. They share basic values and goals with other members of the nursing profession: (1) to provide the highest quality nursing service possible; (2) to incorporate nursing diagnosis, outcome measure, and intervention language of the nursing process with research-based practice; (3) to contribute to the client's achievement of positive outcomes; and (4) to limit the quantity of documentation. They also share a nursing tradition linked to clinical information systems which involves collecting, managing, processing, transferring, and communicating data in a meaningful way (NCNR, 1993).

Nurses in ambulatory and home care settings have unique experiences within their practice settings, especially when compared to nurses in acute and long-term care settings. They have greater access to environmental, psychosocial, and health-related behavior data which dramatically influence a client's history, current status, and future potential. Also available are those data involving family members, friends, and others who serve as caregivers. The knowledge, skill, dedication, and other resources that care givers provide are critical factors for client independence and recovery. Nurses in ambulatory and home care develop a customer-focused attitude when they receive frequent, strong cues that clients as individuals, families, aggregates, and communities are in control of their health and illness rather than the nurse. As a result of working with clients for longer periods of time, nurses are more likely to support a comprehensive approach to health care services and to recognize the need for preventive measures. Because nurses in ambulatory and home care frequently explain benefits to clients, they tend to be well-informed about the costs of services. Nurses usually recognize that the frequency, length, and type of client-contact is directly related to regulations of third-party payers.

How can nurses in ambulatory and home care settings address their data base needs? It is critical that nurses with varied backgrounds and roles are represented on decision-making information system teams. Typically, a team for a specific setting explores hardware options and monitors software development, including planning, system requirements definition, programming, testing, and implementation. Nurses in particular should consider issues related to standardized language, validity, reliability, cost, and control. They also need to address reimbursement regulations and issues of utility specific to their practice and setting. As these issues are resolved, ambulatory and home care nurses can develop or use models and systems having the potential to convert data into useful information and knowledge, the ultimate power of information systems.

The Omaha System

The Omaha System is an example of a practice-based model designed to address the issues that concern ambulatory and home care nurses. Developed by community health nurses to describe and measure ambulatory and home care nursing practice, the Omaha System evolved because of 20 years of effort, 11 years of federally funded research, and the combined work of many health care and data processing professionals (Martin and Scheet, 1992a, 1992b; Martin, Scheet, and Stegman, 1993). Because the System exists in the public domain, it is equally accessible to ambulatory and home care nurses and other potential users.

The Omaha System was developed to consist of three components: The Problem Classification Scheme, Intervention Scheme, and Problem Rating Scale for Outcomes. The Problem Classification Scheme is a taxonomy of client problems or nursing diagnoses that provides consistent language to address client concerns. The Intervention Scheme is a taxonomy of nursing actions or activities that offers a method of describing services provided to clients. The Problem Rating Scale for Outcomes is an evaluation tool designed to measure client progress in relation to specific problems or nursing diagnoses.

The three components of the Omaha System represent an approach to practice, documentation, and data management that is both structured and comprehensive. Because the Omaha System provides a research-based, valid and reliable method for obtaining standardized data, it offers interrelated benefits to clinicians, administrators, nursing students, faculty members, and national researchers (Martin, Leak, and Aden, 1992). Both extensive field testing and national-international use have occurred. The application of the Omaha System in home care, public health, school health, clinic ambulatory care, parish, migrant, and jail programs, as well as by faculty and students, has been described (Martin and Scheet, 1992a, 1992b; Martin et al., 1992; Tully and Bennett, 1992).

Problem Classification Scheme

The Problem Classification Scheme is a taxonomy of nursing diagnoses developed from actual client data by community health nurses that provides holistic language and a flexible structure to define the practice of nursing. This classification system offers a comprehensive method for collecting, sorting, classifying, documenting, coding, and analyzing client data for the clinician, supervisor, and administrator. The Scheme enables users to sort essential from non-essential data objectively and efficiently, and to identify patterns in the data. Thus, the Problem Classification Scheme furnishes a diagnostic bridge between the client data base and client care, and the use of this system can enhance the science of nursing.

The structure of the Problem Classification Scheme consists of four levels: domains, problems, modifiers, and signs/symptoms. Four domains represent the essence of nursing practice: Environmental, Psychosocial, Physiological, and Health-Related Behaviors. A total of 40 client problems or nursing diagnoses are included in the Problem Classification Scheme. Income, Caretaking/Parenting, Circulation, and Substance Use are examples of problems from each of the domains. Two sets of modifiers are used in conjunction with each problem. Problems are referenced as health promotion, potential, or actual, as well as family or individual. When an actual problem modifier is used, a cluster of problem-specific signs and symptoms provides the diagnostic clues to problem identification. For example, the problem, Substance Use, has six signs and symptoms for the selection if the client abuses over-the-counter/street drugs, abuses alcohol, smokes, has difficulty performing normal routines, reflex disturbances, and behavior change. Because the Problem Classification Scheme is intended to be an open system and not exhaustive, "Other" appears at the end of each domain and each sign and symptom cluster.

Intervention Scheme

The Intervention Scheme is a systematic arrangement of nursing actions or activities designed to help nurses and other health care professionals document plans and interventions. The Intervention Scheme is a framework of nursing actions designed for use with nursing diagnoses. It represents an initial research-based effort to link the effectiveness of interventions with diagnoses, an effort not yet accomplished within the nursing profession.

The Intervention Scheme provides the nurse with a tool that includes standard language to guide both practice and documentation in relation to the other components of the nursing process. The Intervention Scheme is of value not only to interdisciplinary clinicians, but also to supervisors, administrators, utilization review committee members, and other record auditors.

The first level of the Intervention Scheme comprises four comprehensive categories: Health Teaching, Guidance, and Counseling; Treatments and Procedures; Case Management; and Surveillance. When viewed collectively, these categories can be used by a nurse to develop a plan or document an intervention specific to a client problem. The second level of the Intervention Scheme is an alphabetic listing of 62 targets. Targets are defined as objects of nursing interventions or nursing activities. Examples of targets are bonding, gait training, and skin care. The targets are used to further delineate a problem-specific intervention category. The nurse selects one or more targets to describe a plan or intervention category specific to a client problem. Because the targets are not intended to be exhaustive, "Other" appears at the end of the list, enabling the nurse to document a word or words that describe a needed addition.

The third level of the Intervention Scheme is designed for client-specific information. Pertinent, concisely worded, or short phrases are generated by community health nurses or other community health professionals as they develop plans or document care provided to a specific client. Although not part of the research projects, VNA of Omaha staff organized its suggestions into care planning guides (Martin and Scheet, 1992b).

Problem Rating Scale for Outcomes

The Problem Rating Scale for Outcomes is intended to measure client progress in relation to specific client problems and to provide both a guide for practice and a method of documentation. The Scale was designed for use throughout the time of client service. When establishing the initial ratings for client problems, the nurse creates an independent data baseline, capturing the condition and circumstances of the client at a given point in time. This admission baseline is used to compare and contrast the client's condition and circumstances with the ratings completed at later intervals and at client dismissal. The comparison or change in ratings over time can be used to identify the presence or absence of client progress in relation to nursing intervention.

A clinician can compare problem-specific ratings to judge the effectiveness of the plan of care. The Scale provides a needed supervisory tool and a data set for agency management. Management personnel can use client data from individuals or aggregates to evaluate the impact of services and agency operations. The same data can be used by researchers to advance the science of nursing.

The Problem Rating Scale for Outcomes is comprised of three summated or Likert-type ordinal subscales: The first subscale for Knowledge, the second for Behavior, and the third for Status. Although the three concepts of the Problem Rating Scale for Outcomes are interrelated, they represent three discrete dimensions of client outcomes. The three dimensions of the Problem Rating Scale for Outcomes are equal in importance, although they may not be equal when used with a specific client.

The ratings have characteristics of ordinal scales: (1) five mutually exclusive classes or categories; (2) each continuum collectively exhaustive; and (3) categories that fit into a specific order or sequence. Based on the scaling pattern devised by Likert, the scale for each of the concepts has five categories or degrees for response. Unlike some Likert-type scales, the Problem Rating Scale for Outcomes does not include a formal set of questions that can be scored and summed to produce a final numeric rating. Instead, nurses and other users are expected to have a knowledge base that allows them to arrive at a final score for each of the three concepts. Users are also expected to recognize that each scale was designed for use with the range of possible clients; sample patterns or examples are available in a manual (Martin and Scheet, 1992b).

Summary

Nurses and other users of clinical information systems and data bases share certain requirements. These requirements involve the ability to describe practice, facilitate documentation of services, integrate clinical data with other components of an information system, transform data into information and knowledge, and retrieve clinical information. Ambulatory and home care nurses have additional, unique data base needs which relate to the setting. These nurses recognize that it is important to include data about the family, significant others, and caregivers as well as environmental, psychosocial, and health-related behavior information. Practice, documentation, and data management in the ambulatory and home care settings are greatly influenced by the requirements of third-party payers and accreditors. Therefore, a service setting's information system must accommodate data collection and transformation that meets the specific requirements of payers and accreditors for that setting and geographic area.

The Omaha System is a model that ambulatory and home care nurses have found useful to operationalize the nursing process and to describe and measure client problems or nursing diagnoses, nursing actions, and client outcomes. The System was developed during a series of three VNA of Omaha research projects and further studied during a fourth project. The Omaha System can contribute to improving professional practice, documentation, and data management. The Omaha System can also contribute to transforming data into information and knowledge and, therefore, increase the power of nurses as they describe and measure their practice.

References

Abraham, I. L., Nadzam, D. M., and Fitzpatrick, J. J. (Eds.). (1989). *Statistics and Quantitative Methods in Nursing*. Philadelphia: W. B. Saunders Co.

Canadian Nurses Association. (1993). *Papers from the Nursing Minimum Data Set Conference*. Ottawa, Ontario, Canada: Canadian Nurses Association.

Donahue, M. P. (1985). *Nursing: The Finest Art—An Illustrated History*. St. Louis: C. V. Mosby Co.

Grady, M. L., and Schwartz, H. A. (Eds.). (1993, May). *Automated Data Sources for Ambulatory Care Effectiveness Research*. (AHCRP Pub. No. 93-0042). Rockville, MD: AHCPR.

Martin, K. S., Leak, G. K., and Aden, C. A. (1992, November). The Omaha System: A research-based model for decision making. *Journal of Nursing Administration, 22*(11), 47-52.

Martin, K. S., and Scheet, N. J. (1992a). *The Omaha System: Applications for Community Health Nursing*. Philadelphia: W. B. Saunders Co.

Martin, K. S., and Scheet, N. J. (1992b). *The Omaha System: A Pocket Guide for Community Health Nursing*. Philadelphia: W. B. Saunders Co.

Martin, K. S., Scheet, N. J., and Stegman, M. R. (1993, December). Home health clients: Characteristics, outcomes of care, and nursing interventions. *American Journal of Public Health, 83*(12), 1730-1734.

National Center for Nursing Research. (1993, May). *Nursing Informatics: Enhancing Patient Care.* (NIH Pub. No. 93-2419). Bethesda, MD: National Center for Nursing Research.

Tully, M., and Bennett, K. (1992, March). Extending community health nursing services. *Journal of Nursing Administration, 22*(3), 38-42.

Werley, H. H., and Lang, N. M. (Eds.). (1988). *Identification of the Nursing Minimum Data Set.* New York: Springer Publishing Co.

Zielstorff, R. D., Hudgings, C. I., Grobe, S. J., and NCNIP. (1993, May). *Next-Generation Nursing Information Systems.* Washington, DC: American Nurses Association/National League for Nursing.

Decision-Support Systems for Nurse Managers

Nancy K. Meehan, Ph.D., RN
Assistant Professor
Department of Nursing Science
Clemson University

Introduction

(The primary emphasis of the health care reform movement is the availability of cost-effective health care for all individuals. To ensure that health care is accessible to everyone, many cost-containment procedures must be instituted. One method of reducing health care costs is the implementation of decision-support systems (DSS).)

Many Hospital Information System (HIS) vendors presently are marketing DSS as a major cost-reduction tool. Since all managerial activities revolve around decision making, the manager is considered first and foremost a decision maker (Turban, 1993). Numerically, the largest group of managers in hospitals are registered nurses; therefore, nurse managers are the primary decision makers of health care institutions.

Several problems limit the nurse manager's decision-making ability, though; currently there is too much health care information available for one individual to process. Turban (1993) states that most individuals are in "information overload"; there is too much information to assimilate. Sinclair (1990) believes that the quality of professional information available has surpassed the human capability for absorption. Since scientific knowledge is said to double every two years, nurse managers will continue to need assistance in processing these immense amounts of data.

Another problem that exists is the delay in relaying information. Nurse managers often have to wait for additional information. Research indicates that most managers work on many problems at one time, moving from one to another as they await for more information on their current problem (Mintzberg, 1973). In the process, much valuable time is lost waiting for information when managers should be at work forecasting future needs.

A final problem limiting the nurse manager's decision-making ability is that necessary information is not always available. Managers may not have immediate access to essential information. Some managers may have access but for various reasons may not be able to organize the information in a useful format.

These problems illustrate that nurse managers spend considerable time managing information problems that arise from the overload of information. A DSS could assist with most information management problems. A DSS can reduce time spent gathering data, time lost waiting for data, and time used for organizing data. A DSS can provide access to information formerly not available. If a DSS can save nurse managers valuable time, then a DSS can reduce administrative costs and increase time savings. One option, then, to reducing health care costs is through use of a DSS.

Purpose

What if a nurse manager decides that the best approach to cost reduction is a DSS? Where should the nurse manager's pursuit of DSS information begin? How does a nurse manager sort through all the available information about a DSS to make purchase decisions?

The purpose of this chapter is to provide nurse managers with essential information about DSS. First, the chapter describes DSS. Second, it identifies how a DSS can benefit nurse managers. Finally, the chapter provides criteria for guiding the nurse manager in any decision to buy a DSS.

Description of Decision-Support Systems

Textbook Description

No consensus exists on what defines a DSS. Some authors focus on defining a DSS by describing the enhanced human capabilities that evolve through the union between an individual and a computer. Keen and Scott-Morton (1978) define a DSS as a system that couples the intellectual resources of individuals with the capabilities of the computer to improve the quality of decisions. Brennan (1988b) describes a DSS as a system that links computer technology with decision-making algorithms to "augment, extend, or replace the judgment of the nurse," (p. 267). Today, however, the role of decision-support tools is to *extend* decision-making abilities, not *replace* them.

Another author describes a DSS by focusing on specific management problems. Turban (1993) defines a DSS as an interactive, flexible and adaptable computer-based information system developed for supporting the solution of a particular management problem for improved decision making. This DSS utilizes data, provides easy user interface and allows for the decision maker's own insights.

Decision Strategy.

Decision-support systems can be classified in many ways. One way is by the decision strategy used to target problems. Brennan (1988a) states that a DSS belongs to one of two categories: Formatting tools or decision-modeling systems. Formatting tools are templates used to organize, analyze and present data. Formatting tools may include spreadsheets and data bases. Decision-modeling systems involve software used to assist individuals in analyzing and understanding their decision making. These systems are used to "model" the way nurses make decisions. Decision-modeling systems include two types: decision-analysis and multiple criteria modeling. Brennan (1988b) states that nurses often use decision-modeling systems to solve problems when, in fact, further analysis, rather than more data, is needed.

Approach.

A second method used to classify a DSS is by the approach to decision-making. Hannah, Ball, and Edwards (1994) describe three major approaches to decision-support: (1) formatting, (2) analyzing, and (3) advising. Formatting tools are described above. Formatting tools approach problems by presenting information visually for decision making; they do not recommend solutions. Analyzing systems approach a problem by requiring the nurse manager to identify all the variables involved. The nurse manager then assigns a specific weight to each variable to determine priorities. Analyzing systems also do not recommend solutions; advising systems recommend solutions to problems. One type of advising system is the expert system. An expert system allows the specific expertise of an individual or group to be captured within a computer system. Basically, expert systems mimic human experts. Application of expert systems to the nursing profession generally is limited to one domain. For instance, PACE (Health Care Expert Systems, Inc., 1991) was developed to support the domain of nursing education. PACE (formerly COMMES) offers an extensive knowledge base and accelerated development of customized nursing care plans. The Pain Management System (Heriot et al., 1988) is unique to the nursing management domain of pain secondary to total hip arthroplasty. CANDI (Chang, Roth, Gonzales, Caswell, and DiStefano, 1988) is described as a system to aid nursing diagnosis. Currently, most expert systems in nursing remain in the development stage.

Output Generated.

A third method used to classify a DSS is according to the output generated (Alter, 1980). This classification scheme is based on the question—To what extent can system outputs directly support decisions? There are two categories: Data-oriented and model-oriented. A data-oriented DSS performs data retrieval and analysis. These systems focus primarily on the data. Examples are file drawer systems, data analysis systems and analysis information systems. File drawer systems permit basic access to data for simple inquiries. An example of a file drawer system is one that provides an answer to the question—Which nursing staff members attended an in-service on updating policies and procedures? Data analysis systems permit ad hoc analysis of data files. A DSS that uses a statistical program for further data analysis of files would be an example of a data analysis system. This DSS could manipulate files containing length-of-stay data and nursing outcome data to explore existing relationships. Analysis information systems also allow ad hoc analysis but these systems involve multiple data bases. One example of an analysis information system is a DSS that programs a special report describing use of computer-based patient records by accessing patient records and MEDLINE literature.

The second category, model-oriented DSS, provides simulation capabilities, optimization, or computations that propose an answer (Alter, 1980). Examples of model-oriented DSS include: Accounting models, representational models, optimization models and suggestion models. Alter's model-oriented systems parallel Brennan's decision-modeling systems in analyzing the process that individuals use in decision making. Accounting models use standard calculations to estimate future results. An example of an accounting model is a patient classification system. The accounting model DSS takes estimates of nursing activity (patient acuity scores) and gives estimates of monetary results (the cost of staffing a unit). Representational models attempt to estimate consequences of particular actions. A DSS with a cancer-risk component could estimate preventive actions. How would maintaining a regimen of a low-fat diet and routine exercise change an individual's cancer risk? An optimization model calculates an optimal solution to a complex problem. A DSS that plans for resource allocation is an example of an optimization model. A suggestion model performs calculations that generate a decision. An example of a suggestion model is an expert system. Alter (1980) describes the suggestion model as inputting a structured description of the situation (patient signs and symptoms) and receiving a suggested decision (treatment plan).

Components.

A fourth method used to classify a DSS is by the components that make up the system. Turban (1993) describes a DSS as comprising four subsystems: (1) data management, (2) model management, (3) dialogue, and (4) knowledge. This method of classification is helpful to nurse managers because it identifies specific software components useful in a DSS. The data management subsystem is a data base that contains relevant data for management situations. An example of a data base pertinent to nurse managers is a personnel file listing all employees, their addresses, continuing education requirements and immunizations. The second subsystem, model management, also parallels the decision-modeling category discussed by Brennan. In addition, Bonczek, Holsapple, and Whinston (1980) describe model management as containing financial, statistical management science, or other quantitative models that provide analysis capabilities. The third component, dialogue subsystem, is the user interface. This subsystem allows the user to communicate with the DSS. The user interface deals with how the nurse manager interacts with the DSS. Characteristics such as ease of use, accessibility and flexibility are dealt with in the dialogue subsystem. This subsystem can be the most important component because a DSS that is inconvenient or difficult-to-use discourages its use. The final component, knowledge subsystem is optional. This subsystem can be composed of one or more expert systems. The knowledge component allows integration of the expert system.

These are just some of the ways that DSS are currently described in the literature. The real confusion lies in a difference between what the "textbooks" define as a DSS and what "vendors" describe and market as a DSS.

Vendor Description

The amount of budgeting and financial information available in today's health care environment is impossible to handle without the aid of computer technology. More and more vendors are listing DSS as a predominant marketing category (Dunbar et al., 1993). Since cost considerations usually drive hospital decision making, vendors see one of their primary missions as assisting hospitals with cost reduction. The need for decision support began in hospitals because budgeting information and financial information are vital to the everyday management of the hospital.

Vendors tend to take a global approach when describing a DSS. In general, vendors discuss a DSS as an integrated HIS, not a stand-alone microcomputer system. These integrated systems have components of the "textbook" DSS, but integrated systems do not function independently of other hospital computer systems. The integrated DSS pulls data from the HIS and plugs the data into a variety of financial, budgeting or accounting formulas. The results of these formulas supply nurse managers with information on which to make management decisions. Most vendor descriptions of a DSS fall within areas where these monetary decisions are made.

Today, nurse managers make general administrative decisions as well as decisions specific to nursing duties. To meet these needs, vendors make use of general management DSS in their products. Many vendors discuss patient classification systems, staffing systems, and budgeting software as types of DSS available on an integrated HIS. Other vendors market software specifically developed for clinical decision-support. For example, *Computers in Health Care* (Dunbar et al., 1993) publishes a market directory of application software. This directory categorizes DSS as either: Clinical decision-support or managerial/financial decision-support. Clinical DSS include systems such as the one operating at Beth Israel Hospital and Harvard University's Center for Clinical Computing in Boston, MA ("Decision support for," 1992). This integrated system helps primary care physicians make therapeutic decisions for HIV care. In this example, the DSS component works with the computerized medical record. A computer program surveys the clinical data base every night for records of patients with HIV. This program triggers electronic reminders to physicians about adjusting drug dosages, ordering laboratory tests, or starting treatments. The physician then decides whether to follow the computer's recommendations.

The second category, managerial/financial decision-support, includes 11 areas: (1) budgeting; (2) case-mix management; (3) cost accounting; (4) DSS; (5) end-user reporting/query; (6) executive information systems; (7) managed-care contract monitoring; (8) marketing/market analysis/planning; (9) financial modeling; (10) payer-mix status; and (11) product-line management. Each of these areas is important for the comprehensive responsibility that nurse managers hold in health care institutions. For instance, case mix software allows the nurse manager to weigh differences in age, sex and morbidity to offer providers and payers a comparison of patient outcomes (Pastemack, 1992). Nurse managers can use this software to reduce costs of health care by comparing patient outcomes of care given by different nurses, doctors or facilities.

Vendors describe DSS in many different ways. One vendor describes DSS by product costing and management costing (HBO & Company). Product costing is the measurement of profit or loss on a service, a DRG, a patient, or a procedure. Nurse managers must have information to know if they are making or losing money; this information is called product costing. The second category is management costing, described as the determination of whether a given level of costs is reasonable based on a given workload produced. Management costing is important in justifying the cost of services. Nurse managers use management costing when they are asked to justify nurses' salaries. Such a query might be: Are the services provided by the nursing staff to the patients justified in the cost of nursing services?

Other HIS vendors describe their decision-support capabilities in distinct ways. One vendor calls decision-support products for nursing managers by the name, InterAct (Medicus Systems, 1992). The InterAct system defines DSS as including software such as Staffing/Productivity, Cost/Budgeting, Quality Management and Scheduling. The focus on Staffing/Productivity includes patient acuity/classification. Nurse managers are constantly faced with the problem of providing adequate nursing resources to meet the complex needs of patients and maintain quality care while containing costs. Patient classification systems are used by nurse managers because they provide a measure of patient acuity that is used to allocate nursing staff and determine the number of positions needed (Buckle, Horn and Simpson, 1991).

Other DS systems are specific to one clinical area or clinical diagnosis. One such system is the Oncology Clinical Information System (OCIS). OCIS is a DSS for the management of patients with cancer. OCIS was developed to assist with the automated collection, storage and access of clinical data information to manage the large amount of clinical data that is needed to make appropriate medical decisions for the care of cancer patients.

Zielstorff (1989) describes administrative systems in much the same way that some vendors describe a DSS. She states that some administrative systems can be useful to collect, summarize and format data that is needed for administrative decision-making. Hannah et al. (1994) describe administrative uses of information systems to assist nurse managers in decision making as management information systems. Therefore, much of the confusion between the "textbook" and "vendor" descriptions lies in the fact that most vendor DSS are defined in a broad sense. Most vendors include management information systems or administrative information systems in their descriptions of a DSS. For vendors, a DSS might be described as software that allows the decision work load to be shared between the manager and the computer system (Halloran et al., 1990). This definition could include broad information system components as well as "textbook" components.

Understanding all the different ways that vendors describe a DSS is not imperative. What is important, though, is understanding how each vendor involved in the purchase process describes a DSS. Since no well-accepted definition of a DSS exists, one could spend much time deliberating whether a particular software application can be labeled a DSS. Nurse managers have many demands on their time. Therefore, nurse managers should focus on the unique management functions that can be assisted by a DSS. Knowing the right questions to ask are of utmost importance.

How a DSS Can Assist Nurse Managers

Today, nurse managers are being held fiscally accountable to their health care institutions. Financial management is now part of the everyday routine of nurse managers, who have to be financially savvy, as they must be able to make decisions based on changing economic conditions. A DSS can help nurse managers use information more effectively to allocate available resources.

To make important financial decisions, nurse managers must have many skills. Nurse managers must be able to manage effectively the productivity of their health care institutions. They must predict the appropriate number of staff required and must forecast costs. Some nurse managers are responsible for the exploration of patient population characteristics. Other nurse managers look for client patterns and make predictions based on these patterns. Some nurse managers set staff performance criteria.

Basically, nurse managers are responsible for decisions that span many areas. To understand how a DSS can be useful to nurse managers, areas amenable to decision-support should be addressed. Some areas considered nurse manager-intensive for making decisions are: (1) quality management, (2) unit staffing, (3) ongoing reporting and (4) allocation and utilization of resources (Hannah et al., 1994).

Quality Management

The first area, quality management, focuses on TQM (Total Quality Management). TQM is a process of establishing and maintaining the quality of care provided to patients. Nurse manager information needs associated with quality assurance include patient care data bases, patient evaluation of care, nurses' notes on the chart, patient care plans, performance appraisals and incident reports.

Unit Staffing

The second category that is considered nurse manager-intensive is unit staffing (Hannah et al., 1994). The category of unit staffing includes patient classification, nursing workload and unit staffing. One of the first nursing management activities to be improved with the assistance of computers was staffing. In the past, nurse managers spent a large percentage of their time with manual scheduling. Currently, providing a schedule for each nurse is not sufficient. The process of unit staffing should include documentation of the relationship between staffing and the quality of care. Nursing management information needs associated with staffing include the merger of patient classification, criteria for determining acuity, nursing workload, levels of expertise of staff, personnel policies and contract elements.

Ongoing Reporting

The third category for making decisions is ongoing reporting (Hannah et al., 1994). Nurse managers report to many different audiences, including the Joint Commission on Accreditation of Healthcare Organizations, the CEO or the patient. Nurse managers need to be able to tailor reports to unique situations and audiences. The most important part of this reporting function is the ability to display data graphically. A DSS that presents a variety of options, such as pie graphs, bar graphs, and plots allows the nurse manager to report data visually.

Allocation and Utilization of Resources

The fourth category is allocation and utilization of resources (Hannah et al., 1994). This category includes human resource management, fiscal resource management and physical resource management. Leung (1991) states that the most supported managerial decision type in hospital nursing divisions and businesses is the planning of personnel (human resource management). Some of the information managers could use include an inventory of the skills and education levels of all nursing employees, job classification and salary level for all staff, dates for performance appraisals, dates for recertification and dates for annual inservice education sessions.

Fiscal resources address the planning, budgeting, operating and controlling aspects of the health care institution. The primary aim of fiscal resource management is to relate the cost of resources consumed to patient outcomes. Managers need information about payroll, supplies, services, patient length-of-stay, and nursing hours per patient day. These data provide defensible justification for making decisions about staffing, scheduling and service delivery.

Another area of resource allocation concern is physical resource management. Physical resource management includes overseeing and maintaining the physical facilities of the patient care unit as well as responsibility for equipment and furniture. This physical resource management also may include inventory control and materials management. DSS can be used to keep inventory control of everything from beds to sheets and can be a major planning device.

Halloran et al. (1990) believe key concerns in contemporary health care include the following areas: (1) epidemiology/demography and case mix of patients; (2) resource availability, allocation, and utilization; (3) performance measures, including output, outcome, quality, and consumer feedback; (4) skill maintenance of staff; (5) monitoring and maintenance of morale; and (6) shaping and maintenance of organizational culture. The areas of epidemiology, demography and case mix of patients require access to specific sets of data such as population characteristics, morbidity data and mortality data. These data sets can be examined for trends or patterns. The category of resource availability, allocation and utilization parallels the category of the allocation and utilization of resources described by Hannah et al. (1994). The third category of performance measures includes: Risk management, research to evaluate nursing care and provision of equitable access to care. These performance measures encompass the topics necessary to determine quality management. The fourth category of skill maintenance was discussed earlier by Hannah et al. (1994) in human resource management. The final categories of monitoring morale and organizational culture are important areas to consider when planning for future decision-support applications.

Other areas amenable to decision-support include workload and productivity management, project scheduling, budget preparation and utilization, implementation of nursing, care plan design, product cost and cash flow, product scheduling and sequencing, long-range corporate planning, ascertaining long-term goals, forecasting use and revenue, and merger-growth and acquisition analysis. McHugh and Schultz (1989) include the nurse manager activities of inservice education, infection control and nursing recruitment as amendable to decision support.

The activities that nurse managers carry out in support of all these areas are similar. Each of the areas mentioned above requires the need to process large amounts of data. The computer's ability to rapidly retrieve, summarize, manipulate and compare large volumes of information makes these areas amenable to decision-support. Decision-support tools are available for solving many information management problems. Nurse managers want a DSS that gives them an edge in making tough decisions. To buy a system that assists the nurse manager in making appropriate decisions based on financial implications, specific selection criteria should be considered.

Essential Criteria for Nurse Managers in Their Purchase Decision

When a decision has been made to purchase a DSS, certain criteria deserve consideration. These criteria are meant to serve as guidelines, not as an all-inclusive checklist. These criteria are intended to trigger thoughtful questions for vendors. Generally, the criteria that are crucial for consideration of today's DSS are software-related. Therefore, these criteria will not attempt to address specific hardware requirements. First, general criteria will be discussed; then specific guidelines are addressed.

Nurse managers requiring assistance with decision-support are dependent on computer systems to feed them information. The most important criterion of a DSS is that the system provide correct and prompt information. Nurse managers need to ensure that the information received is reliable and that it is received promptly (Hefner and Maloney, 1990). If a DSS cannot communicate with an existing system, especially an HIS, then the chances of receiving timely information are reduced.

The second most important criterion required in a DSS is flexibility. Nurse managers must have a system that allows flexibility in the way data are aggregated. If the DSS allows only one way of doing things, then the system is not useful in today's changing health care environment. For example, a manager should be able to use one DSS to predict staffing needs, as well as to calculate budgets and monitor quality. With the changing economic status, nurse managers need to be able to modify the way a system organizes information. They also need to be able to ask for additional information.

Nurse managers need the capacity to make predictions based on existing conditions or expected changes. Ideally, the system should be an information system that allows nurse managers to create and modify algorithms without extensive programming skills. To insure better output, nurse managers should be able to change the input accessed.

When beginning the search process for a DSS, nurse managers should examine certain aspects of their institutions. First, a nurse manager should evaluate and document the health care institution's information needs. Nurse managers should ask questions such as: What does my institution expect from a DSS? How can a DSS increase productivity? What decisions would be facilitated by a DSS? What output would give this institution the best information to increase productivity?

Moore and Chang (1980) include in the characteristics of a successful DSS the ability for future planning and irregular, unplanned use. These two components for evaluating systems are useful to nurse managers because forecasting health care costs is crucial to the success of heath care. The system should be an extension of the user's problem-solving capabilities. The DSS should augment the manager's skills so the nurse manager can control future costs. Since health care institutions work around the clock, the DSS needs to facilitate access at irregular, unplanned intervals.

After a thorough needs-assessment has been completed, the nurse manager can then continue with the purchase process. Vendors respond to questions by stating whether they can meet the manager's information needs. It is not enough for vendors to guarantee that they can address questions or promise access to the information needed. The vendor's solution must be carefully evaluated. The solution should address questions such as: What raw data do the system use and where do these data originate? How does the system organize the data to provide answers?

Next, carefully compare the definitions of terms that the institution uses with the vendor's definitions. Vendors know that most nurse managers need information on productivity so they discuss DSS software that is designed to assist nurse managers in obtaining this information. The problem with this approach is that many nurse managers define such terms as a FTE (full time equivalent) differently. Nurse managers should ask vendors how they define FTE and what formula they use to produce FTE results. Nurse managers should not assume that a vendor defines a FTE the same way that the manager's institution does. An important task for nurse managers is to operationally define the institution's terms for the vendor. Therefore, if you are buying a DSS to help your institution with decisions about productivity, it is important to make sure the software defines terms the same way that you or your institution defines the terms.

Other criteria deserve consideration. Little (1970) states that in order for a DSS to be successful, it must contain the following characteristics: (1) simple, (2) robust, (3) easy to control, (4) adaptive, (5) completely covers important issues, and (6) easy to communicate. Nurse managers must be able to use the DSS with minimal training. The DSS must also allow the nurse manager to determine how a decision was reached.

Summary

Many nurse managers will be faced with the decision to buy a DSS. The criteria given in this chapter may provide some useful guidance in any purchase decision. A major point to consider is that good communication with the vendor is imperative. Many times the vendor's description of a DSS does not match the institution's description. To help nurse managers understand what a DSS can encompass, this chapter presented numerous ways to describe a DSS. By familiarity with these definitions and with the many applications of DSS, nurse managers can make better-informed and well-documented decisions.

References

Alter, S. L. (1980). *Decision Support Systems: Current Practices and Continuing Challenges*. Reading, MA: Addison-Wesley Publishing Co.

Bonczek, R. H., Holsapple, C. W., and Whinston, A. B. (1980). The evolving roles of models in decision-support systems. *Decision Sciences, 11*(2), 337-356.

Brennan, P. (1988a). DSS, ES, AI: The lexicon of decision-support. *Nursing and Health Care, 9*(9), 501-503.

Brennan, P. (1988b). Modeling for decision-support. In M. J. Ball, et al. (Eds), *Nursing Informatics. Where Caring and Technology Meet* (pp. 267-273). New York: Springer-Verlag New York.

Buckle, J. M., Horn, S. D., and Simpson, R. L. (1991). Nursing care classification: A conceptual model. *Applied Nursing Research, 4*, 100-106.

Chang, B. L., Roth, K., Gonzales, E., Caswell, D., and DiStefano, J. (1988, January/February). CANDI. A knowledge-based system for nursing diagnosis. *Computers in Nursing, 6*(4), 13-21.

Decision-support for HIV care via computer. (1992, May). *Computers & Medicine, 21*(5), 6.

Dunbar, C., Laughlin, M., DiGiulio, L., Morris, D. C., Wieners, W., and Zinn, T. K. (1993). 1993 Market Directory. [Special issue]. *Computers in Healthcare, 79*-81.

Halloran, E. J., O'Dwyer, J., Pluyter-Wenting, E., D'Arcy, C., Sermeus, W., Wenn, J., O'Dwyer, I., Barber, B., Cooke, M., Brennan, P. K., and McCormack, R. (1990). Decision-support systems for nursing management and administration. In J. G. Ozbolt, D. Vandewal, and K. J. Hannah (Eds.), *Decision Support Systems in Nursing* (pp. 29-40). St. Louis: C. V. Mosby Co.

Hannah, K. J., Ball, M. J., and Edwards, M. J. (1994). *Introduction to Nursing Informatics*. New York: Springer-Verlag New York.

HBO & Company. *Decision support*. [Advertisement literature]. (Available from HBO & Company, One Ravinia Drive, Suite 1000, Atlanta, GA 30346).

Health Care Expert Systems, Inc. (1991, September). P.S. What is Pace? In *PaceSetter*. [Newsletter]. (Available from Health Care Expert Systems, Inc., Suite 420, 1025 Ashworth Road, West Des Moines, IA 50265).

Hefner, S., and Maloney, S. (1990, Summer). Decision support: What does it do? *Health Care Information Management Journal, 4*(3), 4-16.

Heriot, C., Graves, J. R., Bouhaddou, O., Armstrong, M., Wigertz, G., and Said, M. B. (1988). A pain management decision support system for nurses. In J. G. Ozbolt, D. Vandewal, and K. J. Hannah, (Eds.), *Decision Support Systems in Nursing* (pp. 153-163). St. Louis: C. V. Mosby Co.

Keen, P. G., and Scott-Morton, M. S. (1978). *Decision Support Systems, An Organizational Perspective.* Reading, MA: Addison-Wesley Publishing Co.

Leung, A. (1991). Use of decision support systems in nursing. In V. K. Saba, K. Rieder, and D. B. Pocklington, (Eds.), *Nursing Informatics '91* (pp. 785-790). New York: Springer-Verlag New York.

Little, J. D. C. (1970). Models and managers: The concept of a decision calculus. *Management Science, 16*(8).

McHugh, M., and Schultz, S., II. (1989). Computer technology in hospital nursing departments: Future applications and implications. In V. K. Saba, K. A. Rieder, and D. B. Pocklington, (Eds.), *Nursing and Computers. An Anthology* (pp. 80-89). New York: Springer-Verlag New York.

Medicus Systems. (1992). *Combining the art and science of patient care management.* [Advertisement literature]. (Available from Medicus Systems Corporation, One Rotary Center, Suite 400, Evanston, IL 60201-4802).

Mintzberg, H. (1973). *The Nature of Managerial Work.* New York: Harper & Row Publishers.

Moore, J. H., and Chang, M. C. (1980, Fall). Design of decision support systems. *Data Base, 12*(1 & 2).

Pastemack, A. (1992, January 13). Case mix software tries to match outpatient needs. *Healthweek,* 28-29.

Sinclair, V. G. (1990). Potential effects of decision support systems on the role of the nurse. *Computers in Nursing, 8*(2), 60-65.

Turban, E. (1993). *Decision Support and Expert Systems: Management Support Systems.* New York: Macmillan Publishing Co.

Zielstorff, R. (1989). Computers in nursing administration. In V. K. Saba, K. A. Rieder, and D. B. Pocklington, (Eds.), *Nursing and Computers. An Anthology* (pp. 63-70). New York: Springer-Verlag New York.

Suggested Readings

Brennan, P. (1990). Computerized decision-support. Beyond expert systems. In J. G. Ozbolt, D. Vandewal, and K. J. Hannah (Eds.), *Decision Support Systems in Nursing* (pp. 165-170). St. Louis: C. V. Mosby Co.

Dienemann, J. (Ed.). (1990). *Nursing Administration. Strategic Perspectives and Application.* Norwalk, CT: Appleton & Lange.

Powers, J. (1993, July). Great gravitation: Supporting decisions with mainframe data on PCs. *Healthcare Informatics, 10*(7), 112-114.

Zielstorff, R. D., Hudgings, C. I., and Grobe, S. J. (1993). *Next-Generation Nursing Information Systems. Essential Characteristics for Professional Practice.* Washington, DC: American Nurses Association.

Strategies for Managing Information Systems

Information Systems: Use in Strategic Planning and in a
Managed Competitive Environment 56
Joint Commission on Accreditation of Healthcare Organizations:
Standards for Information Systems 64
Applying Technology Assessment to Information Systems 74
Organizational Impact of Information Systems 83
Choices of Nursing Systems 92
Benefits Management 99
Systems Design and Implementation: Team Building Between
Nurse Executive and Vendor... 108
The Nursing Manager's Role in Successful System
Implementation 116
Training Issues in System Implementation 128

Information Systems: Use in Strategic Planning and in a Managed Competitive Environment

Mary Etta C. Mills, ScD, RN, CNAA
Chair and Associate Professor
Department of Education, Administration, Health Policy and Informatics
School of Nursing
University of Maryland at Baltimore

Barbara R. Heller, EdD, RN, FAAN
Dean and Professor
School of Nursing
University of Maryland at Baltimore

Carol A. Romano, PhD, RN, FAAN
Director, Clinical System and Quality Improvement
National Institutes of Health Clinical Center

Introduction

In today's health care environment of fast-paced medical technology evolution, escalation of health care costs, formation of health care networks and service diversification to non-hospital settings, health care organizations must continually redefine their missions and the means to achieve goals. Efforts to continually lower costs while improving quality and access to care have created pressure on administrators, providers, educators, regulators and consumers to identify new approaches to service organization and delivery. In a rapidly changing high-tech environment, the availability of accurate and timely information in a format that contributes to health care decision making is crucial.

Managed Competition

First adopted as a national health policy strategy through the Health Maintenance Organization Act of 1973, Title XIII of the Public Health Service Act, managed health care was first designed as a prepaid group practice. This capitated system provided prepayment of services at a fixed rate regardless of the frequency of use by the consumer or the cost to the provider. The onus to control cost, therefore, fell on the provider. To remain fiscally viable, each HMO was responsible for coordinating care in a way to eliminate medically unnecessary services and to use the care delivery system efficiently (Miller, 1993).

In 1982, the Tax Equity and Fiscal Responsibility Act enacted by Congress opened HMOs and other eligible managed-care organizations to federal beneficiaries. During the late 1980s, certain sections of the HMO Act were altered to make the inclusion of HMOs in employer health benefits voluntary beginning in 1995. Since that time, new federal health policy reform such as The Managed Competition Act of 1992 (H.R. 5936) has emphasized that an integrated financing and delivery organization provide primary and preventive care as a part of a comprehensive benefit package.

As defined by Enthoven (1993), managed competition is "a purchasing strategy to obtain maximum value for consumers and employers, using rules for competition derived from microeconomic principles...and based on comprehensive care organizations that integrate financing and delivery" (p. 27). The goal of managed competition is to develop provider groups which will compete economically as a result of market forces designed to reward efficient delivery systems. It is not designed to force everyone into clinic-style HMOs but, rather, emphasizes the importance of individual (not employer) choice of plans.

Because of favorable HMO price structuring, the expectation was that employers would send their employees and beneficiaries to lower-cost providers and that consumers would support this effort by seeking providers with the lowest out-of-pocket costs. Still, by 1989, only 18% of medium and large firms had limited their employees' choice of hospitals and doctors, and only 14% offered managed care as the only insurance plan option (Taylor and Leitman, 1989). Current systems include such choices as totally unrestricted access, open arrangements with incentives to use a certain network of providers, and closed systems such as HMOs.

Increased competition and efforts to reduce health care cost have led to changes in hospital organization and diversification of services from hospitals to less costly sites such as outpatient facilities. For instance, many hospitals which were reported as in the process of closing to the American Hospital Association have reopened under different names or management or have merged with other hospitals. In a report by Blendon and Edwards (1991), hospitals were more likely to merge than to close. Between 1980 and 1987, a total of 231 hospitals merged into 111 new institutions (accounting for almost one-half of the reported 558 hospitals closed). During the same time period, a variety of alternative institutions such as free-standing surgical centers were established, eventually totaling almost 600% growth in the 1980s (Blendon and Edwards, 1991).

Changes in legislation, combined with an increasing emphasis on comprehensive health benefit plans, only serve to highlight the increased need for strategic planning. In managed competition, as envisioned under national health policy reform and structured around the formation of integrated organizations, there is a focus on the development of strategic plans which include major organizational change. Not surprisingly, attention to strategic planning between 1980 and 1987 increased by a 71% growth rate in fields such as marketing, advertising and public relations (Blendon and Edwards, 1991).

Strategic Planning

Strategic decision making begins with the explication of a vision for the organization and results in the creation of an operational plan. The strategic plan serves as a directional guide rather than as an absolute map and as such deals with the future of today's decisions. Strategic plans are long term by design—generally projecting five years or more into the future. Such plans take a broad programmatic and environmental perspective rather than concentrating on individual projects.

Each organization exists in a multi-contextual environment of overlapping influences created by regulators, consumers, suppliers and competitors. The nature of strategic planning is, therefore, an externally oriented activity that looks for advantage wherever it can be found in relation to the outside world. A sustainable advantage is one that increases value or lowers cost and is not easily replicated. Domanico (1981) viewed this process as one in which organizations:

> ...assess the total healthcare market and their true competitive position within the market to determine future direction while at the same time addressing community needs and satisfying regulatory requirements (p. 25).

With the growth of health care networks and managed competition, an increasing level of complexity has been added to the arena of health care. This environment has created new health care—and business—partners, weaving together what once were autonomous providers of health care services. In an effort to reduce expensive hospital stays and to utilize lower-cost services such as home health care, ambulatory care and community-based services, new organizational configurations are emerging that require complex planning and forecasting.

These pressures have brought a new emphasis to strategic planning, described by Drucker (1974) as:

> [a] continuous, systematic process of making risk-taking decisions today with the greatest possible knowledge of their effects on the future: organizing efforts necessary to carry out these decisions: and evaluating results of these decisions against expected outcomes through reliable feedback mechanisms (p. 125).

This type of challenge can only be met with appropriate marketing, finance, and management information that is continually revised as economic, political, and social conditions change (Goldsmith, 1980; Halten, 1982). Strategic planning, however, is not just a market-oriented activity; it involves the entire organization. There are key data bases that must be considered within the strategic planning process. For example: *internal data*—descriptive of the range and quality of services; *external source data*—identifying the level of provider excellence or access to capital; *market data*—defining the referral network and patient mix; *operations research data*—measuring the effectiveness and efficiency of service delivery; and *follow-up service measurement data* such as quality of ambulatory care.

Strategic planning requires a transition from the abstract to the concrete (see Figure 1).

At this point of strategy development, the process requires a data base that extends from the retrospective to the prospective; generally this involves a circumscribed path (see Figure 2).

The data requirements for strategic planning indicate that the process is issue driven by the reality of events, rather than cyclical changes. Strategic planning is a continuous process that should result in substantive actions and should involve the people who will have to execute the plan. Further, it must be flexible enough to leave room for change as circumstances require.

Creating Information Systems to Support Strategic Planning

For information-based planning to occur, information systems must be developed that will effectively support strategic planning. As stated by Rheinecker (1993, p. 42), "CEOs have often viewed information systems as an operational cost rather than a strategic investment." In fact, information systems should be created which are capable of answering strategic questions concerning patients, payers, practice patterns and other issues. This type of decision support can provide significant competitive impact to increase market share, raise profitability and add value to health care delivery (Moriarty, 1992). However, health services have lagged behind other industry groups in the strategic application of information technology. Over the past five years, hospitals have invested just 2% of operating costs in the purchase and maintenance of data systems (Winslow, 1993).

Two issues necessary for the creation of valuable strategic information systems are (1) the involvement of the Chief Information Officer (CIO) in the health care strategic planning process and, (2) the development of systems that allow the capture, integration and manipulation of key data.

Figure 1.
Strategic planning process

Mission ➔ Goals ➔ Strategies ➔ Programs

Figure 2.
Data-based strategic planning chronology

Situation Analysis	Scenario Creation	Option Generation	Option Evaluation/Selection	Program Development
Historical trends	Market trends	Options considering markets, costs	Evaluation against criteria	Development of detail
Market position	Future access to capital	Criteria for evaluating options	Reality checking	
Financial position	Cost trends		Integration of information	
Relative strengths/ weaknesses	Technology trends			

Information Systems Manager: Top Level Involvement

The development of effective information systems can only take place within the context of organizational needs. It is essential that the individual charged with responsibility for information systems be a participant in the strategic planning process since systems planning must parallel and support the institutional plan and direction (Sinisi, 1992).

Factors identified as important to the success of a CIO include: reporting to the highest level possible (CEO, COO); having oversight for all of the organization's technology; concentrating on strategic information and long-term strategy rather than day-to-day operations; and, championing a strategic information plan that is synergistic with the corporate long-range strategic plan (Ball and Douglas, 1992).

In a study of Vice Presidents of Nursing (VPN) and Nursing Informatics Specialists, Mills and Braun (1994) found that slightly more than one-third of the Informatics Specialists reported to the VPN. Although VPNs cited strategic planning among their top three priorities for the future, the actual communication between VPN and NIS encompassing systems planning and strategic planning was among the least well-developed (r=.3333; p<.01) interactions.

Increasingly, the changing nature of information systems capability, combined with leadership requirements for data-based decision making, is demanding that managers of information systems be directly involved with the strategic planning process (Dunbar, 1992; Reavis, 1992). Information systems must provide data that allow managers to assess strategic decisions and should give access to information that will help managers identify and pursue broad new goals and directions (Rheinecker, 1993). This can only be accomplished through ongoing communication between key members of the administrative team—including the Information System Manager—regarding organizational needs, priorities, and directions.

Development of Information Systems

Information systems may be viewed as instrumental to changing the way service is provided [strategic systems] or supporting current operations [support systems] (Moriarty,

1992). A Strategic Information System is "any combination of computers, workstations, software systems, and communications technology used to gain competitive advantage" (Morton, 1988, p. 28).

If used in the strategic system context, the information system itself can substantively change the way in which the organization conducts its business. In addition to providing information about issues such as the impact of technology on practice patterns or changes in case mix in terms of patient-type or disease severity, the information system could be used to create new opportunities. For example, linking ambulatory settings at distant locations to one or more hospitals and emergency departments could provide new network opportunities for patient referral, program development and enhanced patient care.

Information systems development should be conducted with both purposes in mind and attention given to ensuring that systems components are integrated and have multi-relational capacity.

Integrated Systems

Relational data bases allow information to be located by searching through all or part of the contents of the data base using search criteria determined *after* the creation of the databases. They permit information from multiple sources to be merged, integrated and/or configured in a way that supports clinical and managerial decision making. As such, relational data bases are increasingly important to the process of transforming data to information.

Data are described as raw numbers, figures, and individual responses collected from a sample or a population. Information results when one set of data is analyzed and used in specific relationship with another set of data (Al-Assaf, 1993). Relational databases function to process, retrieve and manipulate information. They are founded on a structured query language and a standard that allows different data bases to interchange data. As a result, they are not only able to manage words and numbers but voice and image as well.

Future information systems will increasingly have the capacity not only to interchange data but to integrate pictures, maps, sounds, and words. Each of these media offers a different description of the object being recorded. Information systems will utilize the patient care data base, a knowledge base, and a graphical user interface (drawings and schemas) based on hypertext techniques which integrate text and graphics.

At first, finding the relationships that exist among data can be difficult. Finding just which fact within a relationship is the most significant is much harder, yet this will be increasingly important to strategic planning. Clinical information systems design will increasingly permit the automatic collection and processing of data into information supportive of managerial decision making.

The degree of success surrounding the usefulness of information to the planning process will be a direct result of the administrators' ability to identify what questions need to be answered and what data is necessary to answer them. Figure 3 shows examples of clinical data that support administrative decision making.

The integration and transformation of this type of data provides the basis for decisions ranging from case management and clinical outcomes to service, demand projections and the formation of new service enterprises.

Executive Use of Information Systems for Planning

The capability of information systems is expanding exponentially. Reports can be generated to almost any level of detail and data integrated to yield key information. Several guidelines can be offered for the use of information systems.

Figure 3.
Clinical-administrative data transformation

Clinical Data Sources	⇒ ⇒	Administrative Data
Orders		Acuity - Staffing
Assessment		Quality
Diagnoses		Risk Management
Progress Indicators		Patient Volumes
Flow Sheets		Cost - Revenue
Progress Notes		Marketing
Test Results		
Consults		
Discharge Summary		

Knowledge of System Capability

Identify the type of information system(s) in place and the reports they currently generate. Consider which reports you use most and why they are valuable to you. Briefly list the type of information you must frequently—or regularly—compile in preparation for planning. For example: patient acuity; workload productivity; resource use (capital expenditures); patient volumes by service area; shifts in patient care service (i.e., hospital- based endoscopy to physician ambulatory center). Identify whether reporting currently delivers needed information.

Selective Requesting

Selective and specific requesting of information can be the single most important skill in effectively obtaining useful data. This process is twofold. First, identify not only what data is necessary but how it should be displayed (i.e., graphs, charts). Control the process by not requesting or accepting all available data since much of it is detail oriented (e.g., lists of supplies purchased). Request information summaries by an established time frame such as month, quarter or year.

Second, begin to establish data integration requirements. Are comparisons needed between existing reports or seemingly disparate services?. For example, consider the relationship between primary care services availability and emergency department utilization. Also, consider requesting reports that profile given services by information such as average number of patients per year by specialty, diagnostic utilization per visit, outcomes of care, and referral and follow-up after service delivery. Identification of the "right" questions is critical to the process of becoming selective in information acquisition that will support strategic planning.

Intra-organizational linkages

Many health care delivery organizations have multiple geographic locations and multiple service diversification such as hospital services, community-based kidney dialysis, diagnostic and ambulatory centers. Information systems should be integrated to allow a single computer-based patient record to drive data continuity, reduce redundant data collection, and create organizational systems that extend across the patient's health care experience. The availability of this type of system is critical in a managed care environment.

Cost driven versus revenue driven

Integrated clinical and financial data are important to validly track the cost of care delivery. Managed competition focuses on the provision of quality, cost-effective care and gauges the success of the provider organization by the expeditious use of resources (e.g., cost savings). This represents a paradigm shift from an emphasis on revenue production to one of cost reduction. Future strategic planners will require information that indicates current cost and provides projections of future costs using practice scenarios that can be translated into financial models for simulation.

Managerial decision-support systems will be useful to key strategic planning activities such as: choosing objectives; planning the organization; identifying marketing policies; and choosing new product lines or diversifying services.

Future Directions

Managed competition will favor networks of providers able to control costs. Information systems will effectively support efforts to coordinate care and collect information supportive of planning needs. There are already prototypes where information is available beyond the boundaries of single organizations. For example, Cincinnati health care officials ("Cincinnati providers," 1993) are constructing a community-wide health information network to link health care institutions, payers, major employers, some financial institutions,, and as many as 2,000 or more physicians. The major focus of the network will be to provide clinical data but other information such as health claims and wellness information will also be available. The target date for network operation is 1999. This is being viewed as a "managed care product" which will serve to open and interconnect systems. The White House Task Force on Healthcare Reform has called for the nationwide development of this type of system—referred to as Community Health Management Information Systems. Databases would be automatically collected and compiled from the capture of all patient encounter information. The network would:

> monitor and track provider performance and patients over time and integrate input from patients on quality of services, functional status and lifestyle behavior, ...integrate information from employers and other purchasers and aggregate and analyze patient-care delivery, provider activities and billed costs over time (Scott, 1993, p. 23).

The intent of creating this integrated system is to allow an informed Health Insurance Purchasing Cooperative or health alliance to choose the health care provider that would render care at the best price, quality and efficiency. With the advent of this type of comprehensive information collection, future strategic planning will take on a new scope of information retrieval and application.

Senior administrators and managers must keep current on these developments, especially with regard to the type of information that is available for their use in monitoring, comparing, and planning health care delivery services.

In a managed competitive environment, the use of information systems will prove invaluable to strategic planning decision support.

Summary

Managed competition is being formulated within national health policy reform to integrate the financing and delivery of health care. The development of provider groups which compete on price for patient care service contracts is anticipated to create opportunities for the formation of new health care partnerships. Strategic planning will—by necessity—be more complex and dependent on accurate and timely information. Thoughtful use of information systems capable of data collection and integration can support the creation of viable strategic plans.

References

Al-Assaf, A. F. (1993). Data management for total quality. In A. F. Al-Assaf and J. A. Schmele (Eds.), *Total Quality in Healthcare* (p. 124). Delray Beach, FL: St. Lucie Press.

Anderson, K., and Wootten, B. (1991). Changes in hospital staffing patterns. *Monthly Labor Review, 114*, 3-9.

Ball, M. J., and Douglas, J. V. (1992, May). The CIO's key role in healthcare strategic planning. *Computers in Healthcare*, pp. 17-21.

Blendon, R. J., and Edwards, J. N. (1991). Looking back at hospital forecasts. In R. J. Blendon and J. N. Edwards (Eds.), *System in Crisis: The Case for Health Care Reform* (pp. 7-30). New York: Faulkner & Gray, Inc.

Cincinnati providers plan community healthcare network. (1993, July). *Computers in Healthcare*, p. 10.

Domanico, L. (1981). Strategic planning: Vital for hospital long-range development. *Hospital and Health Services Administration, 26*(4), 25-50.

Drucker, P. (1974). *Management: Tasks, Responsibilities, Policies.* New York: Harper & Row Publishers.

Dunbar, C. (1992, May). CEOs—Listen up! *Computers in Healthcare*, pp. 23-24.

Durant, G. D. (1989, March-April). Ambulatory surgical centers: Surviving, thriving into the 1990s. *MGM Journal*, pp. 8-12.

Enthoven, A. C. (1993). The history and principles of managed competition. *Health Affairs, 12*(Supplement), 24-49.

Goldsmith, J. C. (1980). The health care market: Can hospitals survive? *Harvard Business Review, 58*(5), 100-112.

Halten, M. L. (1982). Strategic management in not-for-profit organizations. *Strategic Management Journal, 3*(2), 89-104.

Managed Competition Act of 1992, (The), H.R. 5936, 102nd Congress, 2d sess., 15 September, 1992.

Miller, R. (1993). Managed care as a national strategy: Issues. In K. Kelly and M. Maas (Eds.), *Managing Nursing Care* (pp. 175-189). St. Louis: C. V. Mosby Co.

Mills, M. E., and Braun, R. (1994). Organizational priorities for the nursing informatics specialist. In Grobe, S. J. and E. S. P. Pluyter-Wenting (Eds.), *Nursing Informatics: An International Overview for Nursing in a Technological Era* (pp. 8-13). Amsterdam: Elsevier Science Publishers.

Moriarty, D. D. (1992). Strategic information systems planning for health service providers. *Health Care Management Review, 17*(1), 85-90.

Morton, M. S. S. (1988). Information technology and corporate strategy. *Planning Review, 16*(5), 28-31.

Reavis, M. (1992, May). The role CIOs must play in multihospital strategic planning. *Computers in Healthcare*, pp. 26-28.

Rheinecker, P. (1993, October). Informed strategy. *Health Progress*, pp. 42-45.

Scott, J. S. (1993, July). Community health MIS. *Computers in Healthcare*, p. 22-28.

Sinisi, A. (1992, July). Information services' role in strategic planning. *Healthcare Informatics*, p. 16.

Taylor, H., and Leitman, R. (1989). *Corporate Health Plans: Past, Present, and Future.* New York: Louis Harris and Associates.

Winslow, R. (1993, October 8). Hospitals wake up to the power of computers. *The Wall Street Journal*, p. B1.

Joint Commission on Accreditation of Healthcare Organizations: Standards for Information Systems

Carole H. Patterson, MN, RN
Associate Director for Standards Development
Department of Performance Measures Development
Joint Commission on Accreditation of Healthcare Organizations (JCAHO)

NOTE: The standards discussed in this chapter were published in the 1994 and
1995 editions of the Accreditation Manual for Hospitals (AMH), Volumes I and
II, and are quoted with permission of the Joint Commission.

Introduction

Currently, there are two specific roles envisioned for the use of information technology from the perspective of the Joint Commission on Accreditation of Healthcare Organizations (Joint Commission) [JCAHO]: New standards fostering the use of such technology in patient care and data-driven performance measurement or monitoring systems.

What is the Joint Commission?

The Joint Commission, a private, not-for-profit organization, evaluates and accredits more than 9000 hospitals and other health care organizations and is the nation's oldest and most experienced performance measurement organization. In 1986, a new vision was clarified which began the movement of the Commission toward a performance-focused accreditation system composed of new standards addressing "Patient-Focused Functions" and "Organizational Functions."

The mission of the Joint Commission has been and is to improve the quality of health care provided to the public. That mission is fulfilled by developing standards used to measure health care organizations' performance of important functions against the stated requirements and making accreditation decisions based on the results of surveys conducted by experienced professionals. On December 10, 1988, the Joint Commission's Board of Commissioners approved the following definition of "patient care quality":

> Patient care quality is the degree to which patient care services increase the probability of desired patient outcomes and reduce the probability of undesired outcomes, given the current state of knowledge (JCAHO, 1990).

The mission is also fulfilled by providing both formal and informal education and consultation services to the fields accredited by the Joint Commission: organizations providing ambulatory health care, home care, hospital care, long term care, mental health care services, laboratories, and health care networks.

The Joint Commission's Agenda for Change

In 1987, in anticipation of the inevitable evolution toward a new performance measurement mandate in health care, the Joint Commission launched its Agenda for Change. The broad objective of that Agenda was to create a more modern and sophisticated accreditation process that places primary emphasis on actual performance of organizations. Implementation began in 1994 and provides a comprehensive and objective system for evaluating health care organizations using both performance-focused standards and performance measures or indicators.

The three major initiatives of the Agenda for Change involve:
- •reformulation of Joint Commission standards to emphasize actual organizational performance;
- •redesign of the survey process to provide more interactive on-site evaluation and education; and
- •development of the Indicator Measurement System (IMSystem), a national data base resource to support performance improvement in hospitals and other patient care settings.

Performance-Focused Standards: Management of Information

One of the first seven sets of performance-focused standards developed by an expert Task Force on Information Management was a new chapter of standards on "Management of Information" published in the 1994 edition of the *Accreditation Manual for Hospitals [AMH]* (Joint Commission, 1993, pp. 35-44). The other six sets of standards included "Assessment of Patients," "Medication Use/Treatment of Patients," "Operative and Other Invasive Procedures," "Patient and Family Education," "Leadership," and "Improving Organizational Performance."

A preamble to the new 1994 chapter, "Management of Information," explained the new standards and provided definitions (Table 1) developed by the expert Task Force to assist health care organizations in understanding the new requirements. That preamble is reproduced in part below.

Preamble to Management of Information Chapter

An organization's provision of health care is a complex endeavor that is highly dependent upon information. This includes information about the science of care, the individual patient, the care provided, the results of care, and the performance of the organization itself. Furthermore, many individuals, departments, and services within the organization are providing care, and their work must be coordinated and integrated. Because of this dependency on information and the need to coordinate and integrate services, health care organizations must treat information as an important resource to be effectively and efficiently managed. The management of information is an active, planned function. The organization's leaders have overall responsibility for this function—just as they do for managing the organization's human, material, and financial resources (JCAHO, 1993, p. 35).

Information management as a function—a set of processes and activities—focuses on meeting the organization's information needs. Its goal is to obtain, manage, and use information to enhance and improve individual and organizational performance in patient care, governance, management, and support processes. While the efficiency and effectiveness of information management processes may be affected by the technologies employed (for example, computerization), the principles of good information management (as reflected in these standards) are relevant regardless of the technology used. Thus, while these standards are compatible with current, cutting-edge technologies (and, it is hoped, with future technologies), they are intended to be equally applicable in organizations that are not computerized.

These standards describe a vision of effective and continuously improving information

Table 1.

Joint Commission Definitions Developed by Expert Information Task Force for Use in "Management of Information" Standards.

aggregate Combining of standardized data/info

authenticate To prove authorship, for example, by written signature, identifiable initials, or computer key

bias Effect tending to produce results that depart systematically from the true value (to be distinguished from random)

capture Acquisition or recording of data/information

confidentiality Safekeeping of data/information as restricted to individuals who have need, reason, and permission for access to such data/information

data Uninterpreted observations or facts

data connectivity Ability to link data

data definition Identification of the data to be used in analysis

data parity Equivalency of data

database Stored collection of data

function Group of activities and processes with a common goal

information Interpreted sets of data; organized data that provide a basis for decision making

integrity Maintenance of the accuracy, consistency, and completeness of data

knowledge-based Collection of stored facts models, and information that can be used for designing and redesigning processes and for problem solving. In the context of this *Manual* (that is, the *Accreditation Manual for Hospitals*), knowledge-based information is found in the clinical, scientific, and management literature.

medical record Account compiled by physicians and other health care professionals of a variety of patient health information, such as patient's assessment findings, treatment details, and progress notes

minimum data set Agreed upon and accepted set of terms and definitions constituting a core of data; a collection of related data items

security Protection of data from intentional or unintentional destruction, modification, or disclosure

transformation Process of changing the form of data representation, for example, changing data into information with the use of decision analysis tools

transmission Sending of data/information from one location to another location

validation Verification of correctness

---

management in health care organizations. The objectives related to achieving this vision are:
•more timely and easier access to complete information throughout the organization;
•improved data accuracy;
•demonstrated balance of proper levels of security versus ease of access;
•use of aggregate data, along with external knowledge bases and comparative data, to pursue opportunities for improvement;
•redesign of important information-related processes to improve efficiency; and
•greater collaboration and information sharing to enhance patient care.

For most organizations, achieving all of these objectives will take varying periods of time, perhaps up to five years. Thus, the scoring guidelines and aggregation rules for this information management chapter accommodate the time needed for transition to effective organization-wide management of information.

The standards focus on the key information management processes of organization-wide planning to meet internal and external information needs. The standards also focus on management of patient-specific data/information, aggregate data/information, expert knowledge-based data/information, and comparative performance data/information.

Specifically, the standards address the following:
•identification of the organization's information needs;
•structural design of the information management system;

•definition and capture of data/information;
•data analysis and transformation of data into information;
•transmission and reporting of data/information; and
•assimilation and use of information.

The organization's leaders have important roles and responsibilities if an organization-wide approach to information management will be achieved, maintained, and improved. Also, staff at many levels must be educated and trained in managing and using information.

The performance-improvement framework described in the "Improving Organizational Performance" chapter of standards will be used to design, measure, assess, and continuously improve the organization's performance of the information management function.

Performance-Focused Standards: Improving Organizational Performance

New standards representing the transformation of traditional requirements for "Quality Assurance" (first published in 1953), to "Quality Assessment and Improvement" (published in 1993), to a new chapter of performance-focused standards titled "Improving Organizational Performance" (1993, pp. 51-58), were published in the Joint Commission standards manuals beginning with the 1994 edition. These new standards focus on definitions of performance (Table 2) and the continued requirements (1) to design a process to measure performance along many dimensions and in all functions and (2) to assess those levels of performance that can be improved.

Here are excerpts from the preamble (p. 51) to that chapter:

This chapter represents a significant evolution in the understanding of quality improvement in health care organizations. It identifies the connection between organizational performance and judgements about quality. It shifts the primary focus from the performance of individuals to the performance of the organization's systems and processes ("process" means a single process, multiple processes and/or a system of integrated processes), while continuing to recognize the importance of the individual competence of medical staff members and other staff. And, it provides flexibility to organizations in how they go about their design, measurement, assessment and improvement activities. Thus, this chapter describes the essential activities common to a wide variety of improvement approaches.

Improving performance has been at the heart of the Joint Commission's Agenda for Change since its inception. The focus of this Accreditation Manual is on the important functions of an organization, and the focus of this chapter of standards is on a framework for improving those functions. It should now be evident that:

•performance is *what* is done and *how* well it is done to provide health care.
•the level of performance in health care is:
-The degree to which *what* is done is *efficacious* and is *appropriate* for the individual patient.
-The degree to which *how* it is done makes it *available* in a *timely* manner to patients who need it, is *effective*, is *coordinated* with other care and care providers, is *safe*, is *efficient*, and is *caring and respectful* of the patient.

These characteristics of what is *done* and *how* it is done are called the "dimensions of performance."

•The degree to which an organization does the right things and does them well is influenced strongly by its design and operation of a number of important functions—many of

Table 2.
Definitions for the Dimensions of Performance
I. DOING THE RIGHT THING

The **efficacy** of the procedure or treatment in relation to a patient's condition.

> The degree to which the care/intervention used for the patient has been shown to accomplish the desired/projected outcome(s).

The **appropriateness** of a specific test, procedure, or service to meet a patient's needs.

> The degree to which the care/intervention provided is relevant to the patient's clinical needs, given the current state of the art.

II. DOING THE RIGHT THING WELL

The **availability** of a needed test, procedure, treatment, or service to a patient who needs it.

> The degree to which appropriate care/interventions are available to meet the needs of the patient served.

The **timeliness** with which a needed test, procedure, treatment, or service is provided to a patient.

> The degree to which the care/intervention is provided to the patient at the time it is most beneficial or necessary.

The **effectiveness** with which tests, procedures, treatments, and services are provided.

> The degree to which the care/intervention is provided in the correct manner, given the current state of the art, in order to achieve the desired/projected outcome for the patient.

The **continuity** of the services provided to a patient with respect to other services, other practitioners, and other providers, and over time.

> The degree to which the care/intervention for the patient is coordinated among practitioners, between organizations, and across time.

The **safety** to the patient (and others) with which the services are provided.

> The degree to which the risk of an intervention and risk in the care environment are reduced for the patient and health care provider.

The **efficiency** with which services are provided.

> The ratio of the outcomes (results of care) for a patient to the resources used to deliver the care.

The **respect and caring** with which services are provided.

> The degree to which a patient, or designee, is involved in his own care decisions, and that those providing services do so with sensitivity and respect for his needs and expectation and individual differences.

---

which are described in this Manual.

•The effect of an organization's performance of these functions is reflected in patient outcomes and in the cost of its services.

•Patients and others, based on the patient health outcomes (and, sometimes on their perceptions of what was done and how it was done), make judgements about the quality of the health care.

•Patients and others, by comparing their judgements of quality with the cost of the health care, may also make judgements about the value of the health care.

This Improving Organizational Performance chapter, indeed, this entire hospital Manual, is being issued at a time when the health care field is redesigning its performance improvement mechanisms to incorporate concepts and methods developed by other fields (e.g., total quality management [TQM]/continuous quality improvement [CQI] and systems-thinking) and by the health service research community (e.g., reference data bases, clinical practice guidelines/parameters, functional status and quality of life measures). These standards mesh many of these useful concepts and methods with the best of current hospital quality assurance activities.

For example, health care organizations have begun to adopt some of the many approaches to CQI or TQM that have been successful in industry. Most of these approaches place in the hands of health care organizations' leaders and staffs a powerful array of methods and tools that are useful additions to those already used in health care. Also, most of these approaches highlight the pivotal role of the organization's leaders and the importance of assessing the needs and expectations of patients and listening to their feedback.

While the standards in this chapter (as well as elsewhere in the Accreditation Manual) do not require that an organization specifically adopt a CQI or TQM program, they reflect a selective incorporation of several core concepts of CQI/TQM.

Examples of CQI/TQM concepts that are incorporated into the standards include the key role that leaders (individually and collectively) play in enabling the systematic assessment and improvement of performance; the fact that most problems/opportunities for improvement derive from process weaknesses, not from individual incompetence; the need for careful coordination of work and collaboration across departments and professional groups; the importance of seeking judgments about quality from patients and others and using such judgments to identify areas for improvement; the importance of carefully setting priorities for improvement; and the need for both the systematic improvement of the performance of important functions and the maintenance of the stability of these functions.

The standards do not require adoption of any particular management style, subscription to any specified 'school' of CQI or TQM, use of specific quality improvement tools (e.g., Hoshin planning), or adherence to any specific process for improvement (e.g., the Joint Commission's '10-Step Model').

The standards in this chapter of standards reflect the need for:

•monitoring to understand and maintain the stability of systems and processes (e.g., statistical quality control);

•measurement of outcomes to help determine priorities for improving systems and processes; and assessment of individual competence and performance (including by peer review) when appropriate.

This Improving Organizational Performance chapter has some important linkages to the other chapters in this Accreditation Manual and, therefore, to other important functions of a health care organization. In particular:

•The performance improvement framework in this chapter of standards is to be used to design, measure, assess and improve the patient care and organizational functions identified by all the chapters—including this chapter—of this Manual. The standards in this chapter point organizations to those functions and processes most directly related to good patient outcomes (PI.3.2 through PI.3.4.2.4) and help organizations set criteria for the identification and prioritization of their improvement efforts.

•The leaders of an organization must provide the stimulus, vision and resources to permit the activities described in this chapter to be successfully implemented. Standards in the Leadership chapter identify their role.

•Management of the data required to design, measure, assess and improve patient care and organizational functions will necessitate an organization-wide approach. The standards in the Information Management chapter describe this approach.

•Education of the leaders and staff is key to acquiring the new knowledge needed to effectively lead and participate in improvement activities. The standards in the Staff Orientation and Education chapter and the Medical Staff chapter set the expectations for education and address the elements of this continuing knowledge acquisition process. (In 1995, all staff education requirements are addressed in the "Management of the Human Resource" functional chapter.)

Finally, the scoring guidelines (*AMH*, Vol. II) related to this Improving Organizational Performance chapter have been designed expressly to help organizations envision the long-term goals of the standards and make incremental progress toward those goals. The activities described in this chapter will take varying periods of time to fully implement, require varying types and levels of change, and may require resource acquisition or reallocation. Thus, expectations for full compliance with many of these standards will be phased into the survey and scoring process during the next several years at a pace consistent with the field's readiness.

The standards include language designed to require the health care organization to plan, design, measure, assess and improve organizational performance.

Performance-Focused Measures: The Joint Commission's Indicator Measurement System—The IMSystem

The first set (Table 3) of five perioperative and five obstetrical indicators to be available for optional use by hospitals completed a series of rigorous research and development activities underway since 1987. The ten indicators selected for voluntary use in 1994 are listed in Table 3 (1993, pp. 236-237).

Optional participation for hospitals interested in using the ten indicators was encouraged beginning in 1994, and eventually, as more indicators are added into the Joint Commission's data base, mandatory participation will become a required part of the accreditation process.

The Joint Commission's IMSystem will allow continuous monitoring of performance of the health care organizations in addition to the conduct of surveys for standards compliance activities on both a triennial basis for all accredited organizations and at mid-point (18 months after the triennial survey) for a random sample of all accredited organizations. (Annual surveys are conducted for home care organizations wishing to use the Joint Commission's deemed status relationship with the Health Care Financing Administration.)

Development work continues on both standards and indicators in order to more clearly identify how performance-focused standards relate to other sets of indicators as well as those developed for and placed in the Joint Commission's IMSystem. It is anticipated that in future editions of all the Joint Commission's standards manuals, there will be indicator measures for all functions addressed by the standards.

Additional indicators are in the final phase of Beta testing for addition to the data base in subsequent years. It is anticipated that in 1995, ten more indicators will be selected from those addressing Cardiovascular, Oncology, and Trauma Care.

In 1996, ten additional indicators will complete the rigorous validity and reliability testing necessary to be included in the Joint Commission's data base. Those indicators will most likely come from those related to Medication Use and Infection Control. The final number of indicators in the data base has yet to be determined, but it is expected to contain no more than 30 to 35 indicators to be used as performance measures related to the performance-focused standards found in the Manuals.

Additional indicator sets are in various other stages of development for use in all health care fields accredited by the Joint Commission including, for home care organizations and mental health organizations, those for Perfusion Therapy and Depression. Standards Manuals for those two fields complete the transformation to performance-focused standards with editions published for surveys commencing after January 1, 1995.

Nursing Care Standards and a Focus on Information Technology

In 1989, two Task Forces were working on revisions to Joint Commission standards: the Information Management Task Force discussed earlier and the Nursing Standards Task

Table 3.
Joint Commission IMSystem

1994 List of Ten Performance Measures/Indicators

1. **Focus:** Preoperative patient evaluation, intraoperative and postoperative monitoring, and timely clinical intervention
(Numerator): Patients developing a central nervous system (CNS) complication within 2 postprocedure days of procedures involving anesthesia administration, subcategorized by ASA-PS class, patient age, and CNS- versus non-CNS-related procedures

2. **Focus:** Preoperative patient evaluation, appropriate surgical preparation, intraoperative and postoperative monitoring, and timely clinical intervention
(Numerator): Patients developing a peripheral neurologic deficit within 2 postprocedure days of procedures involving anesthesia administration

3. **Focus:** Preoperative patient evaluation, intraoperative and postoperative monitoring, and timely clinical intervention
(Numerator): Patients developing an acute myocardial infarction (AMI) with 2 postprocedure days of procedures involving anesthesia administration, subcategorized by ASA-PS class, patient age, and cardiac- versus noncardiac-related procedures

4. **Focus:** Preoperative patient evaluation, intraoperative and postoperative monitoring, and timely clinical intervention
(Numerator): Patients with a cardiac arrest within 2 postprocedure days of procedures involving anesthesia administration, subcategorized by ASA-PS class, patient age, and cardiac- versus noncardiac-related procedures

5. **Focus:** Preoperative patient evaluation, intraoperative and postoperative monitoring, and timely clinical intervention
(Numerator): Intrahospital mortality of patients within 2 postprocedure days of procedures involving anesthesia administration, subcategorized by ASA-PS class and patient age

6. **Focus:** Prenatal patient evaluation, education, and treatment selection
(Numerator): Patients delivered by cesarean section, subcategorized by primary and repeat cesarean section
(Denominator): All deliveries

7. **Focus:** Prenatal patient evaluation, education, and treatment selection
(Numerator): Patients with vaginal birth after cesarean section
(Denominator): Patients delivered with a history of previous cesarean section

8. **Focus:** Prenatal patient evaluation, intrapartum monitoring, and clinical intervention
(Numerator): Live-born infants with a birthweight less than 2,500 g, subcategorized by presence or absence of medical indications for the birthing method (cesarean section, medical induction, or spontaneous vaginal delivery)
(Denominator): All live-born infants

9. **Focus:** Prenatal patient evaluation, intrapartum monitoring, neonatal patient evaluation, and clinical intervention
(Numerator): Live-born infants with a birthweight greater than or equal to 2,500 g, who have at least one of the following: an Apgar score of less than 4 at 5 minutes, a requirement for admission to the neonatal intensive care unit within 1 day of delivery for greater than 24 hours, a clinically apparent seizure, or significant birth trauma
(Denominator): All live-born infants with a birthweight greater than 2,500 g

10. **Focus:** Prenatal patient evaluation, intrapartum monitoring, neonatal patient evaluation, and clinical intervention
(Numerator): Live-born infants with a birthweight greater than 1,000 g and less than 2,500 g who have an Apgar score of less than 4 at 5 minutes
(Denominator): All live-born infants with a birthweight greater than 1,000 g and less than 2,500 g

---

Force. Given both the importance of the patient's medical record as the primary means of communication about the patient and the patient's care between health care providers, and the key role nursing plays in the patient's care, it was seen as essential that nursing care data be integrated into the permanent copy of the patient's medical record. Even in 1989, when the Nursing Standards Task Force first convened, there were still a few hospitals that did not keep *any* nursing portions of the patient's medical record when the discharge record was compiled for storage.

Hospital policies and procedures, approved by the hospital authority responsible for medical records, usually describe the mechanism for assuring that nursing information related to patient assessments, nursing care planned, nursing interventions provided, and patient outcomes is permanently integrated into the patient's medical record.

In 1990, an article published in *Computers in Nursing* noted, "The work-in-progress of the Nursing Standards Task Force (convened to revise the nursing SERVICES standards into new nursing CARE standards) considered new language related to the use of efficient interactive data management systems or computers for clinical and other information in the support, delivery, documentation and improvement of patient care is facilitated, wherever appropriate (p. 109). That recommendation for new language was deferred to the Task Force developing the new Management of Information standards.

The Nursing Standards Task Force also considered the sixteen (16) recommendations in The Final Report of the Secretary's Commission on Nursing on how the public and private sectors could work together to address the shortage of registered nurses prompted, in part, by the changing demand for nursing care services. The Joint Commission's new nursing care standards published in 1990 incorporated seven (7) of those recommendations.

Recommendation 3 addressed information technology (New Joint Commission Standards, 1991). The *final* Nursing Care standards related directly to both Recommendation 3 and the need to retain all nursing documentation "in toto" in the patient's final closed record that were approved for the 1991 edition of the *Accreditation Manual for Hospitals* appear below.

Recommendation 3.

The federal government should sponsor further research and encourage health care delivery organizations to develop and use automated information systems and other new labor-saving technologies as a means of better supporting nurses and other health professionals. Health care delivery organizations should work with researchers and manufacturers to ensure the applicability and cost-effectiveness of such information systems and technologies across all practice settings.

NC.1.3.5 Nursing care data related to patient assessments, the nursing care planned, nursing interventions, and patient outcomes are permanently integrated into the clinical information system (for example, the medical record).

NC.1.3.5.1 Nursing care data can be identified and retrieved from the clinical information system.

NC.5.5 The nurse executive, or designee(s), participates in evaluating, selecting, and integrating health care technology and information management systems that support patient care needs and the efficient utilization of nursing resources.

NC.5.5.1 The use of efficient interactive information management systems for nursing, other clinical (for example, dietary, pharmacy, physical therapy), and non-clinical information is facilitated wherever appropriate.

In the 1994 edition of the *Accreditation Manual for Hospitals,* the indicated Nursing Care standards were deleted from that chapter and addressed in the concepts found in new chapters of performance-focused functional standards addressing the Leadership function and the Management of Information function. This carried out the recommended direction and implemented the vision of the Nursing Standards Task Force. The members of the Nursing Standards Task Force were initially charged with the task of developing standards that would serve into the next decade (the 1990s) and into the beginning of the 21st century. Consistent with the concepts envisioned by the Information Management Task Force, those addressed in the new Nursing Care standards were congruent and are now one and the same as written in the new chapter on Management of Information first published in August 1993 for surveys conducted beginning in January 1994.

Summary

This chapter outlines Joint Commission work in the areas of developing both performance-focused standards and performance measures or indicators of quality performance for use in health care organizations. Seven Manuals of accreditation standards are either completed or "in transition" to contain fully developed sets of performance-focused standards to be used for measuring the performance of health care organizations. The health care organizations for which accreditation by the Joint Commission is available include ambulatory care organizations, home care organizations, hospitals, laboratories, long term care organizations, mental health organizations, and health care provider networks. Work on the research and development of performance measures or indicators related to the field-specific sets of standards published in the Manuals of the Joint Commission will also continue. This work is being done in support of the development and implementation of the Joint Commission's national data base of health care organization performance data related to both the processes and outcomes achieved by each accredited organization. In the long term, such information will permit health care organizations to benchmark their own levels of performance of key activities, processes and functions against those organizations who have been validated as exceptional performers related to ever-improving levels of quality.

For information on "up-to-the-minute" progress in either of these areas, contact the author in the Department of Performance Measures Development at the Joint Commission.

References

Joint Commission on Accreditation of Healthcare Organizations. (1993). *Agenda for Change Information,* Oakbrook Terrace, IL: Joint Commission, Department of Communications.

Joint Commission on Accreditation of Healthcare Organizations. (1991). *An Introduction to Joint Commission Nursing Care Standards,* Oakbrook Terrace, IL: Joint Commission, 1991.

Joint Commission on Accreditation of Healthcare Organizations. (1990). "Glossary," *Accreditation Manual for Hospitals* 1991 edition, Vol. I Standards, Oakbrook Terrace, IL: Joint Commission, 1990.

Joint Commission on Accreditation of Healthcare Organizations. (1993). "Improving Organizational Performance" Chapter, *Accreditation Manual for Hospitals* 1994 edition, Vol. I Standards, Oakbrook Terrace, IL: Joint Commission, pp. 35-44.

Joint Commission on Accreditation of Healthcare Organizations (1993) "Joint Commission Indicators for the Indicator Monitoring System," *Accreditation Manual for Hospitals* 1994 edition, Vol 1 Standards. Oakbrook Terrace, IL: Joint Commission, pp. 235-237.

Joint Commission on Accreditation of Healthcare Organizations. (1993). "Management of Information" Chapter, *Accreditation Manual for Hospitals* 1994 edition, Vol. I Standards, Oakbrook Terrace, IL: Joint Commission, pp. 35-44.

New Joint Commission Standards for selecting technology: The nurse's role. (1991, January). *Nursing & Technology,* pp. 1-3.

Quality assurance, control, and monitoring. The future role of information technology from the Joint Commission's perspective. (1990, May/June). *Computers in Nursing,* 8(3): 105-110.

Applying Technology Assessment to Information Systems

Barbara A. Happ, PhD, RN
Senior Consultant in Healthcare Information Services
Hamilton/KSA
Fairfax, VA
This study was partially supported by a grant from Epsilon Zeta Chapter of Sigma Theta Tau.

Introduction

Technology assessment is frequently described as a health care reform measure, which is not surprising when technological advances are said to account for between 30 to 40% of the after-inflation growth in health care spending (Lave, 1993). Without this assessment, the effectiveness of advanced health care information system technologies such as bedside computers is left in question. Do bedside systems really improve the delivery of patient care and increase the productivity of care givers? What is the social impact on patients when care givers use computers in their rooms? The Health Care Technology Assessment (HCTA) framework, which includes evaluation of the safety, cost, effectiveness and social impact, is a practical tool to assist in answering these questions. This chapter describes the framework, and how it was used to evaluate bedside systems located on general medical/ surgical units in three acute care hospitals.

What is Technology Assessment?

The Health Care Technology Assessment framework is an approach to systematically evaluate drugs, devices, medical and surgical procedures, and information systems, in an effort to improve patient care. The results from such evaluations are used for health care policy decisions. Technology assessment was first addressed in 1965 by Congressman Emilio Daddario (D/New York). The Office of Technology Assessment (OTA) was established in 1974 to examine the safety and efficacy of products. In 1993, the Agency of Health Care Policy and Research budgeted 74 million for conducting technology assessments and developing guidelines on the effectiveness of medical technologies. Bedside information systems are technologies that need to be examined because of the cost and rapid diffusion of the technology. Administrators and providers should be aware of the usefulness, risks, cost, and side effects not only of drugs and equipment, but also of information systems used to provide patient care. As a comprehensive research framework, the HCTA can assist with difficult decisions when data on potential benefits and acceptable risks are made available. In contrast, data from HCTA can constrain diffusion and use of technologies which lack effectiveness to guide appropriate use.

The HCTA framework applied to bedside systems includes evaluation of the safety, costs, effectiveness and social impact of the technology. A literature analysis was conducted to explore safety and cost issues. Effectiveness was tested using two measures of quality (patient satisfaction questionnaires and patient care documentation) to describe the social impact of bedside technology (see Table 1).

Table 1.
Application of Health Care Technology Assessment

SAFETY/COST	EFFECTIVENESS	SOCIAL IMPACT
Literature analysis	Two measures of quality	Patient interviews

How is Health Care Technology Assessment Conducted?

Four steps are involved in the HCTA process: (1) identification of what needs to be studied; (2) testing through analysis and trials; (3) synthesis of information to make recommendations; and (4) dissemination of the findings. For bedside systems selection and implementation, the following questions were asked: What is known? What is unknown? What is needed and can be obtained at what cost?

What Are the Methods Used to Perform Technology Assessments?

Methods include testing through random clinical trials; review of case studies, registries, data bases, sampling surveys, and surveillance studies; and/or group judgement methods such as the consensus conferences at NIH (Office of Medical Application Research). Cost/benefit analysis (effects stated in term of dollars) and cost-effective analysis (effects stated in terms of human lives) can also be performed. For information systems selection, a complete literature and vendor review and study (including a cost/benefit analysis) should be performed.

The information gathered must be assimilated, interpreted and recommendations made to be followed by dissemination of the findings and policy formation. Questions to be answered include: Will the information system improve patient care? Is it safe? What are the costs and benefits? What is the expected impact on the patient and care providers?

Literature Analysis

Computers as a Nursing Technology

According to the OTA, the definition of technologies includes drugs, devices, procedures and systems (Institute of Medicine, 1991). Any process of examining and reporting these technologies is considered a technology assessment.

While nurses have dramatically increased the use of technology in their practice, few studies have actually evaluated the impact of nursing technologies such as information systems on patients. Nursing technologies have been examined in terms of positive or negative human responses (Curtin, 1990). Curtin described a trend in which patients related quality of patient care with more nursing time and concern. As computers and communications technology provide faster, safer and more efficient information transmission, nurses should have more time for patient requests for distinct and individually tailored care arrangements.

Pillar and Jacox (1992) examined the relationship between technology and quality of care. These authors indicated that the key point in the control of technology is its transition from experimental to standard care. Health care technologies need to be controlled by effective processes of testing and approval. Similarly, Pillar and Jacox indicated that technology alone does not mean improved patient care. They pointed out that technology is only one factor for improving patient care, and may not be the most important.

Pillar, Jacox, and Redman (1990) studied the impact of technology on patient expectations. These authors noted that the complexity of new technologies challenges the nursing profession in such new areas as educating patients about new technology, and reducing the anxiety surrounding the complex equipment stationed near the patient. Each of these authors studied information systems as major nursing technologies because they affect nursing practice and patient care. The authors brought up many issues that have not been examined thoroughly, such as questions about technology and the quality of care, patient responses to technologies, and the expanded role of nursing to deal with technologies that encompass information systems.

Zielstorff (1993) analyzed all studies concerning evaluation of information systems for health care and found that there were many studies on the effects of information systems on nurses, but few on the effects of these systems on patient care. She concluded that assessment of systems focused on labor savings, cost-benefit studies, and surveys of nurses' attitudes toward computerization. Further, this author indicated that the studies were dated and not relevant to today's technology, and some were inconclusive. Studies did not measure the contribution of information systems in relation to actual clinical outcomes.

Staggers (1988) pointed out the sparseness of studies and the methodological problems in published studies on the impact of information systems on nursing practice. She reported that published studies on the impact of information systems on nursing practice lacked instrument statistical reliability and validity.

Zielstorff and Staggers indicated a gap in the literature which evaluated information systems using empirical studies. Evaluative research on the effectiveness of information systems in nursing has not been focused, nor has it yielded empirically sound results.

While bedside information systems for nurses are new and rapidly emerging tools that seem to offer qualitative and quantitative benefits for patients, nurses and hospitals, descriptive and anecdotal reports have not provided solid evaluative data of their impact. This may be because of the newness of the technology, the variety of systems available, and the lack of a standard evaluation framework. In one study, however, Knickman, Kovner, Hendrickson, and Finkler (1992) did explore nursing innovations to enhance nursing practice and thus improve recruitment and retention of nursing personnel. As part of a larger study of nursing innovations, two types of computer projects were studied together: computers on nursing units and bedside computers. A total of 27 hospitals implemented one or both types of projects. While computerization had a substantial positive effect on recruitment and a smaller positive effect on nurse satisfaction, there was no significant change in patient satisfaction on the 69 units in the study. Patient satisfaction with nursing care did not improve when bedside computers were implemented.

Using the Health Care Technology Assessment Framework

The Health Care Technology Assessment framework offers nursing a tool to structure evaluation of bedside systems in acute care. HCTA is a form of research and analysis which explores the impact of safety, effectiveness, cost-effectiveness and social impact on the individual and society. Several authors have used this framework to evaluate health technologies and their impact on quality of patient care.

Safety

Safety is essential if bedside systems are to operate in a patient environment. The hardware must be electrically safe and able to adhere to hygienic guidelines for cleaning. The electrical standards and hygienic guidelines for bedside systems are neither documented nor discussed in the literature. The design of software to include security, confidentiality, and drug accuracy are also important areas to evaluate. While safety is both a software and hardware concern, a few studies report the benefit of increased accuracy and timeliness in documentation or reporting on adverse drug events. Overall, however, the area of safety evaluation has not been explored in depth.

Cost-Effectiveness

Cost-effectiveness is the dollar value of bedside systems measured by financial return on investment (ROI) or cost recovery on a capital investment, cost avoidance, or cost per patient day. While most published articles and studies seem to indicate that computers at the patient bedside are cost effective, one recent study showed an actual cost increase. A large study of several innovations including health care information systems showed increased cost per patient day (Knickman et al., 1992) on units which had either bedside or other information systems used by nurses.

The delicate preservation of the balance between costs and the quality that new technology engenders is an ongoing discussion (Fitzgerald, 1989; Hendrickson and Kovner, 1990; Sussman, 1991). The cost of new bedside systems can be measured by changes in unit costs, annual dollar benefit projections, pharmacy savings, and estimated ROI studies.

Many studies have attributed considerable time savings in documentation to computer technology (Blank and Bauer, 1991; Byers, Gillum, Plascencia, and Sheldon, 1990), which saves health providers from walking long corridors, and reduces time for unit communication. By using estimates of reduction in agency and overtime costs and converting these into full time equivalent (FTE) nursing positions saved, Herring and Rochman (1990) found that the ROI averaged financial payback in 24 months. In their study of three hospitals using a cost-effectiveness analysis, Hopkins, Harvey, Bell and Agnew (1990) found the time to recover capital costs varied from two years to more than five years. They also found that bedside terminals can be cost effective, particularly when there is an interface to existing hospital information systems. Kahl, Ivancin, and Fuhrmann (1991a; 1991b) further described full-time equivalent avoidance or potential reduction of 28.5 FTEs in their 567-bed facility. In a case study of six hospitals, Abrami (1990) found that users reported the tangible and intangible benefits as outweighing the costs of bedside systems. Conclusions were drawn from subjective self reports of users.

Effectiveness

Asking the question "Does it work?" and measuring bedside systems under average conditions would indicate the level of effectiveness. Qualitative subjective findings abound in the literature for the positive impacts of automation in hospitals (Halford and Pryor, 1987; Hopkins, Harvey, Bell and Agnew, 1990; Knickman et al., 1992; Thomas, 1991). Measurement has included questioning nurse executives (Dunbar, 1992), comparing experimental and control units (Byers et al., 1990; Halford and Pryor, 1987), pre- and post- implementation (Kahl, Ivanancin, and Fuhrmann, 1991a; 1991b), and case studies (Abrami and Johnson, 1990). One study, however, reported no difference in the completeness and timeliness of computerized documentation on units with bedside computers (Marr, 1992). All of these studies showed efficiency and effectiveness improvements due to bedside systems, but strong empirical evidence of the relationship between bedside systems and quality of patient care was lacking.

Social Impact

Although there are few studies on the social impact of computers on patients, Marr (1992) found positive patient perceptions with the use of bedside computers. Several studies reported the impact of bedside systems on patients and staff. Blank and Bauer (1991) found that physicians indicated nurses were reporting patient changes sooner because they were spending more time with patients who had bedside computers. Patient outcomes as measured by patient satisfaction with bedside systems and other computers were studied by Knickman et al. (1992). While initial findings indicated no change in patient satisfaction where either bedside or other nursing information systems were in place, positive impacts on RN satisfaction and nurse recruitment were identified.

Overall, few empirical studies have established the influence of bedside computers on the quality of patient care and the social impact on the patient. Bedside technology is yet an emerging technology, and the HCTA framework offers the structure for a complete evaluation.

Study Design

A descriptive and quasi-experimental study of the impact of bedside systems using a convenience sample of 90 patients on 5 medical/surgical nursing units was conducted in three acute care hospitals in the northeastern United States. A quasi-experimental design was selected because there could be no random assignment of subjects to conditions. A pre-test\post-test design was used to compare units before and after bedside computers were introduced. Finally, a pre-test\post-test with comparison/ experimental units was conducted.

The study included a descriptive component because open-ended patient interviews were conducted. The interview elicited the patient's perception, attitude and opinion about the computer and technology in the patient room.

The main independent variable of the study was the presence or absence of a computer at the bedside. There was one cluster of dependent variables: effectiveness or quality of patient care as indexed by patient satisfaction with nursing care and perception of computer-related/technology-related nursing care, and nursing documentation compliance. The covariates were patient gender, race, age, and computer experience of the patient.

The study assumed that the nursing units in each of the three hospitals selected were matched for patient acuity and staffing level experience, and were therefore comparable. Several proxy measures of comparability included turnover and nursing staff experience. It was also assumed that the study hospitals were comparable and that the convenience sample of patients were representative of all patients on the units studied. Furthermore, patients who had questionnaires read to them and patients who filled out surveys themselves were assumed to respond similarly.

There were several acknowledged study limitations. The study sample was limited to three hospitals with varied bed capacity located in the northeastern United States. These hospitals serve different populations (rural, suburban, and urban) and may not be representative of all U.S. hospitals. Documentation of charts was a proxy, at best, for the indication of the quality of care and was limited to the care that was charted. As a result, it may not have included either all the care which was delivered aspects of the quality of that care.

Bedside System Evaluation

For this study, three different bedside systems were evaluated using the HCTA framework. One system was a mainframe application brought to the bedside and two were distributed clinical systems. Two different computers were used in patient rooms. Their effectiveness was measured using two quality of patient care indicators. Social impact was evaluated through patient interviews. The cost and safety of bedside systems were appraised through analysis of the literature.

The Patient Satisfaction Instrument (PSI) by Hinshaw and Atwood (1982), adapted from Risser (1975), was used. The PSI was a self-administered, 25-item Likert-type scale. It has internal consistency and reliability across many studies; the average alpha coefficient is .785. The coefficient alpha for reliability was .893 for this study of 90 patients.

A Patient Perceptions of Computer-Related/Technology-Related Care Instrument (PPCI) was developed for this study to investigate the patient's perception of computer or technology in the hospital room.

The Joint Commission on Accreditation of Healthcare Organizations' (JCAHO), 1991, 27 item Nursing Care Standard, NC.1. was used for nursing documentation auditing. A convenience sample of 21 patients from the units equipped with computers were interviewed using the Patient Interview Guide. These patients had also answered the PSI, PCCI, had their charts audited and, therefore, were representative of the entire sample of patients in this study.

Definition of Terms

Bedside Computers: These computers are the hardware (computer) and software (application) that allow input, access and processing of patient clinical information at the point of the patient-nurse encounter.

Effectiveness of Bedside Computers: The definition of effectiveness of a technology is the differences in performance under normal conditions (Jacox and Pillar, 1992). For this study, effectiveness was the degree of improvements in the quality of patient care. Effectiveness was measured by patient satisfaction with nursing care and nursing documentation compliance. The instruments used for measuring effectiveness of bedside systems were the PSI, the PPCI, and the JCAHO Chart Audit.

Quality of Patient Care: Donabedian (1992) defines quality in health care as the application of science and technology for improvements in health to include measures of effectiveness, optimality, acceptability, legitimacy and equity. Patient satisfaction and nursing care documentation are measures of quality of patient care (Donabedian, 1980; Hinshaw and Atwood, 1982). For this study, quality of patient care was considered to be consequences or effects related to the presence of the computer in the patient's room. These were measured by PSI, PPCI, and JCAHO.

Nurse, Nursing Staff: For this study, the "nurse" was defined as all direct nursing care givers. The Registered Nurse, Licensed Practical Nurse, Nursing Assistant, Nursing Tech, or Graduate Nurse were the "nurses" or "nursing staff" in the study.

Hospital Unit: For this study, hospital units were general medical/surgical units in an acute-care facility.

Social Impact of Technology: The effects of technologies on society and particularly on the patient were considered social impacts. This may include the psychological, legal, ethical, or political effects and may be described by personal preferences, perceptions of self, locus of control, cultural differences, relationships or coping styles of the patient or care givers. For this study, social impact was the responses or opinions given during the patient interview.

Study Findings

Quality/Effectiveness

Three instruments (PSI, PPCI, and JCAHO) were used to measure the quality of patient care. For each instrument, three tests were performed (ANOVA, TWO-WAY ANOVA,

Table 2.
Effect of Bedside Technology

Instrument	Hospital A		Hospital B		Hospital C	
	Precomputers	Postcomputers	Units without computers	Units with computers	Units without computers	Units with computers
PSI	+	−	+	−	+	−
PPCI	+	−	+	−	+	−
JCAHO	+	−	+	−	+	−

PSI	Patient Satisfaction Instrument
PPCI	Patient Perception of Computer Instrument
JCAH	Joint Commission on Accreditation of HealthCare Organization Chart Audit Instrument
+	positive finding
−	negative finding

and multiple regression). The ANOVA showed significant differences in individual patient care units for all instruments. In addition, lower scores were found on the nursing units that had bedside computers when the TWO WAY ANOVA was performed on the data obtained from the three instruments (p <.05). Two significant predictors were found using multiple regression: Patient race predicted lower JCAHO charting scores and the presence of the computer predicted lower PPCI and PSI scores, along with marginally lowered charting documentation scores.

Although patient satisfaction, patient perception and chart compliance total scores were generally high, the study found that patients on the units without computers were more satisfied with nursing care, and had better chart documentation compliance than patients monitored with computers in their rooms. Nevertheless, most patients were very positive when describing the technology's effect on their care in the room environment. This finding is similar to Marr (1992) who found patient perceptions of bedside computers to be positive in a study at a large medical center.

According to this study, then, the presence of a bedside computer in a patient's room did not improve the quality of patient care (see Table 2). All patients in the study reported high patient satisfaction with nursing care scores, but the patients on units without computers at their bedsides had higher mean scores than patients with the bedside computers. Chart audit scores were higher on units without the bedside computers.

Social Impact
A total of 21 patients were asked to participate in an interview after they filled out the questionnaires to assess social impact of bedside computers. Most of the patients said they liked the computer and thought that it helped the nurses. One patient worried that it might take health care jobs away. A few patients indicated that it did not bother them; the computer was like any other machine in the room. Some contended that when they were sick, machines did not matter.

Discussion and Implications
There are many areas to examine when looking for an explanation of the negative findings for bedside systems.

Both patients and staff may need additional education on the purpose of bringing computers closer to the patient. Examining work processes for possible re-engineering may also be necessary before implementing bedside systems. Process re-engineering examines the work functions which staff perform and evaluates the value of those functions. The study sites had basically automated the paper process of nursing care delivery. The results of the study might have been different if other questions had been asked before systems implementation. For example, asking "Is this a value-added process for care delivery?" may have changed the implementation and use of the bedside system.

More attention should be paid to evaluation of the automation of nursing care delivery. There may be necessary process improvement or redesign before system selection. For example, analysis of the taking and documentation of vital signs on some units could lead streamlining of the process and elimination of this activity as a 4 or 8 hour routine task. For some patients it may only be needed every 24 hours. This type of process redesign is essential before automation. Computerization of obsolete nursing care does not improve the quality of patient care.

In any replication of this study, two factors should receive careful consideration and analysis: (1) a negative nursing attitude towards the presence of computers in the patient room and (2) the physical placement of computers in a patient's room may have influenced the use of the computers in the provision and documentation of care. Bedside computers were placed at the foot of the beds of most of the 90 patients in this study.

Furthermore, a longitudinal study is recommended to measure the effects of beside computers over time. Revisiting the goal of bedside systems would also be important. The effectiveness, cost, safety and social impact of health care technologies must be studied before information technologies are selected and implemented in health care organizations. This study has shown that bedside information systems do not necessarily improve the quality of patient care.

Summary

New technologies are bringing dramatic changes to health care and rapidly reshaping nursing practice. The HCTA framework (safety, cost, effectiveness, social impact) was used to evaluate the use of computers in patient rooms. This descriptive and quasi-experimental study found that while patients had a positive reaction to bedside computers, this new technology did not improve the quality of patient care.

References

Abrami, P. F. (1990). Six case studies. In P. F. Abrami, and J. E. Johnson (Eds.), Bringing Computers to the Hospital Bedside (pp.17-27). New York: Springer Publishing Co.

Abrami, P. F., and Johnson, J. E. (Eds.). (1990). Bringing Computers to the Hospital Bedside. New York: Springer Publishing Co.

Blank, M., and Bauer, A. (1991). Issues to consider before investing in bedside terminal systems. AHA Hospital Technology Series Special Report, 10(30), 1-10.

Byers, P. H., Gillum, J. W., Plascencia, M., and Sheldon, C. A. (1990). Advantages of automating vital signs measurement. Nursing Economic$, 8(4), 244-247, 267.

Curtin, L. (1990, July 7-8). Touch-tempered technology. Nursing Management, 21(7), 7-22.

Donabedian, A. (1980). The Definition of Quality and Approaches to its Assessment. Ann Arbor: Health Administration Press.

Donabedian, A. (1992, February). Quality in Health Care: Whose Responsibility? Paper presented at the meeting of the American Board of Quality Assurance and Utilization Review Physicians, Clearwater, FL.

Dunbar, C. (March, 1992). Nurses want I/S selection power, but do they have it? Computers in Healthcare, pp. 20-24.

Fitzgerald, K. (1989, December). Technology in medicine: Too much too soon? IEEE SPECTRUM, 24-29.

Halford, G., and Pryor, T. A. (1987). Measuring the impact of bedside terminals. In W. W. Stead (Ed.), Proceedings of the Eleventh Annual Symposium on Computer Applications in Medical Care (pp. 359-373).

Hendrickson, G., and Kovner, C. T. (1990). Effects of computers on nursing resource use. Computers in Nursing, 8(1), 17-22.

Herring, D., and Rochman, R. (1990). A closer look at bedside terminals. Nursing Management, 21(7), 54-61.

Hinshaw, A. S., and Atwood, J. R. (1982). A patient satisfaction instrument: Precision by replication. Nursing Research, 31(3), 170-175, 191.

Hopkins, F. D., Harvey, G., Bell, E., and Agnew, C. (1990). Bedside Terminals: A Cost Effectiveness Analysis. Unpublished manuscript.

Institute of Medicine. (1991). The Computer-Based Patient Record. Washington, DC: National Academy Press.

Jacox, A., and Pillar, B. (1992). Health care technology and quality of care. In M. Johnson (Ed.), The Delivery of Quality Health Care. Series on Nursing Administration: Vol. 3. St. Louis: Mosby-Year Book, Inc.

Joint Commission on Accreditation of HealthCare Organizations. (1991). Nursing Care Standards. Accreditation Manual for Hospitals (p. 131). Oakbrook Terrace, IL: Author.

Kahl, K., Ivancin, L., and Fuhrmann, M. (1991a). Automated nursing documentation system provides a favorable return on investment. Journal of Nursing Administration, 21(11), 44-51.

Kahl, K., Ivancin, L., and Fuhrmann, M. (1991b). Identifying the savings potential of bedside terminals. Nursing Economic$, 9(6), 391-400.

Knickman, J., Kovner, C., Hendrickson, G., and Finkler, S. (1992, June). An Evaluation of the New Jersey Nursing Incentive Reimbursement Awards Program: Final Report and Appendix. NYU: The Health Research Program. New York: New York University.

Lave, J. R. (1993, March 15). A crisis of medical success. Business Week, p. 78.

Marr, P. B. (1992, May). NYU study supports community general's stance. Healthcare Informatics, p. 72.

Pillar, B., and Jacox, A. K. (1992). The control of health care technology. Nursing Economic$, 10(2), 152-153.

Pillar, B., Jacox, A. K., and Redman, B. K. (1990). Technology, its assessment and nursing. Nursing Outlook, 38(1), 16-19.

Risser, N. (1975). Development of an instrument to measure patient satisfaction with nurses and nursing care in primary care setting. Nursing Research, 24, 45-52.

Staggers, N. (1988). Using computers in nursing. Documented benefits and needed studies. Computers in Nursing, 6(4), 164-170.

Sussman, J. H. (1991). Financial considerations in technology assessment. Topics in Health Care Finance, 17(3), 30-41.

Thomas, M. (1991, July/August). Computers free nurses for care. American Nurse, pp. 1, 24.

Zielstorff, R. (1993). Methodologies for evaluation effects of nursing information systems. In Nursing Informatics: Enhancing Patient Care, A Report of the NCNR Priority Expert Panel on Nursing Informatics. National Nursing Research Agenda. Bethesda, MD: NCNR. U.S. DHHS, US PHS, NIH.

Organizational Impact of Information Systems

Carol A. Romano, PhD, RN, FAAN
Director, Clinical Systems and Quality Improvement
National Institutes of Health Clinical Center

Introduction

"When . . . a wave of change crashes into society, traditional management, values, cultures, organizational procedures and organizational forms become obsolete" (Sankar, 1988, p. 10).

Many new computer-based information systems are riding the crest of the wave of technological change in our society. Computer-based information systems are defined as automated systems that collect, transmit, process, store, retrieve, and distribute information to various users both within and outside an organization. The purpose of these systems is to support the operations and management of the organization (Ahituv and Neumann, 1990). With this purpose, these systems are a means to an end, organizational effectiveness and efficiency, not an end unto themselves. Becker (1988) notes, however, that the social and organizational context into which such technologies are introduced must be considered if we are to understand the impact of these new developments and to direct the successful implementation of this type of change. The impact of introducing computer-based information systems on an organization and its personnel is in part due to the interaction of such systems with the corporate culture, and with the formal and social systems within the organization.

Cultural Impact

The essence of culture is defined as a set of important unstated assumptions held in common by members of a community that encompasses shared feelings, objects, language, and behavior (Sathe, 1985). Classically, organizational culture is viewed as a combination of beliefs within the organization about the way work should be organized, the way authority should be exercised, and the way in which people are controlled and rewarded (Handy, 1982).

Harvey and Brown (1988) note that beliefs within a culture deeply affect an organization, and in fact, are the major factor to consider when planning to implement any change. When an organization introduces computer-based information systems into the work environment, employees are immediately confronted with new artifacts or objects, a new technical jargon, and an altered system of beliefs, values, and assumptions about their work lives (Gundry, 1985). Such enormous changes will cause a "culture shock" that will require everyone in the organization to undergo a period of adjustment, and such a response should be anticipated and planned for in any major changes within the organization.

Cultural Symbols

A culture is dependent upon the nature of the artifacts it uses or the symbols that manifest its ideals. The artifacts of information technologies are a mixture of hardware, software, work stations, and telecommunications facilities, each with its own jargon and varying levels of required computer skills. A personal computer may be a user-friendly, locally based interface isolated from the rest of the organization, whereas a mainframe computer may be less personal and more corporate-oriented, and very likely, even off-site. A computer system, however, brings to its environment specific rules and protocols not previously in force in the organization. These tools require standard methods, standard formats for results, and some standardization in the work processes (Morieur and Sutherland, 1988). Some organizational members may feel constrained in their use of the new automated systems and may thus continue to function in non-standard ways.

As the symbol of information technology, the computer terminal device itself may signify a cultural change in the assumptions of authority. Gundry (1985) observes, for example, that the computer may be perceived as the "real boss," because information processing requirements need to conform to the system's capabilities, not to workers' computer skills. In addition, with a computer system in place, employee work can be more closely monitored electronically and new methods of performance evaluation are certain to be introduced. How, and if, an employee is to be rewarded for the responsibilities that the new automation requires is unclear and of concern to organizational members.

The artifacts of automation may also symbolize shared beliefs of inflexibility, greater control over workers, or reduced inefficiency. Other values also emerge. Morieur and Sutherland report that "interimness" is viewed as a valued phase of the work process when information technology is used. That is, reports move through an organization in "draft" form as opposed to completed documents. As a result, the report procedure becomes faster and more flexible.

As computer-based information systems invade an organization, a specialized jargon emerges among employees. This points to the language change that needs to become part of the transformed cultural pattern of communications. In addition to artifacts and language, the aesthetic characteristics of computers also affect an organization. The presence of computers require changes in seating, lighting, temperature, and noise conditions in the work place. Physical space and work settings are affected. These required new adjustments in turn change the shared views about the nature of the organization as a place to work (Gorry and Norton, 1989).

Organizational Ecology

Organizational ecology is the study of ways in which the management of the physical setting affects and is affected by values, expectations, and work practices (Farlee, 1978). Traditional organizations make certain assumptions about how space is structured, about peer relations and interactions, and about turf and privacy; however, these assumptions are challenged by the installation of computer-based information systems. For example, traditionally, space is allocated by organizational status; top management is assigned a larger percentage of available space without regard to actual space requirements to perform work tasks.

The introduction of information technology has not created the hoped-for paperless office. Instead, it has stimulated a deluge of paper, the need for desk space for middle and lower-level employees, and the need for continual updating of employee computer skills. These new developments require an addition or redistribution of space to more effectively use the computer-based systems necessary to support work. These needs, however, undermine conventional assumptions about space and its use in our culture to symbolize status and power in the workplace. Therefore, administrators should take into account such long-held, unspoken cultural assumptions, for it is such assumptions that are the most difficult aspect of culture to change (Becker, 1988).

The use of space also affects the possible interaction of employees. Characteristically, highly structured organizational hierarchies tend to discourage communication across departments and projects. Computer-based information systems, however, affect the availability, accessibility, and sharing of information sources at all levels. This, in turn, challenges previous assumptions about internal communication patterns. The demands of automation may require the re-conceptualization of work and suggest the need for multiple offices, project rooms, shared spaces, as well as for private work areas (Becker, 1988).

Sathe (1985) notes that an organization's effectiveness is influenced by its leadership, culture, and systems. In addition to affecting culture as described above, automated computer systems influence the formal systems of an organization as well.

Impact on Formal Systems

Sathe reports that the formal system of an organization centers around the task to be completed, the personnel required to do the task, and the structures in place to support the work. From a systems perspective, the structural subsystem of an organization influences effectiveness (Watlington, 1989). Ford and Slocum (1977) report that considerable research has been directed toward isolating factors that influence organizational structure; three important variables that have been studied extensively are size, environment, and technology. Most research supports that either technology *per se,* or the interdependency created by technology, is central to determining structure.

Organizational Structure

Most researchers agree that the three major dimensions of structure are an organization's complexity, formalization, and centralization. Hage and Akin (1969) discuss these dimensions as the means by which organizations operate. Complexity is the degree of differentiation; formalization is the degree to which rules are specified and adhered to; and centralization is the locus of formal control for decision making.

Although traditionally used for data processing at the operational levels of an organization, computer-based information systems are increasingly employed by middle and upper levels of management. The importance of transforming data into information for purposes of administrative decision making has been recognized (Ahituv and Neumann, 1990). In fact, information systems are designed especially to support the structured and semi-structured decisions required at the middle and strategic levels of an organization (Rogers, 1983). Centralization or decentralization of decision making may result because of this capability, which may be a change from the status quo.

Regarding these three major dimensions of structure, Farlee (1978) reported the implications of an integrated computer-based hospital information system (HIS) as a focus of organizational change in a hospital. She noted that HIS produced an increase in formalization and centralization; theoretically, this should increase productivity and efficiency. Farlee found, however, that these factors were inversely related to employee satisfaction and accommodation to change. There is evidence, then, that acceptance of a computer-based information system is related to such variables as low formalization, low centralization and high specialization or complexity of tasks.

An automated system, however, may be selected precisely because of the organizational need to achieve more conformity to policies and procedures, or more standardization and control over particular roles. Thus, the introduction of this technology may result in an unanticipated change to the established formal system, or the new technology may be introduced as the vehicle to effect this type of change.

Organizational Roles

The roles and responsibilities of personnel/employees in an organization are also part of the formal system (Sathe, 1985). Computer systems may influence how work is done and determine the skills required to accomplish a task. Boddy and Buchanan (1982) explored the effect of information technology on the roles of those employees who were directly affected by the change to a computer-based system. These authors concluded that technology can either replace or complement roles, depending on the capability of the technology and on how work is organized around the technology.

When computer automation is introduced into an organization, certain roles are made redundant and obsolete; others, however, are complemented in such a way that the accessibility of information through an automated system facilitates one's ability to function more effectively within an organization. Surprisingly, middle level management may be the most dramatically affected by automated systems. That is, existing organizational roles that traditionally focused on the movement and processing of information may need to be redirected, since these types of activities are accomplished better through information technology (Ahituv and Neumann, 1990; Gorry and Norton, 1989). Fuchs-Kittowski, Schuster, and Wenzloff (1981) address the substitution of human activity by machines and the effect of this on workers. While automation creates new working places and more challenging tasks, it also creates trivial and monotonous jobs. And although some routine human activities may be replaced, others are created. Operations performed by machines must be suitably integrated into the process of social work. For these reasons, the psychophysical dimension of work cannot be ignored.

Impact on the Psychosocial System

The psychosocial system of an organization involves the interaction of people and their established communication patterns. The introduction of computer-based information systems has the potential to alter the structure and function of communication and social behavior within an organization (Ahituv and Neumann, 1990; Zuboff, 1982). A key factor for the successful implementation of such new technology is to devise technologies that are acceptable to employees. To date, little research has been conducted on the effect that computerized information systems have on the coordination of work within an organization.

Aydin (1989) explored the effect of an HIS on the occupational community of health care professionals in hospitals. Her study showed that, in fact, changes in tasks for nurses and pharmacists increased the interdependence between the two. This new interdependence was accompanied by improved communications and cooperation, factors which provided an opportunity to encourage improved working relationships between these departments. Watlington (1989) also noted that mutual reliance upon a hospital computer-based information system forged increased cooperation among departments linked on the system.

As with any change, however, the threat or fear of the unknown exists; so, too, with the introduction of computer-based information systems into the work environment. At first, anxiety and stress may increase as employees question the security of their jobs, the potential effect on their autonomy, and the potential change in their power base. Administrators should be aware that resistance to such systems may exist and such resistance should be anticipated in planning change (Dowling, 1980).

Resistance

Theories of Resistance

The introduction of computer-based systems, by definition, requires a change in how information is acquired, processed, and managed. Because information and its communication is a critical component of organizational as well as individual work, changes affecting both must be managed if the organization is to be effective. Resistance, though not always fully anticipated, can be viewed as an opportunity to understand oneself and one's role in the organization (Sathe, 1985). The underlying assumptions of change strategies assert conditions for accepting change; hence, they infer factors inversely related to resistance.

Haffer (1986) discusses three change strategies which focus on different targets of change and causes of resistance. Findings include: (1) people will resist change that is perceived as irrational and of no direct benefit to them; (2) people with less power will not resist the plans of those with greater power; and (3) people resist change when it clashes with existing norms and values which direct roles and responsibilities. This framework of resistance is consistent with Sathe's model of organizational effectiveness which asserts that behavior (including changes to behavior) is affected by leadership, formal systems, and culture. While these models are useful, they are not adaptable in dealing with resistance related to information technology.

Markus (1983) proposes three types of theories of resistance related to automated management information system implementation in organizations, and discusses each from the perspective of assumptions about information systems, organizations and about resistance itself. The first theory attributes the cause of resistance to factors internal to people and groups, such as cognitive style or personality. For example, discussions which relate to or explain resistance in terms of analytic versus intuitive thinking patterns are consistent with this people-determined theory. This theory is consistent with Sathe's discussion of the human tendency to resist change.

Second, Markus's system-determined theory relates the cause of resistance to factors inherent in the software application. He cites empirical studies that note technical problems as a factor in implementation failures. While these two theories are divergent, it is realistic to assume that both may operate simultaneously, suggesting that resistance to computer-based information systems is a multivariate problem. The third theory relates resistance to information systems to the interaction between people and systems. The interaction can come from the sociotechnical perspective of the division of labor and its effect on roles and responsibilities. It can also be from the political perspective of the interaction of different sources of organizational power.

From the perspective of these three theories, assumptions about the information system, the organizational context in which it is used, and the nature of resistance can be compared and contrasted. The people- and system-determined theories assume that the purpose of information systems is to achieve organizational goals, such as enhancing decision making, controlling performance, and improving communications. These theories assume that goals are shared by organizational members, and that resistance is undesirable.

In contrast, the interaction theory acknowledges that the purpose of some information systems may be to change organizational culture, the balance of power, or the dependency and control processes, not merely the work flow. This theory assumes that goals differ across the organization, and that conflict is endemic. Resistance from this perspective is a product of the setting, the users, and the system. As such, it is neither desirable nor undesirable. This theory is derived from the non-rational view, or contingency view of organizations, which Harvey and Brown (1988) regard as appropriate in a changing environment.

In considering resistance to change, however, one is cautioned about using the rationalist, traditional model of organizational theory in planning change. Traditional models of an organization's objectives and goals that need to be achieved are not always agreed upon, and in reality may be controversial. Therefore, user resistance may result because the pre-specified ends meet the needs of one group (management) at the expense of another (employees). Strategies for implementing computer-based information systems need to address whether the objectives for the system are perceived as legitimate and are agreed upon. Theoretical approaches to resistance, then, need to acknowledge the non-traditional view of organizations as well as the interaction model of resistance.

No one theory in isolation, however, can adequately describe the complexity of modern organizations nor the dynamics and resistance encountered in organizational change. From the viewpoint of employees, the introduction of computer based-information systems, though, is more than an organizational change: it poses a stronger threat—the introduction of an innovation.

Innovation Models

An innovation is defined as an idea, practice, object or knowledge perceived as new by individuals or groups. While not all change is considered an innovation, all innovations are considered changes. Computer-based information systems can be considered an innovation, and as such, can be reviewed from the perspective of Roger's innovation diffusion/adoption model (1983). This model proposes that innovations are diffused within a social system, and then a decision is made whether or not to adopt the innovation. The diffusion of an innovation is the process by which an innovation is communicated through channels over time among the members of a social system. Adoption of the innovation involves a decision process through which an individual becomes aware of, is persuaded to try, and adopts or rejects continued use, based on perceived characteristics of the innovation. These attributes or characteristics include advantage, complexity, compatibility, trialability, and observability of effectiveness. An adaptation of Rogers' model was developed by Romano (1993) and incorporates organizational theory in proposing predictors of innovation adoption.

From these models, resistance can be viewed as rejection of an innovation based on unawareness, negative evaluation of attributes, or incompatibility with the dynamics of the social system. The models are consistent with Markus's (1983) people- and system-determined resistance theory in that they include variables related to the computer system as well as to the adopter, user, or customer. The interaction theory is also consistent with the social system context of both models. It is unclear, however, whether adoption is synonymous with use or acceptance. Administrators are cautioned against the pro innovation bias which asserts that adoption is always in the organization's best interest.

In summary, a variety of perspectives have been used to address resistance to change in general, and to computer-based information systems in particular. The critical question, however, is how an organization can plan for the systematic introduction of a computer-based information system to enhance organizational effectiveness, efficiency, and employee satisfaction. To this end several strategies for implementing such systems can be considered.

Implementation Strategies

In weighing strategies to successfully implement computer-based information systems and the required behavioral changes, the *methods* of change cannot be considered in isolation. The incentive to change (*motivation*), and the communication and speed of implementing new expectations (*model* for change) must also be factored into the equation (Sathe, 1985). Six approaches for dealing with change have been proposed by Kotter and Schlesinger (1979). These include: (1) education and communication; (2) participation and involvement; (3) facilitation and support; (4) negotiation and agreement; (5) manipulation and co-optation; and (6) implicit and explicit coercion. Each approach has its strengths and weaknesses; administrators are cautioned to carefully match the strategy to the particular situation to be effective.

In addition to considering strategies for behavioral change, administrators must also address the cultural changes required for the implementation of computer systems. An assessment of the magnitude of the change and the effect on the content and strength of the culture is needed to determine the degree of resistance to anticipate. Strategies to address cultural change include focusing on the intrinsic motivations and justifications for behavior, emphasizing cultural communications, and hiring and socializing members with "cultural fit" while removing deviants. Behavioral change without cultural change may be temporary and result in lack of commitment to the change by organizational members (Sathe, 1985).

Haffer (1986) reports three possible strategies of change: (1) to focus on providing the knowledge needed to make a rational choice; (2) to use power to manipulate or force compliance; and (3) to clarify changes to habits, attitudes, and values and to direct the development of new ones. Of critical importance, however, is a focus on participation by the individuals affected by the change. These strategies are consistent with those of Kotter and Schlesinger and Sathe. While the above principles apply to change in general, Dowling (1980) notes that recognizing resistance to computer-based information systems is critical to effectively applying implementation strategies. His study demonstrated five common types of resistance: passive resistance, oral defamation of the computer by complaining and spreading rumors, declaring an inability to learn, actively interfering by sabotage, and overt refusal to use computers.

While the diversity within an organization would seem to require separate automated systems, the commonality desired for sharing data can best be met through the integration or networking of such systems. Integration, however, poses the problems of constraints of the state-of-the-art hardware, space requirements, security, and compatibility of and controversies over the choice of input and output media and devices. These realities need to be addressed in the planned change process (Hejna, Donovan, and Williams, 1982.) Davis and Salasin (1982) propose seven interacting factors which play a part in influencing human responses to change, and are considered both necessary and sufficient to account for responses to change. These factors present a framework to direct and guide strategies in the implementation of computer-based information systems as an innovative organizational change. These multiple factors incorporate the theories of resistance, as well as the change strategies discussed above, and each is discussed in turn.

Commonly, computer systems are introduced into an organization as a solution looking for a problem to solve. While this can be explained in terms of an organization's response to "be modern," it suggests that the first implementation strategy should focus on triggering a felt *need* for the technology or innovation. Next, *awareness* and training interventions are needed to increase clarity regarding what the computer-based system can do and how individuals can use it to meet their needs. A computer system must "fit" the organization's culture or *values* or "way of doing things." Changing the organizational culture may be required. Davis and Salasin (1982) suggest identifying and developing a cadre of zealous participants who can network within and outside the organization, along with adopters to facilitate the spread of the innovation.

Mobilizing and budgeting *resources* to support implementation beyond equipment and set up costs are also required, especially for personnel and training. *Timing* the implementation of computer-based systems with other concurrent changes such as reorganization, arrival of new leaders, or a crisis may also facilitate the change. *Anticipating resistance* by addressing legitimate concerns over unreliable hardware and software, cryptic output, and cumbersome interfaces is invaluable to ensure success. Gradual change softened by peer support, pilot testing and demonstrations of use also help to reduce uncertainty and, hence, resistance. Finally, emphasizing the *benefits derived,* such as advantages to a program area or a resulting decrease in workload or stress, helps to make the benefits more visible and reaffirms new behaviors.

Summary

The introduction of computer-based information systems is acknowledged as a dramatic organizational change and innovation which may affect, either directly or indirectly, all members of an organizational unit. The type and extent of the technology introduced will determine the degree of organizational impact. Administrators of today's organizations need to anticipate the effect that information technology will have on the culture of the organization and its formal and psychosocial systems. Further, they need to understand the principles of adopting and resisting change. And finally, to improve the quality and performance of the organization, administrators must skillfully apply multiple implementation strategies to ensure the successful use of such technologies.

References

Ahituv, N., and Neumann, S. (1990). *Principle of Information Systems for Management* (3rd ed.). Dubuque, IA: Wm. C. Brown, Publisher.

Aydin, C. (1989). Occupational adaptation to computerized medical information systems. *Journal of Health and Social Behavior, 30*(2), 163-179.

Becker, F. (1988). Technological innovation and organizational ecology. In M. Helander (Ed.), *Handbook of Human-Computer Interaction* (pp. 1107-1156). North Holland: Elsevier Science Publishers B.V.

Boddy, D., and Buchanan, D. (1982). Information technology and the experience of work. In L. Bennon, U. Barry, and O. Holst (Eds.), *Information Technology Impact on the Way of Life* (pp. 144-157). Dublin: Tycooly International Publishing.

Davis, H., and Salasin, S. (1982). Computers and organizational changes/factors that influence useful adoption of computer applications. In B. Blum (Ed.), *Proceedings of the Sixth Annual Symposium on Computer Applications in Medical Care* (pp. 371-379). New York: IEEE.

Dowling, A. (1980). Do hospital staff interfere with computer system implementation? *Health Care Management Review, 5*(4), 23-32.

Farlee, C. (1978). The computer as a focus of organizational change in the hospital. *Journal of Nursing Administration, 8*(2), 20-26.

Ford, J., and Slocum, J. (1977). Size, technology, environment and the structure of organizations. *Academy of Management Review, 2*(4), 561-575.

Fuchs-Killowski, K., Schuster, V., and Wenzloff, B. (1981). Working environment-organizational, technological and social problems of computerization. *Computers in Industry, 2*(4), 275-285.

Gorry, G., and Norton, M. (1989). A framework for management information systems. *Sloan Management Review, 30*(3), 49-61.

Gundry, L. (1985). Computer technology and organizational culture. *Computers and the Social Sciences, 1*(3), 163-166.

Haffer, A. (1986). Facilitating change—Choosing the appropriate strategy. *Journal of Nursing Administration, 16*(4), 18-22.

Hage, J., and Akin, M. (1969). Routine technology, social structure, and organization goals. *Administrative Science Quarterly, 14*(3), 366-376.

Handy, C. B. (1982). *Understanding Organizations.* Harmonsworth, United Kingdom: Penguin Books.

Harvey, D. F., and Brown, D. R. (1988). *An experiential approach to organization development* (3rd ed.). Englewood Cliffs, NJ: Prentice Hall.

Hejna, W., Donovan, A., and Williams, F. (1982). Implementation of medical information systems in major medical centers. In B. Blum (Ed.), *Proceedings of the Sixth Annual Symposium on Computer Application in Medical Care* (pp. 381-383). New York: IEEE.

Kotter, J. P., and Schlesinger, L. A. (1979). Choosing strategies for change. *Harvard Business Review, 57*(2), 106-114.

Markus, M. (1983). Power, politics, and MIS implementation. *Communications of the ACM, 26*(6), 430-444.

Morieur, Y., and Sutherland, E. (1988). The interaction between the use of information technology and organizational culture. *Behaviour and Information Technology, 7*(2), 205-213.

Rogers, E. (1983). *Diffusion of Innovation* (3rd ed.). New York: Free Press.

Romano, C. A. (1993). *Predictors of Nurse Adoption of a Computerized System as an Innovation.* Doctoral dissertation, University of Maryland at Baltimore.

Sankar, Y. (1988). Organizational culture and new technologies. *Journal of Systems Management, 39*(4), 10.

Sathe, V. (1985). *Culture and Related Corporate Realities.* Homewood, IL: Richard D. Irwin, Inc.

Watlington, A. G. (1989). Benefits realization at Mercy Memorial results in a changed organizational culture. *Computers in Health Care, 10*(8), 26-29, 32.

Zuboff, S. (1982). New worlds of computer-mediated work. *Harvard Business Review, 60,* 142-152.

Choices of Nursing Systems

Shirley Hughes, RN
Principal
SJ Hughes Consulting
Chandler, Arizona

Introduction

Information systems designed to support the nursing professional are already in wide-spread use today. According to a recent marketing study, 83.7% of hospitals over two hundred beds in size (65.5% of all hospital beds) in the United States have patient care systems of some description in service today (Dorenfest, 1992). In many cases, however, those systems are nursing station-based Order Communication Systems used primarily for requisitioning services and supplies, results reporting and charge capture; therefore, these systems are not really designed to support the nursing process. A growing number of those hospitals (currently approximately 50%), however, also have information systems with nursing applications. In addition, 3 to 5% of all hospitals in the United States have extended their clinical applications to include in-depth patient care documentation with computer terminals placed at the bedside.

The availability and use of automated nursing and clinical information systems is predicted to become even more prevalent over the next several years (Reed, 1993). This is due to several factors, but most notably the advances in information technologies and the influences of health care reform—especially related to automation of patients' records.

Does this mean that nurses can expect to have automated information systems available that actually add value to their professional practice? Can we look forward to improved application of new technologies that really do support the care provider? Will these systems provide opportunities for expanded nursing research? Is it realistic to look for automated nursing decision-support capabilities to be included in these systems? With these questions in mind, this chapter looks at the state of the art in choices of systems for nurses today and at current information systems trends, along with the outlook for the future.

Much of the following discussion focuses on commercially available systems, rather than on development by individual health care facilities. This approach seems appropriate in light of the trend that we have seen in the last few years in which the number of health care facilities developing their own systems has decreased while the number of commercial systems has increased. This is attributable to the high cost of initial development and the long-term commitment of resources required to maintain and keep systems updated with new technologies. It is much more cost-effective to enter into joint projects in which one or more hospitals or health care facilities work with a vendor to define their system requirements and then share costs over time with multiple organizations (Hughes, 1992).

Types of Nursing Systems

A nursing information system is a software system that automates the nursing process from assessment to evaluation, including patient care documentation. It also includes a means to manage the data necessary for the delivery of patient care, e.g., patient classification, staffing, scheduling, and costs. It is not separate, but an integral part of the health care organization's overall information system (Simpson, 1993, p. 11).

In other words, there are a number of different aspects or different types of nursing information systems. Systems used by nurses may be offered in a variety of "packages" that might range from documentation systems to education, financial, and management. For the purposes of this discussion the following categories are used to group nursing systems:
• patient care documentation systems
• patient care decision support systems
• business systems for nursing
• quality management systems
• systems in support of nursing education
• systems in support of nursing research.

Patient Care Documentation Systems

Patient care documentation systems are those systems used in the variety of environments where patient care is provided by nurses, doctors and other clinicians to document activities ranging from the plan of care to implementation of that care and the related assessments and outcomes. The systems in use today for this purpose vary a great deal in depth and breadth and in their integration with other health care information systems. For this reason, it is important that we look at these systems in view of their design focus: (1) those designed as a part of a Hospital Information System (HIS), (2) those designed specifically for the clinical (nursing) department, and (3) those stand-alone systems focusing on a specific application or aspect of care.

Hospital Information Systems

Many Hospital Information Systems vendors provide patient care documentation modules as a subset of their house-wide systems. The applications typically are very highly integrated and often use a central data base for all clinical and financial information. Historically, they have been nursing station-based. Many of these systems evolved from financially oriented order-entry systems with primarily clerical users. Over the past few years, however, many of these systems have been enhanced to include more "clinician friendly" user interfaces and more robust patient care applications. This type of patient documentation system offers the greatest variety of depth and breadth of function from system to system (more so than the departmental or stand-alone systems).

A listing of the general characteristics of HIS patient care documentation modules follows:
• All meet at least minimum documentation requirements.
• Most are "user friendly" in some manner (e.g., user prompts, list selections, alpha name searches).
• Some now offer "point-of-care" options. This is most often in the form of bedside terminals that facilitate documentation and data retrieval at the point of contact with the patient. Some HIS vendors have added new point-of-care applications, but most have simply added terminals to extend the same applications used at the nursing station to the patient room. One HIS vendor, Health Data Sciences (HDS), designed its Ulticare system with a point-of-care focus, using the patient and the patient's care environment as the central focus of all applications.
• Most of these systems use a central architecture—a central computer processor and data base with all terminals accessing this data base.
• Terminals with pointing devices, (e.g., light pen, mouse, trackball) are very common. Some offer the option of using PCs as terminals to add flexibility and enhance usability.

•Most use menu-driven displays in which the user is routed through a series of screens to input data, either by selecting from pre-defined lists or by typing into pre-formatted fields.

•Paper worksheets and reports are used extensively to extend the information beyond the on-line access points.

•These systems are designed to facilitate communication as well as documentation—especially communications among departments within the health care facility.

Applications typically offered with HIS systems include:

Acuity	Order entry/results reporting
Admit/discharge/transfer	OR scheduling/staffing
Budgeting	Patient accounting
Care planning	Patient appointment scheduling
Case management	Patient care documentation
Case mix	Pharmacy
Cost accounting	Quality management
Decision support	Radiology
General financial	Scheduling/staffing
Managed care	Surgery management/scheduling
Medical records	

A list of examples of HIS companies and their patient-care documentation products follows:

Compucare—Affinity	Meditech
First Data—Saint Express	Phamis—Lastword
HBO & Company—Clinstar and CliniPac	SMS—Unity and Invision
HDS—Ulticare	TDS—7000 Series
IBAX—Series 3000, 4000, and 5000	

Patient Care Departmental Systems

Those systems focused specifically on nursing/patient care delivery are typically "point-of-care"-oriented systems. They were designed to be used in the patient care environment, and both applications and placement of (and in some cases design of) hardware and terminals reflect that focus. The intent of these systems is to replace the paper record of the patient's care with an automated version that makes the information much more accessible and useful for making care decisions. The automated version is the legal documentation of patient care as well as a decision support tool. These systems have often been developed for a specific specialty care area initially (e.g., critical care or medical surgical), but over time many have developed solutions to address the needs of other patient care areas. Although these systems are focused almost entirely on patient care documentation, most are at least partially integrated and/or interfaced to one or more of the following systems: patient registration, order communication, laboratory, pharmacy or patient billing systems.

The general characteristics of departmental patient care documentation systems include the following:

•Many use a distributed architecture—multiple processors, distributed data base, and interconnection of work stations or PCs via local area network.

•Almost all offer terminals with pointing devices (mouse or trackball), some use touch screens and bar code readers, and others offer portable options. There is a great deal of interest on the part of both clinicians and vendors, as well as work in progress, to incorporate the technologies available for wireless communications and portable terminals to find the ultimate solution(s) for the clinical users.

• Most systems use some type of windowing displays. Because these systems are designed to be used by the nurses and physicians, the human interface factor is very important and has, for the most part, received a great deal of attention in the system design.

• Fewer paper worksheets are used with these systems as much more data is readily accessible for review and manipulation on-line.

• These systems are designed to facilitate communication as well as documentation—especially among clinicians.

Applications typically offered with clinical departmental systems include:

Acuity	Order entry/results reporting
Admit/discharge/transfer	Patient care documentation
Care planning	Physician documentation/review
Case management	Quality monitoring/tracking
Critical care	Trending/graphics
Decision support (clinical)	

Some examples of patient-care departmental systems listed by departmental focus include:

Med/surg	**Critical Care**
Medtake	Corometrics - NICU-Link
CliniCom - CliniCare	EMTEK - System 2000
	Hewlett-Packard - Careview 9000
Operating Room	**Emergency Department**
Atwork - ORSOS	EmergiSoft
Enterprise - Orbit	
EPIC - Optime	

Patient Care Stand-Alone Systems

Stand-alone nursing applications usually address some specific aspect(s) of documentation (e.g., care planning) or a specific type of care (e.g., home health). These systems are not normally integrated with any other systems.

The general characteristics of stand-alone patient care documentation systems include:

• A single terminal architecture—one self-contained processor and associated data base.

• A standard PC user interface, (e.g., DOS, Windows).

• Paper worksheets and chart documents. (On-line retrievals are not always readily available).

• A focus on documentation, not communication.

Applications typically offered with stand-alone systems include:

Acuity	Patient registration
Nurse care planning	Quality monitoring/tracking
Nurse scheduling/staffing	Time/attendance
Nursing documentation	

Some examples of stand-alone patient care systems follow:

RN Act—used both in home health and acute care

Excelcare

Care Computer Systems—VistaCare (a nursing home system)

Infomed—Stat 2 (a home health care system under development for the Visiting Nurses Association using a pen-based portable terminal)

Patient Care Decision Support Systems

As information systems technology continues to evolve, more and more evidence confirms that computers really can be used to assist the health-care professional to make decisions. In some cases, knowledge rules of varying types have been incorporated into clinical applications with resulting reminders and suggestions automatically presented to the caregiver in the process of documentation and planning care. The 3M-HELP System developed at LDS Hospital in Salt Lake City, Utah, is one of the best known automated information systems equipped with this type of decision-support. Other HIS and patient-care departmental systems are beginning to add decision-support features as they continue to enhance their basic applications. Some examples of the types of decision support capabilities commonly seen in these systems include: suggested nursing diagnosis based on patient assessments; expert reference data bases integrated into the documentation applications (e.g., PACE for care planning, STAT-Ref for information look-ups); and alerts on out-of-range data values or overdue medications. Because of the potential impact these types of applications could have on quality improvement, and the rapidly evolving expert systems technologies, more and more systems are likely to incorporate clinical decision support logic in their product offerings.

Business Systems for the Nursing Unit

Business systems for nursing come in the forms of Acuity/Severity and staffing and scheduling (e.g., Grasp - MIStro, APACHE III, Atwork - Ansos, InCharge); Nurse Recruitment, Budgeting/Cost Accounting (often a part of the financial or HIS systems); Productivity Management (e.g., MECON - Optimis); and Executive Information Systems (EISs) (management decision-support—usually a part of the HIS).

Although EISs are often developed with the Chief Executive Officer and Chief Financial Officer as the targeted users, the nurse executive could realize great potential benefit from the EIS. These systems provide access to demographic, clinical, and financial information and support ad hoc reports and "what if" queries, both of great value to a nurse executive needing to understand the effectiveness of the current operation and what effects a specific change might cause. This kind of information is especially important with the growing influence of managed care on health care delivery organizations. Nurse executives and managers face increasing demands that they be able to evaluate the business of patient care as it relates to costs per case type, and so forth. These new information demands are requiring old management systems to be expanded and may also mean some new modules will be required to identify more specifically the costs of care and compare those more accurately to the severity and outcomes information.

Other types of software that can be helpful in supporting the nurse manager include the generic PC software programs such as word processing, spread sheets, project management, and electronic mail.

Quality Management Systems

Automated patient care systems have made the challenge of identifying lapses in quality much more timely, less time consuming and more accurate. With real-time alerts provided to the care giver, many quality errors can be avoided entirely. The integrated audit tools provided with many patient-care documentation systems allow automated quality audits to be accomplished in a very efficient and effective manner. Once the audits have been performed, the resulting data is often then entered, either via interface or manually, into quality monitoring and tracking systems, some offering the ability to compare an institution's results with those of similar institutions. Examples of these quality-monitoring systems include Code 3/HSI, a product of the 3M Corporation, and Medicus' InterAct system.

Systems in Support of Nursing Education

Computer-Aided Instruction (CAI) has been recognized for some time as an effective learning tool. CAI is offered by several vendors of patient care systems to maximize the effectiveness of training users on the new system in the minimum amount of time and with minimal trainer resources required. In addition, CAI has been used extensively in many learning laboratories in schools of nursing in the form of interactive video disc programs and PC software tutorials, simulations, and testing programs.

On-line literature searches using gateway services, such as Dialog, to search for references and to access various data bases (e.g., Nursing & Allied Health, National Library of Medicine) are available for subscription by anyone with access to a modem-equipped PC.

Patient care documentation systems may also be considered as a tool supporting education of the novice as well as the experienced nursing professional. Help screens and on-line reference manuals (e.g., the department's procedure manual, standard care plans, The Physicians' Desk Reference, Stat-Ref), can be easily accessed whenever needed as care alternatives are considered and care is provided. With many of the patient care systems available today, it is possible to customize the system to include the department's or health care facility's standards of care, to guide the care planning and assessment processes through these standards, and to base the user alerts on these standards as well. Such a patient care documentation system can be a very powerful educational tool for the student or less experienced nurse, as well as a quality improvement tool for all care providers.

Systems in Support of Nursing Research

As in the case of quality management, nursing research benefits immensely when patient care documentation systems are used to capture what nurses do. With an automated record of the nursing process and patient outcomes available, the ability to capture data elements needed for research projects makes the data collection aspect of research an automatic by-product of the documentation system. Many of the patient care documentation systems provide the tools to access the data elements and to "export" this data to external files or reports for data analysis. The difficulty arises, however, when attempting to compare this data across multiple facilities with a variety of systems and data elements. Minimum data sets and data standards are not yet entirely defined, nor are those currently available widely implemented. This deficiency hampers the efforts of the nurse researcher. Because of the work of The Institute of Medicine (Dick and Steen, 1992), professional nursing organizations, and other national health care reform and information systems initiatives, there is a renewed urgency to define data standards for health care. This work will greatly enhance the ability to conduct meaningful research and to learn from the work of nursing professionals. As the profession accumulates this knowledge, it should be much better prepared to define the knowledge rules required for expert systems. Such progress will certainly lead to further incorporation of expert systems into real-time use in the delivery of patient care.

Trends in Clinical Information Systems

Today, significant strides are being made to the benefit of nursing in the information systems market place. The nursing profession, in general, is much better educated in the use of automation and better prepared to articulate systems requirements than ever before. More comprehensive nursing applications and clinical information systems are evolving. There is a greater awareness of the complementary nature of clinical and research applications and therefore more cooperation between the commercial, educational, clinical and research interests. We will see more decision support functions integrated into systems, in the form of both reference data bases and interactive alerts. Newer technologies are being adapted to the clinical environment in the form of terminal options and Graphical User Interfaces (Hughes, 1992). Health care reform will no doubt influence changes in information systems, especially those related to accessibility of patient records across episodes of care. Integration of information across health care networks has become a priority and will soon become a reality. This will not only provide better information for the patient care provider, but could also enhance our efforts in nursing to monitor quality and implement effective research projects. The next few years will be an exciting time for the field of nursing informatics. We will have many opportunities to develop, test, and lobby for new technologies. It is our challenge to make the most of these opportunities so that technology is applied in meaningful ways designed to optimize nurses' ability to use information to enhance professional decision making.

Summary

Nursing information systems software allows automation of nursing process documentation and a means to support clinical and managerial decision making. There are commercially available systems which address varied nursing information requirements related to patient care, business systems, quality management, nursing education and nursing research. In the future, increased systems' integration will further enhance information support of nursing care.

References

Dick, R. S., and Steen, E. B. (1992). The Computer-Based Patient Record, an Essential Technology for Health Care. Washington, DC: National Academy Press.

Dorenfest, S. I. (1992). Hospital Information Systems, State-of-the-Art 1992. Chicago: Sheldon I. Dorenfest & Associates.

Hughes, S. J. (1992). Status of nursing information systems—Snapshots from around the world. In Proceedings of the Nursing Informatics—Today's Reality and Tomorrow's Potential, MEDINFO '92 Workshop (p. 10). Geneva, Switzerland: EMTEK Health Care Systems, Inc.

Reed, W. (1993, July). Trends in healthcare computing. Healthcare Informatics, pp. 26-30.

Simpson, R. L. (1993). The Nurse Executive's Guide to Directing and Managing Nursing Information Systems. Ann Arbor, MI: The Center for Healthcare Information Management.

Benefits Management

Barbara J. Hoehn, MBA, RN
Senior Manager
KPMG Peat Marwick
New York, New York

Introduction

Over the years, hospital administrators have implemented and reimplemented patient accounting software, based upon the premise that the faster clean and accurate billings can be released, the quicker insurance companies will reimburse the hospital. The benefit of purchasing and implementing new and improved patient accounting systems has rested solely on the anticipated increased cash flow to the institution. Clinical information systems (clinical systems), on the other hand, have not been perceived as having as obvious and immediate beneficial effect on hospital operations. Routinely, before hospitals start planning for and selecting clinical systems, efforts are made to cost-justify these systems. In other words, benefits achievable through effective systems implementation in the clinical environment are identified in advance.

Today, with the advent of managed care and other health care reform initiatives, the importance of clinical information can not be overemphasized. Some health care facilities now view the expense of purchasing and implementing clinical systems as a "cost of doing business" and will purchase these systems regardless of whether specific benefits can be identified and realized. Many hospitals, however, still focus on identifying, quantifying and achieving financial and operational benefits from clinical technology. Very often, it is the clinical departments, especially the Department of Nursing, that will be held directly responsible for achieving these benefits.

Benefit Realization

As this is the case, it is important to note that, from the onset of any clinical systems project, *benefits realization does not just happen: It is a process that must be closely managed.* The integration of the *operational and information systems needs* of the health care facility must be the central focus in developing long-range clinical systems strategies, prioritizing applications, developing Requests For Proposals, interacting with the vendors and ultimately to selecting and implementing a clinical information system. If this integrated process does not occur, the end result could be an information system that dictates how patient care is delivered or one that is poorly utilized because it impedes care delivery rather than enhances it.

To achieve maximum benefit, patient care delivery models need to be refined and operational? policies and procedures developed to address any needs that the information system will not meet. Conversely, the information system may need to be modified to support the selected operation model.

This chapter defines benefit terminology, explores why benefits planning is important, discusses why realizing benefits has been difficult in the past, identifies various methodologies to identify and manage benefits achievement, and addresses steps to position health care facilities to effectively manage benefits.

What is a Benefit?

Webster's Dictionary defines a benefit as "something that guards, aids or promotes well being, a natural advantage, an advance or an improvement." This definition proves helpful in examining the potential benefits of implementing clinical information systems.

Before embarking on a benefits realization project, it is important to become familiar with the terminology associated with benefits realization and to learn how different benefits will fit into the scheme of the work of one's organization.

A *benefit* associated with a clinical information system is one that results in a change in an operational process, directly or indirectly produced from the implementation of the clinical information system, that positively affects the resources required to provide patient care (time, people, costs) or the quality of patient care provided. When the benefit is perceived to positively affect the resources required to provide care, it is viewed as a *quantitative* (numerically measurable) *benefit*. When the benefit is perceived to positively affect the quality of care provided, it is viewed as a *qualitative* (service value) *benefit*.

A *potential benefit* is any improvement or positive outcome (quantitative or qualitative) that is possible or likely to occur through the implementation of a clinical information system. The implementation of an order-management system has the *potential* to speed up and improve the communication of clinical orders to clinical support departments such as the laboratory, radiology and pharmacy. While the likelihood of achieving that benefit is dependent upon factors other than just automation, the possibility of acceleration of that benefit is inherent in an order-management system.

An *expected benefit* is an improvement or positive outcome that the health care facility identifies as important to its clinical and business needs, anticipates achieving and actively pursues. In fact, it is often the promise of improvement that is used to justify the purchase and implementation of the clinical system. For instance, a potential benefit of an automated nursing documentation application is a reduction in the amount of time needed to document patient care. If a hospital experiences a high degree of overtime associated with nursing documentation, its nursing executives could *expect,* with the implementation of an automated documentation application, a reduction or elimination in this overtime.

On the other hand, a *realized benefit* is a positive outcome or improvement in clinical or business operations that has actually already occurred. It may be a benefit that the hospital actively pursued, or it may be a benefit inherent in any implementation of automation. In any case, a realized benefit is a measurable improvement in either the quality of care or the amount of resources needed to provide care resulting directly or indirectly through the implementation of a new clinical information system.

Clinical system benefits tend to fall into several specific categories that include strategic positioning, quality enhancement, patient service efficiency, management effectiveness, cost reduction, revenue enhancement and productivity improvement.

Why is Benefits Planning Important?

All too often, participants in a clinical systems project have a "Field of Dreams" attitude (based on a popular motion picture of the same name) towards benefits realization: "If you build it, they will come"; that is, if you implement the system, benefits will happen. Unfortunately, this is not always true. If a clinical system is to achieve benefits from automation, a proactive approach must be implemented to identify potential and expected benefits, establish a game plan for achieving the benefits and a methodology for tracking results against the plan.

Several reasons can be offered as to why is it important to plan and effectively manage towards benefits realization. First, evaluating, selecting and implementing clinical information systems requires a major investment on the part of the facility. A fully implemented clinical information system can cost tens of millions of dollars in hardware, software, communication networks and interfaces. In addition, installation of such a system also requires large expenditures in time and professional staff resources. Without planning for both the change resulting from automation, as well as implementing operational changes in conjunction with the automation, hospitals will achieve only marginal efficiency benefits from the technology, none of which can compare with the cost outlays.

Second, incorporation of information technology into a clinical environment should be viewed as a catalyst for change. Many inefficient processes develop over the years. Automating these inefficient processes merely speeds up their inefficiency; it does nothing to correct it. True benefits realization is dependent upon changing operating practices. Early planning for both automation and consequential operational changes focuses emphasis on improving clinical practices and processes rather than speeding them up.

Third, benefits planning is critical for selecting the clinical system that best meets the needs of the health care institution. All too often, systems are selected based upon what users *want* from technology rather than on what the users truly *need*. Unless an effort is made to visualize what future clinical processes will be, and how they will be supported by information technology, it will be almost impossible to identify the features and functions needed to enhance clinical practice.

Why Has It Been So Difficult Proving Benefits From Clinical Information Systems?

A literature search on benefits realization of clinical systems will reveal numerous articles identifying *potential benefits* achievable through the implementation of clinical systems but few articles reporting success in actually realizing many of these benefits. Three major reasons for this lack of benefit realization are:

Costs are underestimated. One of the major steps in any benefits realization process is to first identify the costs of implementing the system so that they can eventually be compared to the "savings" resulting from the use of the technology. All too often, identification of these costs is limited to the one-time and yearly maintenance expenses of software, hardware, communication networks and vendor/consultant implementation support. While these are the obvious costs associated with system installations, many hidden costs surface after the contract is negotiated and system implementation begins. These include:

• *Customizations and interfaces:* While many hospitals go into a system implementation with the intent of installing the applications the way the vendor delivers them (the "vanilla" system), very few actually do. Refinements and actual changes to both screens and system logic are often required after the implementation starts and additional, unplanned-for costs are incurred. Interfaces are also areas where unforeseen costs can present themselves. All prospective vendors will identify the cost of their portion of any interface to a disparate system. However, it is also important to identify the costs of writing and maintaining the returning portion of the interfaces residing within the alien applications. These interfaces are usually written by the associated vendors or the hospital's own information system department. Either way they are a costly process often not included in cost analyses.

• *User training requirements:* Most vendors will promise user training support during a system implementation. This support often defined as "train the trainer." It implies that a core group of hospital employees have been identified as being responsible for first-time and ongoing user training. The vendor will train these trainers on the features and functions of the systems; then, it is the responsibility of these in-house trainers to conduct all subsequent educational sessions. This results in new roles, responsibilities and personnel costs and requires in either replacing the trainers in their former positions or establishing new job levels for trainers involved in the project.

• *Technical risks:* Many of the "bells and whistles" associated with advanced clinical systems are on the cutting edge of technology. They may be hardware devices (hand-held or portable technology), input media (voice and image) or access methodologies (data bases and graphical user interfaces). Often, it is these very features that make the system attractive to the clinician. These additions are costly and may not have been initially planned when the system was purchased, or they may quickly become obsolete. In the past, as soon as the latest technology has become commercially available, the next generation of technology was announced. Facilities should know that in purchasing cutting edge technology, they are assuming both a technical and fiscal risk in acquiring technology with unproven performance or a short shelf life.

Benefits are unrealistically estimated. The benefits potential of clinical information systems can be likened to the structure of an iceberg. Attention tends to be focused on what can be easily seen while the real impact is often hidden below the surface. Traditionally, when efforts are made to identify potential benefits, several things happen. These include:

• *Obvious benefits are overestimated:* The most obvious benefits associated with clinical information systems revolve around clinical and professional efficiency. Some nursing system vendors promise time savings of 40 to 60 minutes per nurse/per shift through the use of nursing documentation systems. In theory, this time can then be devoted to additional time spent with the patient. Order management application vendors may promise a decrease or elimination of medication errors if medication ordering is implemented. Unfortunately, in both cases, there are unstated assumptions that must be in place if a client is to achieve these efficiency benefits. In the first case, nurses must have specific plans for what additional professional nursing duties will be initiated in the time freed up through the implementation of the documentation applications. If there are no specific plans, this time will most probably be filled with other non-nursing related tasks. In the second case, the unstated assumptions are that an interface to a pharmacy system will be in place, removing the need for the pharmacist to enter the order information into a pharmacy system manually, and more importantly, that physicians will enter the medication orders directly into the system. If physician order entry is not planned for or achievable, the chance for transcription errors associated with medication ordering will not change.

• *Qualitative benefits are rarely identified:* Quantitative benefits of time, resource and cost savings are much easier to measure than are quality service benefits. Quality is difficult to define, for it is a very subjective variable that may mean different things to different people. Therefore, because quality benefits are difficult to measure, users tend to shy away from identifying and targeting them during the evaluation, selection and implementation process. These benefits are also more closely associated with clinical and operational processes than are quantitative benefits. Likewise, they are more dependent upon effective clinical process redesign in order to be realized. The necessary effort to redesign clinical processes is often viewed as an overwhelming addition to an already complex implementation.

• *Identified benefits are not aggressively pursued and therefore seldom realized:* Even when benefits are realistically identified, they are often not aggressively pursued. The perception is that any benefits realization process requires a high level of professional involvement over a prolonged period of time at a definite cost to the institution. The result of this misconception is that most benefits realization processes are only half completed. In some cases, baseline information is collected prior to system implementation and subsequent post-implementation information collection is neglected. In other cases, no baseline values are collected and, after implementation, users attempt to identify the benefits obtained through system use. In either case, vital information needed to truly docu-

Figure 1.
The traditional approach to benefits realization

Cost-Justification Model

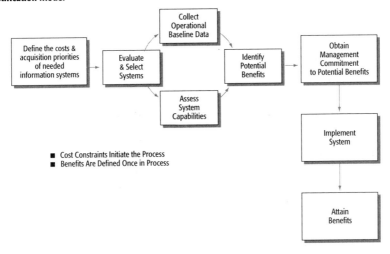

- Cost Constraints Initiate the Process
- Benefits Are Defined Once in Process

ment benefit realization is not collected because of the perceived effort involved in doing so.

Most benefits realization processes do not result in commitment from the system sponsors and senior management. Most benefit realization processes may identify expected benefits but often lack the commitment from the individuals responsible for actually realizing the benefits—the users and senior management. Very often, the benefits realization processes is initiated merely to justify the purchase of the system, and there is little accountability on the part of the users and the vendors to actually achieve these benefits. And finally, many of the clinical systems projects tend to be vendor-driven, technical systems installation rather than process-oriented system implementations. This installation mind set does little to set in place the operational changes necessary to truly realize benefits.

Models

The Cost Justification Model

The traditional approach to benefits realization is the *cost justification model* (see Figure 1). This process is often conducted by the clinical systems vendor or the hospital's information systems department as a mechanism for justifying capital and operating budget funding for the clinical systems project.

In reviewing the steps of a cost justification process, we see the following activities:

1. *System costs and priorities are defined.* The hospital determines, through its long range information systems' master plan, the amount of money it can realistically spend on systems and the priority in which the system portfolio needs to be implemented.

2. *Appropriate systems are selected.* The selection process focuses on user wants and system features and functions. The vendor who can best meet the system requirements with the most cost effective business proposal is the selected vendor.

3. *Collect operations baseline data and assess system capabilities.* After the vendor is selected, baseline operational data is collected. Users examine the selected applications in

Figure 2.
Cost justification Methodology

Benefit	Number of Occurrences	People/Resources	Time Involved (minutes)	Cost Involved	Cost/Time Savings
Reduction in medications being delivered to the wrong unit	Two times per unit per day (approx.); 20 nursing unit hospital	Pharmacist Nurse Transport Staff Member Unit Clerk	20 10 15 10	$10.00 $10.00 $3.33 $4.60	
TOTALS	2 x 20 x 365 = 14,600/year		55 minutes per occurrence	$27.93 per occurrence	$407,778/year 13,384 hrs/year

detail so that potential benefits can be identified.

4. *Define benefits.* Potential benefits, based upon the features of the selected system, are identified and validated with the appropriate departments. General assumptions are documented, potential savings are determined and extrapolated for a fully installed system. (Figure 2 is an example of a cost-justification methodology that can be utilized to help identify benefits).

5. *Obtain management commitment to potential benefits.* Senior management agrees to the benefits identified through the cost-justification process and acknowledges its expectations that these benefits will be realized.

6. *Implement the system.* The clinical information system is implemented based upon the vendor/hospital developed system implementation workplan.

7. *Attain benefits.* After a pre-determined time period, post-implementation data collection, identical to the initial departmental data collection is conducted so that before and after data can be compared and realized benefits identified.

The shortcomings of this approach are numerous. This model is cost driven and initiated *after* a vendor application portfolio is selected. Because it tends to focus on potential cost savings that are common to all hospitals implementing the chosen vendor's applications, it ignores significant benefits that may be institution-specific. It also tends to emphasize the productivity savings resulting from eliminating manual efforts and improved efficiency from speeding up transactions. Another shortcoming to this approach is that benefit calculations which result from this type of process, while hospital-specific, tend not be realistic. This is because the calculations do not take into consideration the implementation schedule, current operations, job descriptions that may change, minimal staffing levels needed to be in place or the probability of actually achieving the benefits.

Benefits Management Model

The Benefits Management approach to benefits realization (see Figure 3) is a continuous process that identifies realistic benefits, targets them effectively and positions the hospital to actually realize the benefits identified as expected through system and clinical process integration.

The following activities comprise the benefits management approach:

1. *Obtain senior management sponsorship for the benefits program.* All participants in the clinical systems project understand that benefits realization is an *ongoing* process. As system enhancements are implemented and as operational processes change, users will be expected to seek continual benefit from the information technology. In order for the users to be able to accomplish this, senior management must buy into the concept of an ongoing process and allocate the time, personnel and funding needed to effectively conduct the process.

Figure 3.
The benefits management approach to benefits realization

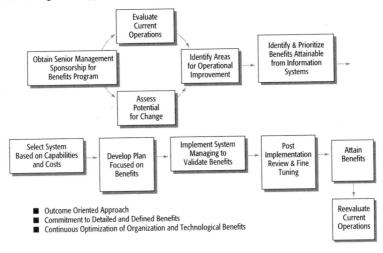

■ Outcome Oriented Approach
■ Commitment to Detailed and Defined Benefits
■ Continuous Optimization of Organization and Technological Benefits

---

2. *Evaluate current operations and assess the potential for change.* Any information system project must be viewed as a change in current operations. To simply automate current processes will result in minimal, if any, value. Therefore, it is important to assess current clinical and business processes, identifying those that are productive and worth maintaining and those that are counter-productive and need to be changed. Before initiating any change, it is imperative that the potential for successfully implementing change be judged.

3. *Identify areas for immediate operational improvement.* It is important to immediately start implementing clinical process changes that are identified as needing change, even before addressing system issues. There are two primary reasons for doing so at this point in the process. First, improving processes at the onset of the project allows those participating in the clinical system evaluation and selection to visually see the "future" environment into which the automation will be integrated. Second, the process of evaluating, selecting and implementing systems can be a protracted one. Participants need to see change and improvement throughout the process so that enthusiasm, participation and momentum can be maintained.

4. *Identify and prioritize benefits attainable from information technology.* After the current and future clinical and business environment are defined, system features and functions needed to support these settings are identified. During this process, potential and expected benefits are also identified. Most importantly, the expected benefits are prioritized. During a benefits management process, it is acknowledged that all benefits are not immediately attainable. By prioritizing the order of expected benefits realization, the process becomes a continuous one and realistic, achievable successes are formulated.

5. *Select the system based on system capabilities and costs.* Now that the operational settings are defined and associated features and functions detailed, system evaluation is focused on user needs rather than user wants and wishes.

6. *Validate benefits.* No health care facility has ever purchased the exact system they initially defined. Once a vendor of choice is identified, the benefits management team needs to validate the initially identified benefits against the capabilities of the vendor's

software. Some benefits may no longer be valid; others not previously identified may become expected benefits.

7. *Develop an implementation plan focusing on benefits achievement.* A system implementation focused on benefits achievement is not a technically driven system installation, but a process-driven operations and system integration. Both clinical process redesign and system implementation activities must be incorporated into the project workplan.

8. *Implement the system managing to validated benefits.* Just as no hospital has ever purchased the system it thought it wanted, no hospital has ever "gotten" the system it thought it purchased. As the implementation process proceeds and users become more familiar with the system's capabilities and functionality, new benefit potentials may surface and previously identified expected benefits may fall by the wayside. As the implementation progresses, it is important to continually validate the benefits being targeted.

9. *Post-implementation and fine tuning.* One of the reasons why hospitals often cannot validate benefit achievement is because the project team collects post-implementation data too soon after going "live" with the production system. Any system takes a while for the learning curve to flatten, for the system to be accepted, and appropriately and effectively utilized. An appropriate amount of time should pass before going back to determine if benefits have actually been realized.

10. *Identify attained benefits.* Identify and document both those expected benefits achieved and those not realized. Determine why benefits were not realized and make appropriate efforts to address these reasons in future benefit realization cycles.

11. *Reevaluate current operations.* The process recycles back to the beginning. The clinical and business environment currently in place will most likely not resemble the environment first defined at the initiation of the clinical system benefits management cycle. The current environment should be analyzed and the next wave of prioritized benefits realization should begin.

This model differs dramatically from the cost-justification model. The benefits management model is initiated at the point of system planning rather than after system selection. This allows benefits to drive the prioritization of information system initiatives. It includes defining operational changes, system requirements and expected benefits throughout the process rather than at any single given point. The implementation plan includes milestones for periodic assessment and revisions as needed. The benefits monitoring concept turns into a cyclical assessment which is sustained after the initial system activation.

The final and most distinguishing difference between the cost justification and benefits management model is that the benefits management model can be initiated at any point in the life cycle of a clinical systems project. While the cost justification model starts after the system is selected and before implementation begins, the benefits management model can begin during the system planning, selection, implementation or post-implementation phase. The 11 detailed steps of the benefits management model can be consolidated into six interrelated steps (see Figure 4).

At any point in the system project, benefits from process redesign and system integration can be identified, validated and prioritized. Clinical process can be re-engineered and associated benefits monitored. At the completion of the cycle, benefits realization is confirmed and the process starts again. One of the key steps in successfully achieving benefits is the ability to monitor all the activities associated with benefits realization. A benefits worksheet can be a critical tool to monitor these activities. It identifies the targeted benefits, the system features and functions influencing this benefit potential, the assumptions under which the benefit was defined, the critical success factors that must be in place to achieve the benefit and the roadblocks that will have to be overcome to be successful. It

Figure 4.
The benefit management cycle

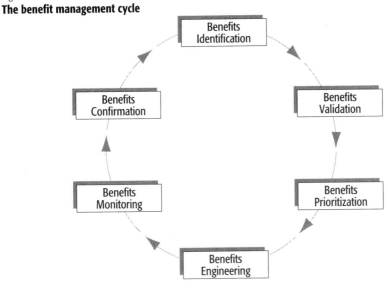

also identifies and tracks the required operational changes that need to be implemented, the implications if the system functionality is not implemented, the estimate of the potential benefit impact, any reassignment of resources required and the measurement against which benefits realization will be determined.

Summary

A benefits realization process can result in maximizing the benefits achievable through the integration of clinical process redesign and information technology. While the cost justification model may be appropriate at certain times, it is the benefits management process that will truly position the health care facility to effectively achieve long-term benefits from clinical systems. The key steps to successfully conduct this process include the identification of realistic quantitative and qualitative benefits, targeting benefits through the integration of process redesign and information technology, managing the change process focusing on improved patient outcomes, and committing to a continuous process of benefits identification, monitoring and achievement.

Systems Design and Implementation: Team Building Between Nurse Executive and Vendor

Linda Edmunds, MS, RN
Director of Design
Highland Reserves Inc.
Atlanta, Georgia

Introduction

A joint-development project involves a contractual agreement between a vendor and a client to plan, design, develop, and implement a software application or hardware device. Both the client and vendor contribute resources—staff and money—to the joint effort. The vendors' goal is to build a marketable product. They seek client-partners when a proposed product is complex, "leading edge," and costly. Clients generally underwrite this type of arrangement when a required product is not available in the marketplace. This chapter describes how systems design and implementation can be accomplished through the combined team efforts of the nurse executive and vendor.

The Changing Nature of Vendor-Client Teams

There are important differences between a joint-development project team in which vendors and clients contribute as equal partners and the vendor-client teams that have worked together in the past to develop and implement software for a health care facility. In a traditional vendor-client implementation team, the vendor's staff lead the detailed specification process, design and build the product, and guide the customer through the installation process. The customer's function is to communicate requirements, pay for licenses and services rendered, test any new code on site, and complain if the installed product does not meet contractual expectations.

The traditional vendor-client relationship is not a true collaboration between two equal partners. The underlying assumption is that the major portion of the expertise needed to build or install the software or hardware rests with the vendor. Vendors, in fact, often regard their clients as amateurs in the business of envisioning, describing, and developing clinical software or hardware. In turn, hospital staff members tend to distrust anyone, even professional peers, who work in the marketplace. As Simpson (1991) notes, ". . . nurses are downright hostile and suspicious of anything to do with vendors, considering them the 'enemy' rather than a possible ally—or even better, as partners committed to solutions" (p. 22).

Fortunately, the current health care and data-processing environments are forcing vendor-client teams into true collaborative partnerships. Such cooperation is necessary because building software is much more complicated now than in the past. Nurse executives, who are very aware of the changes and uncertainties in health care delivery, should also be familiar with the rapid upheavals in the data processing industry, particularly in that portion of the industry which develops health care products.

Health Care Computing Today

The most significant change today in health care computing is that the industry is moving away from centralized mainframe or mini-computer solutions. The direction of most data-processing shops is towards distributed data bases and client-server applications linked by local and wide-area networks. Workstations are replacing "dumb" terminals but the hardware installed in many institutions tends to be mixed. Mac, PC, and UNIX proponents each assert that their favorite technology is the only logical choice to support the needs of users. IBM, Microsoft, Apple, Novell, Sun, and NeXT compete fiercely with one another for a market share.

Object-oriented programming languages, such as C++ and Smalltalk, are attempting to replace the procedural languages, such as COBOL and C, that most programmers are familiar with. Alternative methodologies for designing systems including rapid prototyping, business modeling, and structured system analysis, are being championed as a more efficient way to create and maintain software, particularly if CASE (Computer Assisted Software Engineering) tools are employed. Analysts and designers are scrambling to become proficient in these new ways of defining requirements.

Modalities such as imaging, voice and handwriting recognition, natural text processing, and multimedia are becoming practical to integrate into system design but are expensive and not as mature as they eventually will be. Portables and bedside devices are being requested by clinicians, but the products available have technical, functional, and financial limitations. Standards and lexicons for health care data are still being actively debated. Data integration and application interfacing, essential for patient care, administration, and research, remain an expensive and slow proposition. The existence of legacy information systems in which clients have huge investments further complicates new development and marketing strategies for the vendor.

Benefits of Joint Development

A joint-development project may be initiated by customers who cannot find the software that they know is technically feasible but not yet currently available in the marketplace. The primary benefit of such a partnership to the customer, therefore, is assuring the availability of a software product that is needed by the institution. There are also secondary benefits to the facility and its staff as well.

A health care facility that becomes a showcase for innovative software may enjoy enhanced prestige both locally and nationally, and sometimes even internationally. If a system is exciting or new, it may be an attraction for nursing staff and physicians. It may also attract visitors from around the country, as well as elicit invitations to write journal articles and deliver presentations at professional meetings. These requests may be addressed to the executives, the managers, the technicians, and the clinical staff. Participants in a joint-development project team may gain experience and skills that are both useful and marketable in their professional careers.

From a financial standpoint, client-partners may share in product royalties or be reimbursed for their investment. At the very least, the amount invested in the project should be less than what future customers expect to pay for licensing and implementing the product. Finally, if more than one health care facility is involved in a vendor partnership, the sharing of information, ideas, and strategies among institutional personnel may bring benefits that extend beyond the project at hand.

Vendors seek joint-development contracts to share risk—which usually entails financial risk. If a product is going to be costly to develop, the involvement of several client underwriters can ensure that vendors break even or at least keep their own capital investment within an affordable range. The expertise that the client contributes to a project also minimizes the vendor's risk of building products that are not needed or poorly designed.

The second major benefit to vendors in a joint-development project is the accelerated availability of a site where they can bring potential customers. Vendors know that nothing sells software or hardware better than a successful site visit, which would require that software be up and running, with enthusiastic users, and representatives from the facility who are well-informed about health care delivery and the product. No one is better at convincing a vice president of nursing that a product is useful or that a company has integrity than another vice president of nursing. Similar credibility is given to a clinical specialist, a staff nurse, or any other clinician. Those facilities that have invested time and resources in a development effort are motivated to deliver the product to their users and to realize the return on their investment.

Minimizing Risk: Negotiating the Contract

The best way for a health care facility to minimize risk when embarking upon a joint development project is to develop a contract that defines in as much detail as possible the objectives of the undertaking, as well as the process and contributions expected from each party. In addition to clearly defining the project, the contract protects the facility from changes that may occur within the vendor corporation. These include corporate buy-outs or mergers, internal reorganizations, and the departure of key staff who have made commitments on the vendor's behalf.

Simpson, writing in a column for *Nursing Management* in 1991, points out a number of areas that require particular attention when contracting with a vendor for any type of data-processing product (p. 22). These include protection against third-party conflicts, a definition of intellectual property, and handling of system maintenance and upgrades. In addition to these items, a joint-development contract should also address the following:

Objectives.

The contract should specify what will be developed, the hardware and software platforms, and the tools that will be used. If part of the team effort is to define methodology and technology, then timeframes for making these decisions should be settled before the project starts.

Assumptions.

Any assumptions on the part of the client or vendor should be listed in the contract so that disparities can be explored. For example, the client may expect that the proposed product will be operational without additional interfacing to existing systems. On the other hand, the vendor may assume that interfacing is unique to each institution and therefore the responsibility of the client. Prior mutual agreement on assumptions in the contract will reduce misunderstandings between partners.

Financial arrangements.

In addition to delineating how much capital clients will contribute to the project, the contract should also specify how profits will be distributed. Partial-product ownership, license royalties, discounts on future services or maintenance, and credits for hosting site visits are some of the ways clients may receive a return on their investment.

New-product development usually requires team members to use new tools. The costs of software tools, and the necessary hardware should be estimated. Whether the client or vendor is to pay for tools used at a client site should be stated in the contract.

Personnel resources.

Both vendor and client will provide personnel to the project team. The number of staff contributed by each should be specified, as well as their required skills and time commitment. In determining staff requirements, each phase of the project should be considered separately because the staffing needs may change as the project moves through its life cycle. It may be appropriate to identify the actual personnel who will fill key project positions such as project manager or account executive.

Geography.

The contract should describe the exact location where each phase of the project work will be completed. Clients may require that some vendor personnel are permanently assigned to their site to coordinate vendor-client efforts. This is particularly useful in the design and implementation phases. The vendor may want some client personnel to work at its corporate headquarters to ensure that company design and coding standards are adhered to. If meetings are to be held, or work is to be done away from the client site, or if vendor staff are based at the client's facility, the contract should specify who is responsible for travel and per diem expenses.

Other participants.

A vendor may want to include several dissimilar institutions, such as a northeastern university medical center, a community hospital located in the South, and a West Coast HMO, as partners in a development effort. This is important in the design phase because it helps the vendor to distinguish generic requirements from those that are unique to a particular facility because of its size, location, patient mix, and regional practice patterns. Having several institutions implement new application code also facilitates the debugging process and helps implementation specialists to judge how long and how best to install the product when it becomes generally available. If a development effort involves several clients, the relationship between the clients must be specified, as well as the relationship between client and vendor.

Problem resolution.

Joint development teams include staff from many disciplines and multiple enterprises. They are likely to have differing personal styles, professional values, and organizational agendas. With this mix, conflicts and issues are certain to arise that cannot be resolved within the working subgroups. The contract must specify how the problem resolution process will work. This is particularly critical when a number of clients work with one vendor. If a formalized process for resolving disputes is not established early, and adhered to, the project will probably stall.

Communication.

The contract should include guidelines about the communication process between vendor and client and between client and client if more than one client is involved in the project. If vendor and client staff are not working in the same location, a variety of methods can be used to maintain open communication. Teleconferencing is very effective but expensive. Conference calls scheduled at frequent intervals can be almost as useful in building team relationships and keeping the project on course. E-mail and fax machines can speed up the exchange of designs and documentation. Vendor access to the client's in-house computer network, and vice versa, can facilitate development. To allay concerns about the privacy of patient data and the security of vendor files, policies and procedures for computer networking should be discussed and documented as part of the contract process.

A decision should also be made about how communication between different locations will be channeled. Will exchanges always be made through the project manager, or will they occur informally between team members at different sites? A formal communication process can assist in keeping players at all locations equally informed about project status and issues. On the other hand, when all communication is funneled through one person, misunderstandings, biases, and inefficiencies can be introduced. Good communication is critical to project success, and the most effective method may not be discovered until after the project is started.

Schedule.

A project plan must be part of the contract. If it is too early to devise a detailed schedule, then major milestones and deliverables should be listed with estimated timeframes and criteria for finalizing due dates. For example, it may not be reasonable to estimate coding time until the detailed functional specifications are complete. Once the specification is complete, however, this estimate should be available within a specified number of weeks.

Project milestones should include, but not necessarily be limited to, requirements definition, tool selection, prototype development, detailed functional design, technical design, code or device delivery, acceptance testing, pilot installation and full implementation. Because many pieces of the project completed by one subgroup will require review by other members of the team, guidelines setting timeframes for the review process should also be defined. The contract should also identify the dates of major meetings, particularly if several client-partners will meet together with the vendor.

Detailed specifications.

A major reason that development projects fail to meet the initial objectives is that insufficient time is spent on the design process and/or the process is not formalized. It is critical to define in detail what will be built, especially when projects are complex and a team is large and possibly geographically dispersed. This provides the user community and the technical community with a blueprint both can review. Revisions can then be made *before* money is invested in development. Just as in building a house, the earlier changes are made to the blueprint, the cheaper it is to make the modification.

Detailed specifications can take many forms (Edmunds, 1992). Prototypes that allow the end-user to view the interface components of a proposed product are superb for communicating to professional groups and eliciting feedback. Data and process models, which are the outcome of discussions between clinical experts representing all of the partners, delineate the data and process requirements generic to all sites. Detailed functional specifications that include descriptions and drawings of every feature of the proposed product reduce omissions and logical inconsistencies in the design. The ability for clinicians and technicians to review prototypes, models, and specifications prior to the start of development, will help to keep unmet expectations at a minimum and the project on schedule (Covvey, 1985).

Sign-offs.

Each project milestone should end with a formal sign-off on the deliverable. A requirements document is a deliverable. A data model is a deliverable. A prototype is a deliverable. A detailed functional specification is a deliverable. Formal sign-offs on major milestones serve to focus attention on the importance of the review process and the necessity for reviews to be completed on schedule.

Implementation.

Eventually, the product will be ready to implement. The vendor may want the client to commit contractually to installing the product within a prescribed time after acceptance testing. The client may need to retain flexibility in scheduling because most facilities have multiple commitments that cannot always be met simultaneously and successfully. The timing of both the pilot installation and the full implementation should be addressed to eliminate disagreement later on.

The client will probably want the vendor to commit on-site resources during the first few weeks of implementation since unexpected problems are common with a new product. Most vendors will usually concur with this request because of their desire for a smooth installation.

Marketing.
Vendors generally expect their development partners to assist in their marketing efforts by hosting site visits. Welcoming and educating visitors can be very resource intensive, particularly if the vendor has several regional offices and many enthusiastic sales people. An arrangement about the amount of time the client will contribute and whether client time is reimbursed or credited towards services or license fees needs to be worked out in advance. If clients are to be present at user groups or at professional conferences, a contribution from the vendor to offset these expenses may be appropriate and negotiable.

The Role of the Nurse Executive

Be realistic
The nurse executive who decides to participate in a joint-development project should be realistic about what this commitment entails. Building new products is never simple, nor is it a straightforward effort. Despite earnest attempts to write a contract that fully defines the objectives, the assumptions, the process, the schedule, and each partner's contribution, a joint-developmental project is generally landmined with obstacles.

Some of the obstacles that must be hurdled are inherent to any technical development project. It requires time for a staff to master new methodologies, technologies, and tool sets. As a result, progress at the beginning of a project can be agonizingly slow. Finding design solutions that are sufficiently flexible to meet multi-site user requirements requires not only collaboration but also creativity and compromise. Patience is a prerequisite for this part of the process. Finally, the technical problems that arise as the design is converted to the final product may often seem unending and insurmountable.

Surprisingly, it is not these expected obstacles that usually sabotage a joint-development effort. Conflicts that arise among team members because of mismatched institutional values, differing professional agendas, personal preferences, and clashing egos are much more likely to undermine success. Friction between project participants and non-participants within a client facility can dampen enthusiasm for what is being developed. Further, the project can also deflect necessary financial and personnel resources from other institutional activities. If the product is built, internal opposition can obstruct the implementation process and prevent the institution from realizing the fruits of its investment. In short, the political and personal issues that may revolve around a development project are often more difficult to resolve than technical obstacles. It is in these areas that the nurse executive must focus attention and management skills.

Managing innovation
Romano has pointed out that managing innovation requires a specific set of skills (1990). The first of the required skills, she notes, is the ability to use power to mobilize people, to create coalitions, to orchestrate effective communication, and to bend the organization's rules when necessary. Second, managing innovation requires managing participation, which is often a balancing act between having management control and providing opportunities to team members. Finally, managing innovation requires "constructing" change.

This includes:

. . . selecting the right people—the ones with the ideas that move beyond established practices. It involves creating the right places—the integrative environments that support innovation and encourage teams to support and implement the visions. Constructing change encompasses determining the right times—the moments in an organization's history or in a society when one can reconstruct reality in order to shape a more productive and successful future. (p. 102)

Much of the effort of nurse executives who are involved in supporting a vendor-client development partnership should be targeted towards obtaining solid support at their own institution. This means communicating, educating, updating, and selling the value of the partnership and the project to the board of directors, senior administrators, middle management, and staff in both nursing and other departments.

In selecting team members, the nurse executive would be wise to avoid choosing staff members who are unduly discomforted by uncertainty, by questions that cannot be immediately answered, by decisions that have to be revised, by timeframes that may be adjusted, by divergent opinion or by strong personalities. Client-vendor teams should be made up of the imaginative, the cooperative and the resilient. Participants should also be risk takers who perceive the unknown as the opportunity to chart new territory and obstacles as an impetus for rapid personal growth.

Understanding the vendor perspective

It cannot be restated often enough that a client-vendor partnership is, from the vendor's point of view, a business relationship. Vendor companies are run by business executives whose primary concerns are their shareholders and their profit margin. They are as intellectually committed to the value of enterprise as nurse executives are to their concerns for quality patient care. When negotiating with business executives, nurse executives and those who represent them should remember to put forward their ideas, suggestions, and opinions in a way that stresses financial benefits for both the vendor and for the provider. While vendor executives understand that a product must improve the quality of care delivery, they respond more intuitively to arguments based on resource savings.

Product flexibility is a critical design component from the vendor perspective. To recoup an investment, a product must be marketable and implementable at a variety of facilities. These may include small, medium- and large-size institutions; teaching and community facilities, general care and specialty sites. One product cannot meet the requirements of all types of sites; it should, however, be useful at many. Team members must be reminded that their particular view of health care delivery may be biased by a limited range of workplace experiences. Vendor personnel tend to have a broader picture of client requirements because they, as a routine part of their job, are exposed to multiple sites. It is in the best interest of a client-partner to support the vendor's focus on product flexibility for two reasons: first, their own institutions will evolve and a flexible product can evolve with them; and second, a product that is purchased by many sites is more likely to be enhanced and maintained by a vendor than one that fits only a few clients.

Valuing the contribution of nurse clinicians

Vendor attitudes towards nursing professionals have changed significantly over the past 20 years. Initially, it should be noted that nurses, and their input, were ignored by the corporate health care computing industry. Nurses were neither a valued part of a vendor staff nor targeted as decision makers during the marketing process. Hospitals were the first to realize the tremendous contribution nurses could make during system implementation. Many facilities formalized and expanded the role of nurses by identifying nursing coordinators who ran interference between the data processing department, the nursing department and other ancillaries. At about the same time, during the mid-1980s, there was an enormous growth in the number of conferences, continuing education programs, and published literature about information systems and their impact on the nursing profession. In regard to technology, nurses often were the most educated and experienced clinical group in the hospital. Vendors began to hire knowledgeable and experienced nurses to market their products and to participate in requirements' definition and design.

At the current time, the opportunity for nurses in the vendor environment continues to expand. Nurses experienced in both what the market wants and also what really works in a health care environment are assuming high-level positions in product management, which can include strategic planning, functional design and product marketing. Vendors have become cognizant of what nurses' contributions have to offer to their company's profit margin (Ball and Douglas, 1988; Hersher, 1988).

Unfortunately, nurses who fill vendor positions as product managers or designers are quickly removed from the daily operations of health care facilities. It is difficult, when sitting in a corporate tower, to remain fully conversant with the details of health care delivery when practice patterns change rapidly. Products that do not address detail may look impressive during design and coding, but fail during implementation. The contribution that active clinicians can make towards the success of a development project by focusing attention of the team on workplace realities is inestimable. When negotiating with high-level vendor executives in the health care computing industry, always keep in mind the value that nursing staff bring to a joint endeavor.

Summary

Undoubtedly, it is more of a gamble to participate in a joint development-project than to purchase previously installed, well-tested, off-the-shelf software or hardware. But the risk must be balanced against the potential for institutional benefits, as well as the possibility of advancing professional practice. If nurse executives embrace the opportunity for partnership with vendors, they may be able to influence what major vendors build, as well as the future use of computers in clinical health care.

References

Ball, M. J., and Douglas, J. V. (1988). Integrating nursing and informatics. In M. J. Ball, K. J. Hannah, U. G. Jelger, and H. Peterson (Eds.), *Nursing Informatics—Where Caring and Technology Meet* (pp. 12-17). New York: Springer-Verlag New York.

Covvey, H. D. (1985). *Concepts and Issues in Health Care Computing* (pp. 171-182). St. Louis: C.V. Mosby Co.

Edmunds, L. (1992). Methodologies for defining system requirements. In *Proceedings from a MEDINFO '92 Workshop—Today's Reality and Tomorrow's Potential*. Printed from EMTEK Healthcare Systems, Inc., Tempe, AZ.

Hersher, B. (1988). Careers for nurses in health care information systems. In M. J. Ball, K. J. Hannah, U. G. Jelger, and H. Peterson (Eds.), *Nursing Informatics—Where Caring and Technology Meet* (pp. 12-17). New York: Springer-Verlag New York.

Romano, C. A. (1990). Innovation—The promise and the perils for nursing and information technology. *Computers in Nursing, 8*(3), 99-104.

Simpson, R. L. (1991). What you need to know about negotiating contracts. *Nursing Management, 22*(9), 22-23.

The Nursing Manager's Role in Successful System Implementation

Patricia A. Abbott, MS, RN
Clinical Specialist
Geriatric Research Education Clinical Center
Baltimore Veterans Administration Medical Center

Introduction

System implementation is a challenging time for nurse managers. It is during this period that the employment of the system is imminent and activities are focused and intensified within the target environment. The nurse managers' involvement during the implementation phase is critical: as change agents, knowledge sources, leaders, and facilitators.

Implementation brings with it responsibility, opportunity, risk, and *change*. Nurse managers can develop strategies to promote innovation (change) based on an understanding of the behavioral aspects of change and the human decision-making process. Everett Rogers' (1963; 1983) Adoption of Innovation Theory provides a framework for identifying human response patterns to change and will be utilized throughout this chapter to guide the development of implementation strategies.

System implementation may progress in a step-by-step fashion with activities such as site preparation, installation, system testing, piloting, and conversion. In actuality, not all implementation projects will follow this linear approach. The implementation environment, the complexity of the system, and the importance attached to the project may alter the path of progression through the implementation stage. Therefore, a general implementation framework will be offered to assist the nurse manager in understanding and planning for the activities that commonly occur as part of a system implementation.

Implementation requires intensive planning and advance groundwork to prepare users both technically and psychologically. The psychological aspects of implementation are *process* oriented, dealing with the human factors that facilitate or inhibit innovation and change. The technological preparation is *task* oriented, with implementation broken down into step-by-step phases which are focused and manageable. This is not to imply that task and process operate independently of each other. On the contrary, system implementation is a close intertwining of the two, mandating a comprehensive understanding of both technological and psychological aspects by the nurse manager.

This chapter focuses on three areas: (1) identifying behavioral characteristics related to change; (2) understanding and influencing the human decision-making process; and (3) an implementation framework. Each of these areas are integral components of system implementation, and strategies for dealing with implementation are best formulated by melding the concepts of all three. The intent of this chapter is to broaden the nurse manager's knowledge base in these three areas to stimulate critical thinking, contribute to comprehensive implementation planning, and encourage the consideration of psychological as well as technological interventions.

Definitions

Implementation is defined "as the process of putting something into effect according to or by means of a definite plan or procedure (*Webster's New World Dictionary*, 1989)." When specifically applied to information systems, implementation is the actual installation of the information application into the organization, focusing on a mix of issues such as training, testing, file conversion, and procedural changes (Ahituv and Neumann, 1990). Denger, Cole, and Walker (1988) describe system implementation as a diverse and resource-intensive process that combines careful planning, interdisciplinary teamwork and accountability, change management, and a synergistic relationship with the vendor.

Implementation involves working to facilitate the adoption of innovation by planning for and managing change. Planned change is defined by Lippitt (1958) as an intentional, conscious, and collaborative effort to improve the operations of a human system through the application of valid knowledge. Lewin (1952) describes planned organizational change as a deliberate rather than an inevitable, sudden change which uses strategies to decrease the forces of opposition to change. Everett Rogers (1963) defines the adoption of innovation as the decision to continue the use of an idea (which is perceived as new) by the individual. Rogers' theory describes and classifies individual variations in response patterns to change by utilizing "adopter categories," as well as describing steps in human decision-making identified as the "Innovation-Decision" process.

Mobilizing for Change

The degree of impact experienced by the implementation of a system into the operational environment is dependent upon the magnitude of the change. The initial introduction of automation into a facility is considered a radical change, and the most challenging for managers to facilitate. If the proposed implementation is a modification to an existing system, the change is generally less threatening and somewhat easier to manage. Regardless of the magnitude, the nurse manager must be prepared to take charge of change to achieve positive results.

Effective communication is an essential tool for the nurse manager when preparing for change. A decrease in unrealistic expectations and miscommunications will be evidenced by effectively communicating with staff, other disciplines, management and vendors. Increased awareness of the mutual dependence of departments in the operational environment and the laying of initial groundwork for the formation of cooperative partnerships will also emerge. Within the nursing domain, communicating nursing concerns and needs to appropriate sources is crucial. The sense of ownership, involvement, and commitment of users can be attained, though, by making the entire process responsive to those it serves.

Change as part of system implementation will be widespread and affect a broad spectrum of individuals. A reasonable assumption may be that upper management would be accepting of the proposed innovation; however, change agents may find themselves working with upper management as well as staff to facilitate the adoption of the system. The support of upper management is crucial to the success of implementation; assessing the degree of support and then influencing upper management to accept the innovation must be a high priority for the nurse manager. Across the spectrum of those affected by the change, nurse managers can develop strategies to promote innovation based on an understanding of the behavioral aspects of change, and the human decision-making process as described by Rogers (1963; 1983).

Adoption Categories

Rogers uses a classification scheme titled "adopter categories" to reflect the inherent differences between individuals relating to the rate of adoption of innovation. Each category contains individuals with similar degrees of innovativeness. The categorization assists the nurse manager in identifying those quick to accept change and those who are resistant. Change strategies to target each group can be subsequently designed and implemented. The five groups consist of: *innovators, early adopters, early majority, late majority, and laggards.*

Innovators are venturesome and eager to try new ideas. Innovators are risk takers and their heightened interest in exploration leads them away from local peers. In general, the change agent will not have to focus on convincing the innovators to accept a new idea, only in getting them to accept the constraints of the proposed innovation. Innovators are not reference persons for other staff members as they have a tendency to travel in different circles and are generally regarded as revolutionaries by staff members. The nurse manager or change agent should not view the innovator as an influential person in enticing others to adopt the innovation; however, they are very useful as members of steering, planning or equipment committees due to the nature of their personalities. Bushy and Kamphuis (1989) assert that the ideas of the innovator warrant attention, especially post-implementation, because innovators are already looking ahead to enhancements, modifications, and creative uses of the technology.

Early Adopters are generally very integrated into the social structure of the target environment; and are usually the first members of the group to "buy-into" the innovation. Early adopters have the greatest influence with colleagues and are looked to as opinion leaders and role models within the structure. Potential adopters look to the early adopter types for advice about the new idea and rely heavily on that advice when making the decision to accept or reject the innovation. A concentrated effort by the nurse manager in the early adopter group will be invaluable, for a positive impact upon the early adopters will trickle down to other members of the staff. Bushy and Kamphuis (1989) found that early adopters served as excellent role models and troubleshooters during system implementation, not because of their technological savvy but their status among peers.

Early Majority members adopt new ideas just before the average individual. While these members are not viewed as leaders, and have a tendency to delay the full adoption of an innovation, they are determined followers of the early adopter group and thereby play a powerful role in the adoption process. The nature of "following" emphasizes the importance of a positive influencing process with the early adopter group. Nurse managers can persuade members of this group individually and through the early adopters.

Late Majority members are the skeptics of the group who adopt new ideas after the average individual. Generally, the adoption comes as part of a mandate, as part of an economic necessity, or due to peer pressure. If the previous groups choose to reject the innovation, the late majority will be more than happy to oblige. However, if the innovation is adopted, it must be well accepted into practice before the late majority is convinced. The members of this group do not communicate well with others, which contributes to their position on the outer perimeters of the social circle. Intense communication and a deliberate facilitation of user involvement by the nurse manager are warranted with this group, with the understanding that positive results may be delayed.

Laggards are the very last type of individual to adopt an innovation. Members of this group are traditional in their views and are very distrustful of change, change agents, and new ideas. Laggards usually buy into a new idea *after* it has been replaced by a newer innovation, which contributes to a chronic problem of outmoded work practices. Members of this group may sometimes be labeled as saboteurs who deliberately undermine the system and encourage others to do the same. By determining the source of the resistance and negotiating or modifying the innovation or strategy being used to gain the support and trust of these individuals, the implementation process can be positively affected.

A primary responsibility of the nurse manager in preparing for implementation is to assess the readiness of the psychological environment. The intent of the previous section is to encourage the use of Rogers' categorization by nurse managers to assess the characteristics of the users, thereby opening avenues for the subsequent design of customized strategies to facilitate the adoption of innovation.

Innovation-Decision Stages

Influencing the change process is another challenge for nurse managers. Therefore, in conjunction with understanding the differences between individuals related to innovativeness, the nurse manager should have an awareness of the mental processes that occur as individuals evaluate change. The nurse manager can influence behaviors to enhance the adoption of innovation by working through these mental stages.

Rogers (1983) defines the innovative-decision (adoption) process as the mental stages an individual progresses through, from the initial introduction of an innovation to the final decision to adopt or reject the idea. The five stages in the innovative-decision process are: *knowledge, persuasion, decision, implementation, and confirmation.* Particular behaviors are present in each stage, which in turn contribute to the succeeding phase.

Knowledge begins when the individual is exposed to the innovation and a functional understanding of the idea is formed. The exposure to an innovation arises from a need. For example, in the medical center, exposure to information-handling technologies may originate from the need to improve patient care, enhance cost effectiveness, or as a mandate of professional performance standards. Exposure to innovation may also come as a random event, such as when an individual stumbles upon a novel idea. Researchers are quick to point out, however, that individuals will seldom (if ever) expose themselves to ideas if there is not an underlying need.

The beginning phases of adoption can be enhanced by heightening the perception of need for change. For example, the nurse manager may point out the excessive amount of paperwork and clerical activity required of nursing staff to process an order. Managers should challenge existing practices and offer suggestions for streamlining the process while emphasizing the benefits of the new application. The change agent has thereby injected a need for innovation by pointing out the necessity of change and the desirable consequences of new ideas.

Persuasion deals with the psychological or affective nature of the innovation. The individual forms an attitude (favorable or unfavorable) toward the innovation. An active seeking of information related to the innovation occurs and the person may mentally apply the idea to current practice to evaluate possible acceptance. Attitudes which are exhibited during this phase are those directed towards the innovation itself and as a general attitude towards change as a process. The attitude towards change is influenced by previous encounters with innovation, which depending on the perception of success or failure, will affect the activities of the change agent.

In the persuasion phase, individuals are actively seeking information about the proposed innovation, therefore access to knowledge sources should be supported. Special attention should be paid to those in the early adopter category during this period in deference to the informal communications which are particularly active in this phase. It is very important that these opinion leaders are persuaded to the benefits of the proposed implementation. A pro-change attitude can be facilitated by providing material about information-handling technologies in settings similar to the implementation site and inviting speakers who share related positions, experiences, and who have recently incorporated similar change into practice. The exposure to such messages may enhance the creation of favorable attitudes to change which will facilitate the adoption of new innovations.

Decision occurs as the individual partakes in activities which influence the choice to accept or reject the innovation. Generally, the individual tests the innovation in the given environment as a means to reduce the perceived risks of adoption. This testing can occur either mentally or in reality if the ability to test the idea is present. The ability to physically test the innovation speeds up the innovation-decision process and contributes to a favorable response from individuals. By providing multiple opportunities for "hands-on" sessions during implementation, both formally and informally, the adoption process can be enhanced. Potential users can evaluate the innovation by visiting a pilot unit, another facility using the system, or by experimenting with a test system provided by the vendor. They should be encouraged to see the system in action and evaluate its abilities.

Implementation occurs when the individual makes the decision to accept or reject the innovation, puts the innovation into use, and incorporates the change into practice. Behavioral changes occur as the new idea is embraced and the person is actively seeking "how to" information on the use of the new idea. The nurse manager's responsibility at this point will be in the provision of technical assistance and guidance as the individual begins to use the application.

Confirmation occurs as the individual seeks reinforcement for the decision which has been made. It is important to note that the decision to reject or accept is not final; people deal with change in varying styles and degrees. Occasionally the persons most resistant to the system will convert and become proponents of the innovation. After acceptance, individuals will need positive reinforcement, and if the person does not experience benefit or receive the reinforcement, the decision to reject may occur. This is important to note when implementing a system; the process does not end with the "go-live" date. The users must see an enhancement to practice and hear generally positive messages about the system to encourage the full adoption of the innovation into normal operating procedures. Nurse managers need to provide encouragement (even during controversy) for an extended period of time following implementation. The presence of a positive system environment can contribute to creative and comprehensive utilization of the technology, rather than the focused use of mandated system attributes.

Thus far in this chapter, Rogers' categorization of individuals based on the degree of innovativeness (adopter categories) and the processes by which individuals make decisions (innovative-decision) have been discussed. Complex problems cannot be solved until they are understood; it is by comprehending the dynamics of social behaviors, personal characteristics of innovativeness, and the human decision-making process that the nurse manager can design situation-specific strategies to promote system implementation. Several suggestions for strategy development were provided based on these process-oriented psychological factors. The third step in the comprehensive plan for implementation moves to incorporating the task or technically oriented approach of an implementation framework.

Implementation Framework

A step-wise progression in the implementation phase is common. A standard cycle of implementation is proposed: Planning, Hardware/Software Installation, Implementation Task Force Education and Training, Modification or Customization, System Testing, Documentation Development, User Education and Training, Parallel Testing, Go Live, and Post-implementation Reviews/Evaluation. Contemporary circumstances may alter the path of progression, necessitating either the addition, deletion, or re-sequencing of certain phases. In addition, when using a standard implementation cycle, consideration must be given to the previously discussed relationship of task and process. The implementation framework, while task oriented, cannot be used successfully without consideration of human factors and psychological processes.

Each stage during the cycle produces documentation: a scripting of activities, plans, and modifications which have occurred. The documentation is used by subsequent phases to facilitate continuity throughout the implementation cycle. Administrators, managers, or steering committees may also use the documentation for formative evaluation purposes. Decisions to modify the system or process based on document review may occur as the phases of the implementation proceed. The phases in a standard implementation framework are discussed below.

Phase One: Planning

An implementation team is formed, commonly comprised of end users, nurse managers, physicians, administrators, senior management, and other interdisciplinary representatives. Nurse managers should assure adequate nursing representation on this team. Individuals particularly suited for the implementation team are the "early adopters." The interdisciplinary nature of the team will lead to a co-ownership of decisions, a sense of teamwork and common goal attainment, and a breaking down of service boundaries. The implementation team should also include personnel who have been involved in previous stages of the system development. "Seasoned" personnel, in conjunction with the documentation produced in preceding activities, will facilitate a proper sequence of process and planning as the implementation phase progresses.

Efforts are directed towards promoting an understanding of the current environment with a review of the rationale for system procurement and implementation. An overview of the system is provided to team members to enhance a conceptual understanding of the functionality and benefits. A realistic and flexible work plan will be developed which includes a delegation of responsibilities across the team and a realistic timeframe for implementation. Implementation cannot be rushed. Frederick Brooks (1982) discusses timeframes for implementation in large-scale automation projects and states: "When a task cannot be partitioned because of (its sequential steps), the application of more effort has no effect on its schedule. The bearing of a child takes nine months, no matter how many women are assigned."

Planning for a change in process and workflow should be addressed and implemented very early during this phase. The transition to a new system can be made less traumatic if changes in policy and procedures across all involved units/departments are phased into normal activities. For example, if the method of ordering drugs from the pharmacy will change drastically with the implementation of the new system, model and standardize the "new" method. Plan to document, distribute, and incorporate the "new" method into normal operating procedures far in advance of the "go live" date. Finally, the determination of the type of conversion such as a parallel, phased/modular, pilot, or crash (see Phase Eight for detailed explanation of conversion), and planning for system education and training will occur at this time.

Phase Two: Hardware/Software Installation

In advance of actual installation, decisions are made about the location and type of system hardware. Prior to installation and in conjunction with the system installers, a walk-through should be scheduled. Team members will visit and re-evaluate the appropriateness and safety of the installation site. During the walk-through, space, cooling, and electrical requirements will be re-assessed for adequacy and adherence to electrical code and vendor specifications. Personnel such as physical plant engineers, IS personnel, and electricians must be present and consulted during the walk-through.

The location of printers, terminals, and/or workstations is examined. Users must be consulted in determining the proposed location of clinical hardware. The printers must be appropriately located in relation to noise production. The terminals/ workstations should be installed in logical and easily accessible areas with sufficient lighting. Adequate electrical outlets and telephones in close proximity to the hardware are necessary. The physical security of the hardware, software, and data bases must be assured.

After the installation of hardware and software (which is generally done by an installation team), a complete system demonstration should be provided by the vendor. This is not meant to be an in-depth training session (Phase 3 is devoted to this); however, the software should operate smoothly and major features should be highlighted.

Phase Three: Implementation Task Force Education and Training

Education and training are not the same. Training focuses primarily on the skills necessary to master the system while education clarifies the strategic IS plan, unfreezes attitudes, heightens awareness of mission and organizational objectives, and assists learners to understand the impact of the system on work practices.

The implementation team is educated about the system goals and benefits, including the rationale for installation, proposed enhancements to work practices, and organizational/IS strategic plans. The team will also need to understand the system limitations. What is the system capable of doing? What happens during a system failure? How long is the response time? Who is responsible for various problems, i.e., hardware failure, software bugs, network malfunctions? Education will serve to lessen unrealistic expectations and enhance cooperative problem solving.

Training focuses on the actual use of the system. In most circumstances, vendors will provide training for designated staff. While it is not necessary for the team members to understand all of the intricacies of the system, a comprehensive knowledge of overall functionality is desirable. It is during this phase that team members may notice areas of potential conflict, errors, or areas for modification.

Phase Four: Customization/Modification

During the beginning phases of system implementation, and based on formative evaluations, areas for modification may be found. The team will be responsible for examining these areas, reviewing the necessity of modification, developing the specifications for modifications, testing the modifications, and then incorporating these modifications. In many cases, the full effect of the system cannot be demonstrated until the system is fully functional, which is why many software vendor contracts require a 3 to 4 month trial period before additional programming is undertaken.

During this phase, the team may provide input on customized components of the software. For example, the team may make suggestions on the design of forms which are to be preprinted by the computer and specify contents and layout of selected customized reports. In conjunction with others, the vendor will be implementing security measures within the system at this time.

Phase Five: System Testing

After the system (or module of the system) is installed and operational, testing of the system is done in two phases; system testing and acceptance testing. System testing is done by a professional team, while acceptance testing is completed by users in conjunction with the project developers.

In system testing, individual modules are tested independently prior to their integration into the system. After the individual modules or programs have been tested (or if the system is not modular), the entire system should be examined. The system should be completely tested using realistic scenarios. Particular attention should be paid to the interfaces between programs, especially with the transfer of data between modules/departments. Output should be validated and the flow of data must be tracked.

Acceptance testing is verification of the operating procedures of the new system by the performance of a checklist of activities (Ahituv and Newmann, 1990). The test is specified by the users, and performed along with the project developers. It is comprised of a series of conditions that may occur during normal operating procedures, such as heavy utilization, data entry and retrieval, accessing integrated and/or interfaced modules, as well as extraordinary events such as a system failure. The success of an acceptance test is seen as the milestone where the new system "belongs" to the user and the project development team releases the system for operation.

Phase Six: Documentation Development

In this phase of implementation several forms of system and program documentation are being generated by the vendor. The preparation and provision of educational materials for both basic and advanced classes, including handouts and quizzes, should be provided by the vendor. In addition, user and operator guides will be assembled and distributed. Operator guides should include flow charts, program specifications, backup and recovery procedures, table and record layouts, operational procedures, and a dictionary of terms. User guides generally focus upon the operational aspects which relate to specific functions and tend to stay away from technical references. User guides should be provided in sufficient quantity to allow for ready access by system users.

Phase Seven: User Education and Training

Education precedes training and should be initiated as part of the preparation for change process as discussed in relation to Rogers' theory. Education clarifies the strategic IS plan, unfreezes attitudes, heightens awareness of mission and organizational objectives, and assists learners in understanding the impact of the system on work practices. Education also serves to lessen resistance, encourage user acceptance, and fosters true involvement. Instructional sessions which support an open forum where concerns can be voiced and misconceptions dispelled will assist users in the adoption of the new system. Users of the system must be educated about (and personally experience) benefits from automation.

Organizational and functional implications related to system implementation warrant discussion during educational sessions. Will management structures change? Will the changes result in shifts in authority? What are the implications of these shifts? Reporting structures, human roles and activities, and communication patterns may be altered as a result of system implementation. The education of users decreases the mystique of the information system impact, thereby rendering it less threatening.

It is during this time period that nurse managers can apply their knowledge of Rogers' Innovative-Decision process to influence the acceptance of the system, to heighten the perception of need, provide understandable and plentiful information, and allow the users time (private and structured) to experiment with the technology. Especially beneficial to designing educational strategies will be the advance knowledge of the individuals' degree of innovativeness as determined by Rogers' Adoption Categories. Concentrate initial efforts with the early adopters. If the early adopters are convinced, use them as educational assistants, for their influence with others is powerful. Be prepared to devote extra resources with the laggards, as they will require increased educational effort to combat resistance. Resistance or rejection across the categories may be evidenced-not as a reaction to change, but as a direct response to a perceived system failure or error. By heeding and addressing user concerns early in the education process, the nurse manager can promote a collaborative working relationship with the users, foster a sense of ownership, and influence the adoption of innovation.

Training, in an operational sense, familiarizes users with components of the system that relate directly to specific activities. Users may not need to know the finest details of the system, but they do need to know how to interact with all components which contribute to system functionality. Training sessions not only contribute to the acquisition of formal knowledge, but also assist in building helpful rules of thumb.

Training is resource-intensive and requires advance planning by both nurse managers and training staff. Vendors frequently will "train the trainers" who will then assume responsibility for the overall user training. As mentioned in Phase Six, the vendor should provide training manuals, handouts, and quizzes which the trainers will use during sessions. Minimal disruptions to normal activities must be emphasized; staffing coverage (and budgeting) must be predetermined. Training is most beneficial when completed as close as possible to the "go live" date; training that is provided and not able to be practiced will soon be forgotten. Denger et al. (1988) suggest that training begin 2 to 3 weeks prior to the go live date. A review of the literature seems to demonstrate that short segments (1 to 2 hours) of training class provided in multiple sessions is most effective. Denger et al. (1988) discussed differences in the time and complexity of training by focusing on the varying needs of different user groups. For example, nurses received additional hours of training in nursing functions, the entry of orders, and the charging of supplies. Personnel of other departments were trained according to the degree of activity required for successful interaction with the system. The challenge of presenting information to a variety of users with differing educational backgrounds is discussed by Zielstorff (1976). Readers are referred to her work.

Phase Eight: Parallel Testing

Parallel testing involves a test run of the system simulating normal operating procedures. User involvement is encouraged to simulate real-time activity. Procedures for the use of the system are evaluated for comprehensiveness and accuracy by the users and team. The performance of the system is critiqued and the data integrity is determined. If the system passes the parallel test, the "go live" date is set.

Phase Nine: Conversion and Go Live

Going live is the most demanding phase of the implementation process. The system (or module) is fully operational at this point and will be integrated into normal work practices during this phase. Going live occurs as conversion is completed. Conversion is the method by which the previous system is replaced with the new; each approach has its strengths and weaknesses. There are several methods to consider.

The *parallel* approach is viewed by many as the optimal choice, albeit expensive. A parallel conversion will see the new and old system run side by side for a period of time. The old system is "live" while the new system functions in a test mode. The new system begins to take over increasing amounts of real processing, while the old system continues to run in the background. Eventually the new system takes over all processing, and the old system is used for backup and verification. Only after full testing and satisfactory operation is the old system removed. Needless to say, the cost of this type of conversion is very high.

A *modular or phased* approach is used when the system is compartmentalized or able to be broken down into modules. Each module is brought into service and incorporated into practice. When the module is deemed to be satisfactory, the next component or module is added and the process repeated until the project is complete.

The *pilot* method involves choosing a site which adequately represents the installation environment and treating this site as a controlled laboratory. If the system performs satisfactorily in the pilot site, a full-scale conversion in the target environment is undertaken.

A *crash* implementation is deemed to be the most undesirable, but at times necessary. The crash implementation is an instant conversion from old to new. A go live date is scheduled, and at a precise moment, the old system is shut down and the new system takes over. An example of this method is that of Sweden changing its driving laws from driving on the left side of the road to driving on the right. The conversion occurred at a set date and time, and all drivers were expected to radically change driving methods instantaneously. It is obvious why other methods of conversion would be inappropriate in this scenario. In a crash system conversion, the new system must be able to handle the entire operation it is intended to automate from the very moment of the go live. Intense planning and testing must occur prior to the crash, for there is little room for conversion error. The operational cost of crash conversion is minimal; however, the potential for a dangerous system failure or error is present.

At the completion of the conversion, the system is considered live. The go live period is characterized by on line, real-time data handling by the system. The time commitment by team members, system implementors, vendors and managers is intense. Be prepared, for this phase will require 24 hour-coverage by the implementation team for the first few days, with round-the-clock, on-call support for the following few weeks. In addition, the IS Department must provide immediate response (24 hours) for technical problems during the go-live. If a modular or phased approach is used, the experiences from each go-live session are evaluated and incorporated into subsequent go-lives. The sharing of these experiences will contribute to the sense of teamwork as the organization moves towards full-scale implementation. The strengths and weaknesses of the implementation process thus far will be evidenced in the go-live. The post-implementation review will examine these elements, as well as the operational characteristics of the new system.

Phase Ten: Post-Implementation Review

The review serves to examine the implementation process as well as the overall performance of the system. Various team members (implementation, project development, steering) as well as objective users should be invited to participate in the review. The experience and knowledge that the team members possess in combination with the objectivity of users will contribute to a comprehensive and realistic evaluation.

The review will serve to illustrate the weaknesses of the implementation process; however, care must be taken to prevent the review from becoming a witch hunt. The outcome should be a straightforward and impartial evaluation of implementation successes and failures. The lessons learned in the past will be used to improve future endeavors. Each phase, including both technical and psychological aspects, of the implementation process should be investigated. Was the concept and importance of change addressed early and completely? Were all disciplines adequately represented during the planning phase? Were appropriate suggestions by users heeded? Was the acceptance testing sufficient and were concerns by users handled properly? Did the education and training sessions sufficiently prepare users?

The use of the system must also be reviewed. Were the objectives of the system met? Did the system adhere to the specifications set forth in the original plans and contracts?

Aspects related to the functionality of the system must be addressed such as reliability, accuracy, and efficiency. An examination of information flow pre- and post-implementation may assist in the evaluation of system benefits, while the investigation of the functionality and user critiques may lead to system modification.

During this phase, plans for ongoing system evaluations (sometimes referred to as post-audit or post-installation reviews) are made. The first review of this type occurs six months after the implementation is complete. These reviews are generally focused upon technical operations, operating costs, and modification processes as determined by users. In addition, a detailed examination of direct and indirect benefits produced by the system, evaluations of the information generated by the system, and evaluations of system personnel (including vendors) are undertaken.

In practice, the implementation process may vary somewhat from what has been presented in this section. Steps may overlap, change sequence, or be eliminated totally. Systems being installed may be small in scope or as part of a huge conglomerate; regardless, the framework presented has applicability in a wide variety of settings.

Summary

Implementation is about uncertainty, risk, innovation, and opportunity. It has been the intention of this chapter to prepare the nurse manager to take that opportunity and deal with the risks and challenges of implementation. Linking the ideas of categorization, human decision making, and the implementation framework will create a knowledge base from which the nurse manager can work to decrease the risk and challenges to facilitate the adoption of innovation. A summary of the major points and implications for nurse managers follows:

1. Health care is in rapid change; creating a pro-change environment which readily assimilates new ideas and activities into practice is imperative.

2. The approach to the change inherent in system implementation should be evolutionary, not revolutionary. Preparation for change should begin as soon as the organization begins to consider the purchase of a system and should continue indefinitely.

3. Determine individual innovativeness and influence human decision making as a part of the preparation for implementation. Apply these psychological aspects to the task-orientated approach of the implementation framework.

4. Foster collaboration. Consult and work with a variety of users such as staff, other health care providers, management, IS personnel, and vendors.

5. Communicate and educate to lessen miscommunication, mistrust, and resistance.

6. Assess and secure top-level support for the system. Do not assume that upper management either understands or accepts the innovation. The nurse manager must work to influence and gain the support of other managers who are either uninformed or undecided.

7. Secure representation during all stages of system planning. Assuring that nursing needs are being met and a responsiveness to voiced concerns contributes to building a sense of ownership and commitment.

8. Identify your innovators. Invite participation in the beginning phases of implementation—committee formulation, research, and site visits. Look to the innovators, particularly during the evaluation phase.

9. Identify the early adopters within the implementation environment. Concentrate early and positively with these individuals, recalling that early adopters strongly influence others in the environment. Using early adopters as system trainers is a particularly powerful strategy.

10. Listen to user concerns. Resistance may not relate to change as a process, but may signal a serious problem with the operation of the system.

11. Individuals who resist change do so for a reason; investigate and address the sources of resistance to the system.

12. Changes in workflow and processes should begin far in advance of the "go live" date. The "new" methods should be incorporated into practice with documented policies and procedures before the introduction of the technology.

13. Careful assessment and allotment of resources are necessary for the implementation phase. Attention to training and education of evening and night shifts and the additional resources which may be required to work with system resisters is necessary. The policy to change and implement must be complemented by a decision to provide resources to make the policy effective.

14. A primary responsibility of the nurse manager in system implementation is influencing others to adopt the system. Work through the five stages in the Innovative-Decision process. Stimulate a need for *knowledge*, utilize knowledge sources and 'create a pro-change environment to *persuade*, arrange hands-on system testing to influence *decision*, provide technical support to *implement*, and provide positive feedback and demonstrate benefits to facilitate *confirmation*.

Conclusion

The successful implementation of an automated system requires the nurse manager's involvement from inception, a tremendous amount of advance planning, and a solid knowledge base from which to direct and manage. The nurse manager has the unique opportunity to combine psychological as well as technical interventions to positively influence the adoption of the system. It is in seizing this opportunity and maximizing the effect that the nurse manager's pivotal role in successful system implementation is evidenced.

References

Ahituv, N., and Neumann, S. (1990). *Principles of Information Systems for Management* (3rd ed.). Dubuque, IA: Wm. C. Brown.

Brooks, F. (1982). *The Mythical Man-Month: Essays on Software Engineering.* New York: Addison-Wesley Publishing Co.

Bushy, A., and Kamphuis, J. (1989). Rogers' adoption model in the implementation of change. *Clinical Nurse Specialist, 3*(4), 188–191.

Denger, S., Cole, D., and Walker, H. (1988). Implementing an integrated clinical information system. *Journal of Nursing Administration, 18*(12), 28-34.

Lewin, K. (1952). Group decisions and social change. In G. E. Swanson, T. M. Newcomb, and E. L. Hartley (Eds.), *Readings in Social Psychology.* New York: Rinehart.

Lippitt, R. (1958). *Dynamics of Planned Change.* New York: Harcourt, Brace & World.

Rogers, E. (1963). *Diffusion of Innovations.* New York: Free Press.

Rogers, E. (1983). *Diffusion of Innovation* (2nd ed). New York: Free Press.

Webster's New World Dictionary. (1989). New York: Warner Books.

Zielstorff, R. D. (1976). Orientating personnel to automated systems. *Journal of Nursing Administration, 6*, 14-16.

Training Issues in System Implementation

Rita D. Zielstorff, MS, RN, FAAN, FACMI
Staff Specialist, Patient Care Information Systems
Department of Nursing
Massachusetts General Hospital

Introduction

Effective training is a critical aspect of successful system implementation. The benefits of effective training have been well-documented (e.g., Messmer, Kurtyka and Kelley, 1992; Tiano and White, 1990), along with examples of the costs of poorly designed programs (e.g., see "System failures," 1992).

Over the past three decades, considerable scientific knowledge and conventional wisdom have accumulated about how to achieve effective training for automated systems (Merrow, 1991). For example, we have learned that software demonstrations alone are not enough, and that opportunities for hands-on experience with the system are essential (Bolesta, Andersen, and Zeni, 1988). We also know that training should be provided as near as possible to the system start-up time, because the user retention period of newly acquired skills is short. We have learned that training busy adult professionals, often in the workplace, is quite different from educating traditional students. Because of this experience, several principles of adult education should be considered in designing an effective training program (Mast and Van Atta, 1986).

The most frequently reported method of delivering training on a large scale is the train-the-trainer, group-session approach (Merrow, 1991). With this method, system experts (who may be provided by the system vendor or developer) instruct trainers (who are usually employees of the agency implementing the system). These trainers then conduct classroom sessions with six to ten trainees, imparting what they have learned. With no more than two trainees per terminal, each trainee is led through pre-defined exercises on a "practice" system to learn the essential skills. Training may take as little as one hour, or as long as a week or more, depending on the number and complexity of functions to be learned.

Proficiency may be judged by trainer observation or by satisfactory completion of specified exercises.

Group sessions may be used to impart more than just the skills needed under the new system. Objectives of system implementation, explanation of policies, and response to trainees' concerns about new job functions can be covered in group sessions, tailored to the needs of the group (Flaugher, 1986).

Inadequacies of the Traditional Method

While the method just described usually yields satisfactory results, the traditional approach is far from perfect. One drawback is that it is resource-intensive. Training a large number of personnel as close to implementation time as possible requires many concurrent sessions, which necessitates that many trainers must be prepared. Usually these staff are recruited from existing personnel who are diverted from their normal duties for several weeks before and after implementation.

Considerable variation in the training delivered may result , due to the fact that trainers may not have gained sufficient expertise in all areas, and due to other factors such as fatigue and individual delivery style.

Staff must also be diverted from their normal duties to acquire this training. This may require scheduling additional staff coverage at overtime pay, or hiring per diem personnel to cover the units, or paying staff overtime to come in on off-duty hours to receive training (Tiano and White, 1990).

Group sessions involving busy professional personnel tend to be inefficient, because unforeseen events on the units often lead to significant no-show rates, with the necessity to re-schedule. Even when staff members are able to come at the pre-scheduled time, their attention may be more focused on the clinical situation they left behind on the unit than on learning new skills that may not be required for days or weeks (Axford, 1988).

Group sessions must be designed to the median level of computer proficiency. Therefore, those who are computer-proficient must go at a slower pace than they might wish, while those who have difficulty may need to return for a repeat session. The necessity to accommodate different learning styles of individual trainees, and to control for difficulties in trainer/trainee interaction, is challenging.

Finally, the enormous effort required to design and carry out a large-scale training program can be quite disruptive to the agency's central mission: patient care.

Is Technology the Problem or the Answer?

Training to use new technologies can be effectively accomplished using the technology itself. Computer-based training (CBT) is a form of self-administered instruction that uses specially designed courseware to teach needed skills. Well-designed, computer-based instruction programs have two major characteristics: they are interactive, and they are self-paced (Gery, 1987).

Interactivity means that the computer-based program engages the learner in a dialogue in which the computer presents material, and the learner is asked to respond. The learner is often in control of the dialogue, by making choices from menus, asking for more explanation, or requesting exercises to practice skills. Another aspect of interactivity is that the computer provides feedback based on the behavior of the trainee. Corrective feedback is provided in the case of incorrect keystrokes, and diagnostic feedback is provided in the case where length of time or requested repetitions indicate that the trainee is having difficulty. This is different from "page-turner" CBT programs, where the user simply presses a key to progress from one page of explanation to the next. "Page-turner" CBT programs, while simple to develop and maintain, are much less effective as training devices.

Self-paced programs permit trainees to progress as quickly or as slowly as they like. Learners may choose a "fast track" that skips certain modules, or they may choose the fullest complement of modules available, depending on their level of interest and expertise.

While relatively novel in health care organizations, CBT has been used in other industries for many years. The editors of Training magazine have been tracking the use of CBT in industry since 1985. In 1993, a total of 58% of U.S. organizations with 100 or more employees were using CBT, according to the survey conducted by Training (Froiland, 1993). While many of these computer-based tutorials are designed to teach computer-related skills, many companies use CBT for other training, such as technical skills not related to computer operations. Some companies even use CBT for training non-technical skills such as management, sales and interpersonal skills.

Health care system vendors and agencies are catching on to the trend. Several large computer-system vendors such as TDS (Farrel, 1988), Hewlett-Packard ("Hospitals seek," 1991), and HBO (Coulon, 1993) now offer automated packages that train personnel on how to use their products. There are also reports of individual agencies recognizing the benefits of CBT for large-scale system training, and developing CBT courseware with in-house resources or with the aid of consultants (Bush, 1993; Kelly, 1991; Zielstorff, 1992).

Advantages of Computer-Based Training

Computer-based training is especially appealing in the health care environment, for several reasons:

• More consistent with adult learning principles. CBT is particularly suited to adult learners. It can accommodate different learning styles by presenting various amounts of explanation, as the learner desires. It can accommodate the sensitivity of adults about making mistakes in front of their peers by offering individual private sessions of whatever length desired (some programs can even be placed on diskette and used on the trainee's home computer). CBT can be problem-focused, mirroring the reality of the work situation, rather than focused on the functions around which the computer system is designed. And finally, CBT allows the learner to be in control of his own learning by controlling the timing as well as the length, depth and number of sessions needed in order to reach proficiency. This is particularly appealing in an environment where employee shifts include evenings, nights, holidays and weekends, and where staff are diverse in terms of their existing computer skills (Downie and Basford, 1991).

• Permits consistent delivery of material, can assure proficiency. Unlike human trainers, CBT never gets tired and never "forgets" to make certain points. Proficiency tests can be built into the CBT that incorporate the essential functions as they will be carried out on the unit. Failure to pass the proficiency tests can be remedied by recommending that the trainee repeat specific parts of the tutorial.

• Less clinical "downtime." Several reports exist that show the same amount of training can be delivered in less time with CBT than with conventional classroom training (Perez and Willis, 1989; Zielstorff, Heller, Fitzmaurice, Ives, and Millar, 1991; "Computer-based training," 1993). Coupled with the capability of being decentralized to individual care units, this results in less time away from the clinical unit, and less disruption of the agency's primary mission of providing patient care.

• More effective. The characteristics described so far result in better learning, more retention, and more capability for review to "brush up" on skills.

• Automatic data management. The CBT system can contain a data management module that provides appropriate training to each individual, tracks training taken and records proficiency acquired. Reports can be automatically produced for those responsible for personnel training.

• Cost-effective. Until recently, the cost of developing CBT was prohibitive. Currently, several high-level microcomputer-based authoring and prototyping packages are available that permit rapid development of attractive and easy-to-use tutorials. In addition, there are reports that CBT can result in as much as 50% or greater savings in time to impart the same amount of training that would be delivered in conventional classroom settings ("Computer-based training," 1993; Perez and Willis, 1989; Schulman, 1989; "The shadow knows," 1989; Zielstorff et al., 1991). Multiplied by hundreds of employees, the time saved can result in substantial cost avoidance in replacement or overtime pay. The same CBT can be used to orient incoming personnel long after the initial training period is over, at no additional cost. If the costs of CBT development are amortized over the months or years during which the CBT is used, the CBT can eventually result in substantial cost savings, completely apart from the other benefits described (Perez and Willis, 1989).

Limitations of Computer-Based Training

Although there are many benefits of CBT, it is important to recognize what CBT cannot do. There are aspects of orientation that are broader than the skills needed to use the system, and CBT may not be the best medium for imparting them. For example, marketing the system to employees is an essential component of installing a system. Agency leaders must make known that they support the installation of the system, and must communicate the goals and objectives of implementing the system. There may be concern among employees about changes in roles and functions, or about potential job reductions resulting from greater efficiency. Such possible repercussions on employees cannot be handled with CBT. Finally, CBT is currently not suited to answering questions that were not anticipated in developing the program. For these types of issues, person-to-person contact, even in a large group forum, is more effective than CBT.

Other limitations of CBT include the immediate up-front costs and the relative difficulty of altering the program to reflect system changes as compared to training programs delivered by humans.

One Hospital's Experience

Massachusetts General Hospital implemented the first clinical application of its Patient Care Information System (PCIS) in Summer, 1990. The application used Laboratory Results Inquiry, which was both eagerly awaited and easy to use. Still, introducing the first application of the hospital's new information system on all 52 patient care units, including many that would also be moving to a new building at the same time, and at the time of year when new residents would be arriving, was a complex challenge. In addition, many of our 2,500 clinical personnel were unfamiliar with computers, and none knew very much about the characteristics of the system we were co-developing with a vendor.

In an effort to facilitate the coming changes, a Clinical Advisory Committee that represented the major user groups (physicians, nurses, unit support personnel) and the Information Resources group developed a multi-pronged approach to manage the major change. Four areas were targeted: User Interface, Marketing/Publicity, Terminal Deployment, and Training.

The Training Committee reviewed the requirements and the available resources, and developed a proposal for administrators that compared the costs and benefits of traditional classroom training versus CBT (Zielstorff, Heller, Fitzmaurice, Ives, and Millar, 1993). Decentralized CBT was selected, with one modification: administrators worried that staff who had no prior computer experience would have difficulty with self-directed CBT. They decided to recruit volunteers from among leadership personnel who could monitor group sessions in a central classroom where the same tutorial would be used, but the volunteer would be available to answer questions, and to assist with keyboard issues.

The tutorial was designed with in-house expertise. We contracted outside the hospital for the programming, in an effort not to divert existing programming staff from their main objective of readying the Lab Results system for implementation. The entire tutorial was designed, programmed and deployed in three months.

A CBT microcomputer was placed on each care unit two weeks prior to implementation, and removed 2 to 4 weeks after implementation. Microcomputers were also placed in various physician lounges and libraries. Each person was responsible for finding the time to complete the tutorial. No one was granted a password to use the hospital information system until that person had passed a "proficiency check," the final part of the tutorial.

Personnel who didn't feel comfortable using the computer-based tutorial without help could schedule themselves to take the same tutorial in a classroom which was monitored by one of the volunteers. A total of 30 volunteers each contributed 4 to 6 hours to monitor the group classes. About 300 of our 2,100 nurses took advantage of this opportunity, compared to fewer than a half dozen physicians. Among the 300 nurses, it should be noted, many were individuals who came not because they felt they needed assistance, but because there was only one CBT computer on each care unit. On occasions when the workload was light, two or three nurses from one unit sometimes came down to use the CBT computers in the classroom.

Massachusetts General Hospital selected a program called Dan Bricklin's™ Demo II™ for development of the tutorial itself. The designers of the program also developed an administrative program that permitted us to capture user registration data and tutorial usage information. For the administrative program, we used another high-level package, Fox Software's FoxPro, a DBase III Plus compiler. Each software package cost less than 500. Each package allows for unlimited reproduction of the applications that are developed, so there were no licensing fees required. We budgeted for ten weeks of programmer time to complete the tutorial.

Design of the Tutorial

The tutorial consisted of an administrative segment and a training segment. The administrative segment captured registration data (name of the user, hospital ID number, and clinical service), and usage data such as length of time at the computer, modules used and completed, and score on the proficiency check.

The training segment consisted of a total of nine modules: the first seven modules each taught a discrete task related to Results Inquiry. As these modules were designed for the computer-naive user, a considerable amount of didactic material was presented in each module. These modules required from one to four minutes each to complete, and each built on knowledge acquired in earlier modules.

A Quick Review module covered all the material in the first seven modules. This enabled the computer-naive learner to reinforce and integrate material from the individual modules. However, for the computer-proficient user, the Quick Review, which took 10 to 15 minutes to complete, was enough to learn the application.

The Proficiency Check was the final module. This Check provided a simulation of the real system, and asked the user to complete certain information retrieval tasks as they would in the real system. Correct keystrokes were rewarded with points, while incorrect keystrokes caused points to be deducted from the total score. Users were informed at the beginning of the Check that a tally of the score would be kept on the screen (similar to the style of a video game), and that a minimum score of 50 (out of a possible 100) would be required to pass the Check. It took about 10 minutes to complete the Proficiency Check.

Passing the Check allowed users to receive a password to use the live system. Persons who did not pass the check, or who were not happy with their final score, could take this module as many times as they wanted—the system only stored the highest score. About 7% of the staff took the Check more than once.

After passing the Check, users were asked their opinion about the usefulness of CBT to teach Laboratory Results Retrieval, and whether they would recommend using CBT for future PCIS applications.

The program was very attractive visually, with good use of color. The tone of the didactic material was kept light, even humorous at times, and interspersed encouraging feedback based on user responses.

Use of the Tutorial

Between May 15 and August 22, 1990, approximately 2400 personnel completed the tutorial and passed the proficiency check. Among all those who registered, the average user spent 24 minutes total at the tutorial; the median was 17 minutes. Among those who completed the tutorial, physicians as a group spent significantly less time at the tutorial than other groups did, and did better in average score attained on the proficiency check.

Asked their opinion of whether they felt that CBT was a useful way to learn Results Inquiry, 68% of those who completed the tutorial gave a positive response, and about 7% responded negatively (25% stated "no opinion", or did not respond). To the statement "Computer-Based Training should be used for future PCIS applications," 70% agreed, 5% disagreed, and 25% stated "no opinion," or gave no response.

Use Beyond Initial Orientation Effort

The computer-based tutorial continues to be used for training incoming staff, and for orienting personnel as additional hospital departments receive access to Laboratory Results Inquiry. Ten microcomputers are installed permanently in various locations around the hospital. When a new department is brought on line to Results Inquiry, a training microcomputer is placed temporarily in an accessible area in that department, and staff are given the responsibility to take the tutorial. Since the initial orientation period, over 2,500 additional staff have been trained via the tutorial, with minimal expenditure of human resources. There are no staff dedicated to ongoing training of Results Inquiry, yet over 5,000 personnel have been trained in this function since May 1990.

Effectiveness of the Tutorial

Passing the Proficiency Check may be taken as one measure of the effectiveness of the tutorial (99.5% of those who took the check passed it, with only 7% repeating the Check more than once). But a more objective measure is whether staff were able to use the live system without difficulty. The Information Systems Department maintains a 24-hour Help Desk where users can call for help in using the PCIS. The Help Desk reported that in the weeks following implementation of Results Inquiry, the number of calls increased by about 700 per week. Most of the calls had to do with keyboard problems (such as the Caps Lock key being on when it should be off), and with confusion that arose when the monitor's power saver feature regularly caused the screen to go blank. (The tutorial has since been modified to cover these types of issues.)

Maintenance of the Tutorial

In 1991, the tutorial was modified to include a module for a newly added laboratory. Since that time, new laboratories are simply described in special newsletters and handouts made available at each terminal. The tutorial was substantially modified in 1993 to delete modules that were seldom used, and to add a module that taught a major new function. A separate tutorial has also been created that teaches clerical personnel how to verify and edit registration data for patients coming in to the ambulatory care center.

Cost Savings

Table 1 shows our estimated and actual hours for developing and delivering CBT for Results Inquiry, comparing the estimates for traditional and computer-based methods with

Table 1.
Estimated vs. Actual Costs in Hours to Train 2400 Personnel on the Use of CBT

	Traditional (estimated)	CBT with Optional monitored classes (estimated)	CBT with Optional monitored classes (actual)
Develop content, Deliver training	734	714	888
Trainee time	3000 ($1^1/_4$ hrs/trainee)[a]	2275 (approx. 1 hr/trainee)[b]	1189 (approx. $^1/_2$ hr/trainee)[c]
Support costs (clerical support for scheduling, technical support for computer set-up, etc.)	1060	764	716
TOTAL HOURS	4794	3753	2793

[a]Includes 20 minutes travel time to central classroom for 2400 personnel.
[b]Includes 20 minutes travel time to central classroom for 500 personnel who were estimated to want monitored training.
[c]Includes 20 minutes travel time to central classroom for 300 personnel who actually used monitored training.

the actual hours expended. We estimated a 22% savings in hours using the computer-based tutorial, but we actually experienced a 42% savings over the traditional method estimate. This was largely due to three factors: (1) because we placed training terminals on each care unit, the 20-minute travel time was eliminated for all of the trainees, except the 300 who went to the central classroom; (2) because most personnel didn't leave the units, but took the tutorial in small segments of "down time," there was no need to schedule additional coverage or to bring in per diem personnel; and (3) personnel only spent on average less than 30 minutes on the tutorial. We would have designed a 60-minute traditional method group session for teaching this function, and we estimated that personnel would spend about 60 minutes on the computer-based tutorial as well. Trainees were obviously able to get through the material and pass the proficiency check with much less time at the tutorial than we anticipated, an experience that others have also reported.

This experience has convinced us that for applications where several hundred users need to be trained, and where the application is relatively stable, CBT is the method of choice.

Is Computer-Based Training for You?

Jane Schulman, a consultant in computer-based training, offers a set of questions that organizations can use to help them determine whether CBT is appropriate for their specific training situations. Among them:

• Are people who need training geographically dispersed?
• Must the same training be delivered repeatedly?
• Is the subject matter relatively stable?
• Are computers and other delivery equipment already in place?
• Is standardization and consistency an important factor?
• Is record-keeping for attendance, performance results and certification a critical task?
• Is the audience diverse?

•Will privacy and self-pacing enhance learning?
•Is scheduling training a frequent problem?
•Does training involve hazardous activities or expensive equipment? (Schulman, 1989, pp. 20-21).

According to Schulman, the more times a "yes" response appears in this list, the more likely it is that CBT will be an appropriate medium for delivering the training. Even when convinced, however, administrators many find that there are significant barriers. Trainers themselves may be threatened by the new technology, and may offer many reasons why human-delivered training is essential. It may be difficult to find the human resources to develop the training courseware. Simply providing a current trainer with an authoring package and a mandate to develop courseware is not a solution. At least some instruction in courseware development is needed. Contracting with consultants is expensive in the short run, but this approach may be the best long-term strategy to gain some experience and bring some expertise to currently employed training staff. Ordering demonstration disks of courseware is another way to see how the professionals do it, and to give current staff ideas of how to proceed. A careful cost comparison of current or projected training costs, compared to costs of developing and delivering the CBT, is also essential, to justify the up-front costs of the CBT. Table 1 might be helpful as a model, with dollars attached to the hours, as appropriate for your organization. If the CBT can be used by all departments whose personnel will be using the system, it may be possible to consolidate support for the idea, and share the cost among the departments.

One cautionary note: CBT is not a "magic bullet." Post-training audits should be done in the same way that they should be conducted for traditional training methods. Staff's proficiency with the actual system, their comfort in using the system, and their perception of the training experience are among the important post-training parameters to measure.

Summary

Potent forces are combining to mandate the installation of clinical systems to control costs, to promote quality of care, and to support the provision of a variety of health services to patients in many different settings (Corum, 1994; Johnson, 1994; Witonsky, 1994; Zielstorff, Hudgings, Grobe, and the NCNIP Task Force on Nursing Information Systems, 1993). New, more efficient, and cost-effective ways must be found to ease the burden of training employees to use these systems. CBT, effectively developed and deployed, is a promising means to this end.

References

Axford, R. L. (1988). Implementation of nursing computer systems: A new challenge for staff development departments. Journal of Nursing Staff Development, 4(3), 125-130.

Bolesta, R. G., Andersen, S. C., and Zeni, M. E. (1988). Planning for success in systems implementation: Key factors in the conversion equation. In R. A. Greenes (Ed.), Proceedings of the 12th Annual Symposium on Computer Applications in Medical Care (pp. 848-852). New York: IEEE Computer Society Press.

Bush, A. M. P. (1993). Computer-based training: Training approach of choice. Computers in Nursing, 11, 163-164.

Computer-based training gains convert. (1993, November). Healthcare Informatics, 29.

Corum, W. (1994, January). JCAHO standards & systems integration: Five years & counting down. Healthcare Informatics, 22-28.

Coulon, A. (1993, November). Automated training for system users. Healthcare Informatics, 28-29.

Downie, C., and Basford, P. (1991). How to use computer-based training. Nursing Times, 87(37), 63.

Farrel, A. (1988, February). Computer-based training: Support for cost containment and productivity. Healthcare Computing & Communications, 42-43.

Flaugher, P. D. (1986). Computer training for nursing personnel: Suggestions for training sessions. Computers in Nursing, 4, 105-108.

Froiland, P. (1993, October). Who's getting trained? Training, The Human Side of Business, 53-64.

Gery, G. (1987). Making CBT Happen. Boston, MA: Weingarten Publications.

Hospitals seek cost-effective training. (1991, May). Nursing & Technology, 4-5.

Johnson, G. (1994, January). Computer-based patient record systems: A planned evolution. Healthcare Informatics, 42, 44, 46, 48, 50, 51.

Kelly, J. (1991). High-tech teach-in. Nursing Times, 87(48), 59-60.

Mast M. E., and Van Atta, M. J. (1986). Applying adult learning principles in instructional module design. Nurse Educator, 11, 35-39.

Merrow, S. L. (1991). Factors associated with effective and cost efficient computer training for hospital staff nurses. In E. J. S. Hovenga, K. J. Hannah, K. A. McCormick, and J. S. Ronald (Eds.), Nursing Informatics '91: Proceedings of the Fourth International Conference on Nursing Use of Computers and Information Science (pp. 479-483). Berlin: Springer-Verlag.

Messmer, P. R., Kurtyka, D., and Kelley, C. P. (1992). A theory-based computer training program. Journal of Nursing Staff Development, 8(3), 136-138.

Perez, L. D., and Willis, P. H. (1989, July). CBT product improves training quality at reduced cost. Computers in Healthcare, 28-30.

Schulman, J. (1989, September). Getting your feet wet with CBT: How to keep the process orderly. Interactive Technologies: Supplement to Training, 19-22.

Systems failures. (1992). Nursing Times, 88(22), 19.

The shadow knows. (1989, September). Interactive Technologies: Supplement to Training, 11.

Tiano, J. J., and White, A. H. (1990). Effective training of nursing staff enhances hospital information system efficiency. Journal of Continuing Education in Nursing, 21, 257-259.

Witonsky, C. (1994, January). Healthcare reform and its impact on information systems. Healthcare Informatics, 18-20.

Zielstorff, R. D., and Altshuler, S. S. (1992). A computer-based tutorial for H.I.S. orientation: Laboratory results retrieval. In M. E. Frisse (Ed.), Proceedings of the 16th Annual Symposium on Computer Applications in Medical Care (pp. 953-955). New York: McGraw-Hill Book Co.

Zielstorff, R. D., Heller, E. E., Fitzmaurice, J., Ives, J., Millar, S. (1991). Costs and benefits of traditional vs. computer-based training for H.I.S. orientation. Nursing Economic$ 9, 444-447.

Zielstorff, R. D., Hudgings, C. I., Grobe, S. J. and the NCNIP Task Force on Nursing Information Systems. (1993). Nursing Information Systems: Essential Characteristics for Professional Practice. Washington, DC: American Nurses Association. Pub. No. NP-83.

Strategies and Support for Managing Clinical Information

The Computer-Based Patient Record 138

Technology and Case Management 144

Information Systems to Measure the Cost/Quality of
Patient-Centered Outcomes 153

Using the Computer to Measure Outcomes of Nursing Care 167

Electronic Networking for Nurses 174

New Electronic Health Care Community. The Denver
Free-Net 181

Quality Improvement via Clinical Information Systems 193

The Computer-Based Patient Record

D. Kathy Milholland, PhD, RN
Senior Policy Fellow, Research and Databases
Department of Practice, Economics and Policy
American Nurses Association

Barbara R. Heller, EdD, RN, FAAN
Professor and Dean
School of Nursing
University of Maryland at Baltimore

Introduction

As demands for access to patient data continue to grow, soon traditional record-keeping and information management practices of the health care industry will no longer suffice. Computer-based patient records (CPR) are a recognized solution to this problem, yet despite more than 30 years of research, development and implementation of computer systems in health-care settings, the majority of patient records continue to be paper-based. Such a time lag is incompatible with survival in the 21st century. If the health care industry is to succeed, nurse management must have available up-to-the minute financial and patient data.

The computer technology to render these data available to nurse managers is now available. Already, entrepreneurs and developers have created or are now designing systems to support every conceivable application to patient records.

CPR is here, and the only acceptable level of quality, say those who have been charting a course back to competitive excellence, is 100 percent. Such a goal will require the total utilization of CPR as soon as possible. In recent years, the issue of health care quality has become a growing national concern, and the industry is facing increasing pressure to measure the effectiveness and efficiency of care. Providers, practitioners, employers, unions, insurance companies, and government regulators express an interest in "quality of care" for various reasons. Computerization of the patient record should support patient care and improve quality.

The current concern for "quality" is so great that various agencies are now regulating quality in health care. The Health Care Financing Administration contracts with Peer Review Organizations to monitor and control the quality of care provided to Medicare recipients. The National Practitioner Data Bank maintains and offers selected access to the history of malpractice and professional misbehavior by physicians and other health care practitioners. The Joint Commission for the Accreditation of Healthcare Organizations (JCAHO) surveys and accredits hospitals and other providers. Since 1990, the JCAHO uses "quality" standards in the accreditation process. State Health Departments issue licenses for all health care facilities.

According to Richard Davidson, President of the American Hospital Association, some large metropolitan medical centers now have more than four million patient records, which must be stored for up to 25 years, depending on state laws (Davidson, 1992). Because the majority of patient records are currently kept on paper, they are clumsy to access, vulnerable to error and misplacement, and are often illegible. As a result, duplication of these records is common and decision-making is painfully slow.

This was of little concern in earlier times when patients were treated by one health care provider. Today, the delivery of health care is highly specialized; different kinds of care have emerged, including ambulatory care, emergency care, and preventive care. Elimination of fragmented information distributed among various health care providers can help all practitioners reach a whole new level of productivity.

Studies indicate that on average, previous patient records are unavailable at least 30 percent of the time. As a result, in perhaps 70 percent of emergency room situations, the emergency room staff has no information on the bleeding patient in front of them, at a time when seconds count.

The purpose of this chapter is to discuss the CPR: what it is, and which attributes potentiate its success; its benefits in general and for nursing in particular; and some strategies for preparing staff for this rapidly developing practice technology.

Definition of Computer-Based Patient Records

Computer-based patient records can be defined as an electronic patient record which resides in a computer system specifically designed to support users by providing: accessibility to complete and accurate data, clinical alerts, reminders, clinical decision-support systems, links to health-care knowledge, and other aids (Institute of Medicine, 1991). CPR is envisioned as enabling the development of a longitudinal, comprehensive health care record which will provide access to important clinical, financial, and research data. Therefore, more efficient and effective health care will be possible through: (1) collection, maintenance and universal access to lifetime health data on a timely basis; (2) support for continuous quality improvement in health care; (3) ready access to knowledge bases for clinical practice, administration, education and research; and (4) enabling patient participation in health status documentation, wellness, and disease prevention (Computer-based Patient Record Institute, 1992). This vision of CPR extends beyond automation of the current paper-based patient record. Automation of record retrieval, maintenance and use are insufficient. Rather, the CPR must meet the expanding information needs of the health care environment now and into the future.

The traditional content components of the paper—based record (history, physical, plan of care, and test results), are part of the CPR. However, the technology and design of CPR offers additional attributes which assure its success:
- Complete and accurate data and a patient problem list are available at all times to all authorized users.
- The record contains practitioner-oriented clinical reminders and alerts of adverse patient conditions that need to be addressed. Clinical practice guidelines that inform the caregiver of the best and most effective treatments for particular conditions will be easily and readily accessible.
- Decision analysis tools to determine the best course of action for the practitioner to take, along with an assessment of the risks involved, and the probability of risk for the individual patient are available.
- The computerized record provides links to local and remote scientific knowledge, literature, bibliographic, and administrative data bases.
- A lifelong record of an individual's health events is maintained. In other words, a record that encompasses all health care encounters across all settings and across all providers from the time an individual is born through his/her death is available.
- Selective retrieval and formatting of health care information by caregivers with custom-tailored "views" of information which meet each caregiver's unique needs is provided.
- The CPR supports video, graphics, electronic mail, voice, and other technological ad-

vancements as they occur in addition to the recording of text.

• Detailed patient records are transmitted reliably across long distances while maintaining confidentiality, thus assuring access whenever and wherever the patient may be.

Benefits of Computer-Based Patient Records

The patient record of the future is certain to have many more users than it has at present. Then, the needs of all users will be met to an extent not possible with current record systems. The benefits of CPRs are numerous, reducing administrative costs, enhancing health care research, and most significantly, improving patient care.

Administrative costs, too, are reduced by CPRs through a variety of means. These include:

• *Reduced redundant data entry.* This means that once data are entered, such data are immediately available to all who need it. Staff have more time, errors are fewer, and information more timely.

• *Electronic claims submission.* Requests for payment from third-party payers are rapidly transmitted, along with checking for format and content errors. Paperwork is reduced as fewer claims are rejected for clerical errors.

• *Improved risk management.* Information about errors of commission and omission, delays in treatment, and adverse events are available on-line as soon as recorded (manually by provider or automatically by an interfaced system). CPR provides the ability to investigate individual occurrences and evaluate aggregate statistics. Trends can be identified early and preventive actions instituted. Even more importantly, CPR reduces the incidence of adverse situations through its ability to apply error-checking algorithms to almost every aspect of patient care (e.g., medication ordering and administration, evaluation of risk for *patient falls.*

• *Reduced malpractice premiums.* The timely availability of critical patient data, the integration of practice guidelines into decision support capabilities, and the improved quality of documentation provide incentives for insurance carriers to lower their premiums.

• *Reduced storage space.* CPR technology allows for electronic storage of the entire patient record, including the lifetime health record for all patients who receive treatment in a health care facility. Electronic storage (e.g., computer disks) is more compact, thereby saving on physical space required.

• *Faster retrieval time.* Because data and information are stored electronically, recall of those data are rapid, seldom calling for additional personnel. That is, the person requiring the data can ask for it directly and get it immediately. Only in the case of off-line records (e.g., those saved from pre-CPR times), would additional assistance be necessary. Thus, CPRs contribute to savings in time and staff resources.

• *Improved provider productivity.* Health care information is rapidly available, without unnecessary duplication, on demand. Providers can spend their time in patient care or related activities, not in retrieving data. Additionally, the decision support and data analysis features of CPR means that the time spent thinking about patient care problems and solutions is more productive because the information is correct, comprehensive, and quickly available.

• *Provision of financial decision-support.* The wealth of health care delivery information in the CPR can be linked with the costs associated with that care delivery. Product line performance, case-mix and variance analysis provide managers with information for daily and long-term planning. CPR technology enables these data to be retained as long as necessary and to incorporate new decision-support tools as they are developed.

• *Closer connections between provider and patient.* By providing rapid access to all health care data, the provider and the patient can spend their time together discussing treatment plans and the patient's response to treatment instead of once again collecting patient history.. Direct access to the CPR from a variety of locations enables providers to discuss the patient's problems knowledgeably at any time. Also, viewing the information along with the provider gives the patient a stronger sense of mutual participation in the health care process.

Health care research, too, is greatly enhanced by the CPR. Research may focus on patient problems (illness, responses to health problems), delivery of health care (practitioners, systems) or outcomes of care (individuals, groups, the public health). The CPR, because it contains data from individual practitioner-patient encounters, entire treatment or illness episodes, and information on a person's health over his/her lifetime, offers a wealth of information for researchers. For example, patient outcomes might be studied in the context of lifestyle, environmental, or hereditary factors. Practice pattern analysis can be done within an institution or for individual practitioners in the community. Longitudinal studies are much easier when the data are collected and stored in the CPR. Results of clinical and health systems research can be used to refine existing practice guidelines and to develop new ones.

As noted, CPR benefits are most significant for the patient.

• *CPRs improve quality of care.* The CPR positively affects quality of patient care via increased access to patient health data and more specifically by the ability to integrate information over time and between care settings.

• *CPRs provide access to health care knowledge and decision support.* Patient data is readily accessible to health care practitioners, i.e., physicians, nurses, therapists. Access to health care knowledge and decision support includes such items as external references and full-text literature, research outcomes, and up-to-date treatment guidelines for illnesses.

• *CPRs eliminate duplicate tests and diagnostic workups.* A patient problem list is available at all times to all authorized users thereby reducing the need for repeat lab tests, and x-rays.

• *CPRs reduce delays in obtaining test results.* Patient data is readily accessible to health care practitioners because of real-time or "as it's happening" updates.

• *CPRs enhance clinical decision-making capabilities.* Health care practitioners are able to instantly retrieve, display, and synthesize whatever information would be most useful in making clinical decisions. Data can be accessed via anatomical part, body system, specialty, date, symptom, or problem, or any combination of variables.

• *CPRs focus on wellness and disease prevention.* The CPR provides an opportunity to gather data on diet, environment and lifestyle with the ability to link these data to health outcomes. This enables practitioners to address health maintenance issues with their patients.

• *CPRs provide linkages of protocols, patient information and health care knowledge.* Such linkages provide a true patient care *management* system. These linkages allow the computer to suggest additional tests to confirm diagnoses and recommend treatment plans that have the highest success rate on patients with similar conditions.

• *CPRs improve communication between providers.* All CPR users have immediate access to patient information via integration of data from various health care settings (i.e., inpatient hospitalization, outpatient testing or therapy, and provider offices), if they have the appropriate security or "rights" to the information.

• *CPRs organize patient data.* The CPR utilizes a consistent format for terminology and record content, yet allows users to custom-tailor their retrieval and formatting of information.

• *CPRs provide timely data capture.* The CPR ensures that data and information are captured while events are occurring.

√ Implications for Nursing

The use of computer-based patient records will have significant impacts on the practice and profession of nursing. The content of the patient record determines to a great extent what a profession is known for; i.e., what it does. The patient record influences payment for services, assessment of quality, allocation of resources, policy development and so forth. To realize its full potential, the profession of nursing needs to be able to name what it does in a consistent and reliable fashion (American Nurses Association, 1992). Already, much progress has been made in this direction. In fact, nursing is one of the few professions to have identified a minimum data set—the Nursing Minimum Data Set (Werley and Lang, 1988).

The American Nurses Association Steering Committee on Databases to Support Clinical Nursing Practice recognizes nursing vocabularies for incorporation into a unified nursing language system (UNLS). The elements of the UNLS provide the basis for defining core data elements of the CPR which will reflect nursing practice. These nursing vocabularies include: the diagnoses of the North American Nursing Diagnoses Association (NANDA, 1992), Saba's Home Health Care Classification (Saba, 1992), the Omaha System (Martin and Scheet, 1992), and the Nursing Interventions Classification (Bulechek and McCloskey, 1992).

In addition to fostering the naming of what we do, the advent of CPR has implications for nursing productivity and improved clinical decision making. Nursing productivity is enhanced through reduced documentation time, rapid access to information, a restructured nursing report process that provides essential information to all staff simultaneously, better workload analyses and more appropriate assignments. When the nurse manager has access to the care requirements of all patients in her/his domain, these data can be linked with information about care providers. The unit cost for specific treatments and nursing interventions can be identified and analyzed. The impact of nursing diagnoses on length of stay and other cost parameters are rapidly assessable. Knowing the care requirements and knowing the care providers available allows the nurse manager to make patient care assignments with more insight.

Clinical decision-making also is enhanced with the CPR. Nurses can function as data analysts, not data clerks. CPR supports electronic collection of data from multiple devices, as well as reducing the entry of redundant data. The integrated patient data base means that there is better coordination of care. All providers know what the plan of care is and what has been achieved. Decision support tools at the point of care enable nurses to analyze, plan and implement appropriate interventions. Point-of-care access to knowledge resources, including full-text articles, provides each practicing nurse with the most current information. Access to such information is necessary to meet the demands of complex patient care situations.

Strategies for Preparing Staff

What can be done to prepare individual nurses or nursing units for the fully envisioned CPR? A variety of activities can be started now. Nurse managers can:

• Work to assure that nursing is well-represented on all committees that address information management. The current JCAHO standards require that the Chief Nursing Officer or a delegate be a participating member of an institution's executive level information systems committee. Nurse managers and staff must participate in similar committees at their organizational level.

• Encourage staff to "own" their current and future information systems. This can be done by encouraging staff to be involved in selection, implementation and evaluation of the system. Make sure that staff members have a real voice in the decisions that will affect them.

• Provide staff education, beginning now, on CPR concepts through formal and informal classes, newsletters, discussion groups and other techniques.

• Analyze the current clinical information management processes in your institution with the goal of improving the existing manual processes. Identify what processes need to be kept or discarded.

In addition, nurse managers can become involved in national groups working to achieve that vision of the CPR, and can encourage their staff to also become involved. The Computer-based Patient Record Institute (CPRI) is a leader in this arena. CPRI has several work groups which are addressing issues such as coding systems, criteria for evaluating a CPR, confidentiality and privacy, and education of the public and health care professions. CPRI publishes a newsletter to keep members and interested parties apprised of progress and CPR events.

A total CPR is still mostly a vision, but this is a concept whose time has come. Significant progress is being made through current technologies, technologies that are improving all the time. CPR is truly a multi-disciplinary, multi-professional, multi-user project. With imagination, commitment and patience, the CPR will be the keystone of modern health care.

Summary

The problems of the predominantly paper-based patient record are identified and used as a foundation for explaining the emergence of the CPR. The CPR is defined and attributes of the CPR which ensure its success are identified. CPR benefits, such as reducing administrative costs, enhancing health care research, and improving patient care, are discussed. Implications of the CPR for nursing, the major health care discipline involved in collecting and managing health care information, are delineated. Several strategies for preparing staff for the fully envisioned CPR are provided.

References

American Nurses Association. (1992). *National Databases to Support Clinical Nursing Practice.* Train the Trainer Consultation Development Workshop. Washington, DC: Author.

Bulechek, G., and McCloskey, J. (1992) *Nursing Interventions Classification (NIC).* St. Louis: Mosby-Yearbook, Inc.

Computer-based Patient Record Institute. (1992). *Membership Brochure.* Chicago: Author.

Davidson, R. (1992, November-December). Computerized patient records. CPR—The key to health reform. *Health Systems Review,* 18-22.

Institute of Medicine. (1991). *The Computer-Based Patient Record. An Essential Technology for Health Care.* Washington, DC: National Academy Press.

Martin, K. S., and Scheet, N. J. (1992). *The Omaha System: Applications for Community Health Nursing.* Philadelphia: W. B. Saunders Co.

Saba, V. K. (1992). The classification of home health care nursing diagnoses and interventions. *Caring, 11*(3), 50-57.

Werley, H., and Lang, N. (1988). The consensually derived nursing minimum data set: Elements and definitions. In H. Werley and N. Lang (Eds.), *Identification of the Nursing Minimum Data Set* (pp. 402-413). New York: Springer Publishing Co.

Technology and Case Management

Roy L. Simpson, RN, C
Executive Director, Nursing Affairs
HBO and Company
Atlanta, Georgia

Carol Falk, MS, RN
Professional Nurse, Case Management
Carondelet St. Mary's Hospital and Health Center
Tucson, Arizona

Introduction

In an age of health care reform, skyrocketing costs, an aging population and ever more acutely ill patients, case management is becoming an increasingly popular strategy for coordinating health care. In fact, many in the health care professions view case management as an increasingly viable strategy to help improve quality and contain costs.

The American Nurses' Association defines nurse management as a process of care that includes assessing, delivering, coordinating, and monitoring services and resources to assure that patient needs are met. More specifically, case management can be defined as a clinical system that focuses on the accountability of an identified individual or group for coordinating the care of one or more patients across a continuum; ensuring and facilitating the achievement of quality, clinical and cost outcomes; negotiating, procuring and coordinating services and resources needed by the patient/family; intervening at key points (and/or at significant variances) for individual patients; addressing and resolving patterns in aggregate-variances that have a negative quality-cost impact; and creating opportunities and systems to enhance outcomes. In other words, when it involves nursing care, nurse case management is the process of assessing a patient's needs and then coordinating and integrating the appropriate health and supporting services over a period of time.

The goal of case management is care over the continuum. Care delivered and tracked beyond the walls of the acute care facility requires an immense amount of information management. Indeed, managing patient care over the continuum means managing a wealth of information, a task that can be accomplished only through information technology. However, most existing health care information systems are based on "event" management episodes rather than care over the continuum. Emerging technologies such as the information superhighway and the electronic patient record promise to bring case management to a more sophisticated and effective level.

This chapter reviews the basic components of case-managed care in the guise of a community-based model and reviews the technological requirements necessary for achieving the true vision of case management.

Community-Based Case Management

Nurse case managers trace their origins to public health nurses from the turn of this century and to models of case management that began within the discipline of social work (Lamb, 1992). Since the mid-1970s, nurses, social workers, and others have used case management to increase client participation in preventive services and, more recently, to gain Medicaid reimbursement for traditional services offered under new funding guide-lines (Erkel, 1993). There are three major models of nurse case management: (1) hospi-tal-based case management, in which individual nurses or teams of nurses ease transitions across units within the hospital for high-risk individuals (typically does not extend beyond the hospital walls); (2) hospital-to community models, in which case managers work with patients moving from acute care to long-term care settings; and (3) community-based models, in which nurse case managers work with individuals primarily in their homes and other community settings (Lamb, 1992). The community-based model is increasingly be-coming a point of focus for caregivers who wish to have a long-lasting impact not only on patient care, but on quality of care, patient quality of life and overall cost containment.

The Carondelet Health Care Model

The Carondelet St. Mary's model of community-based nurse case management was insti-tuted in 1985 in response to the nursing profession's concern over reduced length of hos-pital stays and the need to coordinate nursing services in the hospital with other programs across the care continuum. In the model of nurse case management used at Carondelet, located in Tucson, Arizona, nurse case managers establish short or long-term relation-ships with clients unrelated to a particular health care setting. Intensity and length of the nurse-client relationship vary based on client need. Goals for each client are individualized and mutually determined, often with interdisciplinary input.

At Carondelet, nurse case management emphasizes the importance of empowering in-dividuals to maximize self-care capabilities and to continue to develop their potential for well-being. Stimulus for the program has included: (1) cost containment; (2) the need to coordinate the transition from inpatient to outpatient services; (3) the increasing shift to ambulatory services; and (4) the appropriate use of health care services.

The difference between mainstream, hospital-based health care models and the case management model is the difference between restorative care and maintenance/preven-tive care. In today's economic climate where the average length of stay in a hospital is 4.2 days, health providers have little time to do more than initiate health restoration. Nurse case management at Carondelet focused on "Wings of the Community"—care beyond the acute illness episode or hospitalization stay—to help patients recover, convalesce or cope with a chronic illness.

Carondelet's target populations included those patients with chronic illnesses, those who temporarily needed community services for recovery from acute illness, and those who required support in coping with terminal illnesses. Clients with the following charac-teristics were specifically targeted: high recidivism; medically complex, frail individuals; chronically ill, terminally ill; cost and/or length of stay outliers.

Shifting the focus on these types of clients from health restoration episodes to health maintenance or health promotion involved three primary goals:

1. **Quality**
   Client-focused process
   Enhance quality of care
   Emphasize quality of life issues
   Needs response model (match client's needs with resources available)
   Match services to needs
2. **Access**
   Maximize access
   Enhance provider continuity
   Appropriate resource utilization

Figure 1.
The Nursing Network

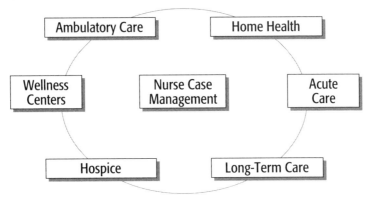

Reprinted with permission of Carondelet St. Mary's Hospital and Health Center, Tucson, AZ

3. Cost

Cost effectiveness: For user, provider, payor

From an illness model to a health/wellness model

Care over the continuum

These goals are highly integrated. For example, in working with patients to educate and inform them about their disease process, many are empowered to take greater responsibility for their health and initiate accessibility into the health care system earlier, at a lower acuity level. Lower acuity means the use of fewer resources, resulting in cost containment.

At some point in the development of a case management program, administrators at most institutions or organizations struggle with the task of determining who is the best case manager for each patient. Professionals in different disciplines may vie for the position of being the patient's or client's *point person*. To solve this problem, the Carondelet model made a decision to place nurse case managers into the community because these professionals were trained to perform thorough physical assessments and could provide greater value in patient education and monitoring.

Integrating Nursing Services into a Network.

√ Carondelet developed a professional nursing network, based on a nursing and health care delivery model, using the environmental resources of both the Carondelet system and the broader local community. Nurse case managers form the central core of the professional nursing network. The components of the model and the flow of interactive relationships are shown in Figure 1.

The various components of the network were designed to create an integrated system of nursing care in which nurses maintain accountability for cost-effective, access to care, and quality of care. The network links services across settings and positions professional nurse case managers to move with clients throughout the network. Other disciplines are incorporated into the network when indicated for individual clients.

The professional nursing network model extended beyond institutional boundaries to include community-based services. Community Health Centers were established as an outreach program for the assessment and evaluation of health needs of older adults. The nurse-run centers provide services such as health status evaluation, health screening, education and referral.

Carondelet refers to the nursing network as a "dancing relationship." For example, when a client is in a hospital, the acute care nurse and all other acute care players become the client's partners. When the client moves to another level of service, such as home health or long-term care, those providers become the client's partners. In cases where the patient is at home but does not qualify for home health care, a case manager is called on the patient's behalf to provide some care. Also, the case manager can help gather documentation to give review processors the information that the patient may need to qualify for home health care status.

As part of its program, Carondelet developed community health centers in volunteer agencies, libraries, banks and other buildings, staffed by seven nurse practitioners. The goal was to offer free, intermittent services such as health screenings, health monitor and illness prevention education for patients who had left the acute care facility with the need of any additional nursing or health care services.

This holistic approach in working with clients across the continuum involved *collaboration,* in terms of establishing an initial partnership in response to the goals of the client; honoring the client's *choice* in regard to compliance (as long as the client understands the consequences of his or her choice); *patterns* of decisions and choices, of utilization and of lifestyle and health choices/outcomes.

Benefits of the Community-Based Case Management Program

Evaluation of the Carondelet program suggests that nurse case management has a direct impact on increased client satisfaction, decreased hospital admissions and emergency department visits, decreased costs and acuity of hospital stay, minimized hospital revenue loss, increased job satisfaction for nurses and decreased job stress for nurses. In a study of hospital utilization patterns of 270 high-risk seniors receiving care within the Carondelet case management program, more than 50 percent experienced fewer hospitalizations and shorter lengths of stay following the introduction of nurse case management and other nursing services (Ethridge, 1991). Total savings continue to be tracked by Carondelet as hundreds of patients receive the education to assume more responsibility for their health care and well-being. Overall, the program brought clients into the system earlier, resulting in shorter lengths of stay while simultaneously improving quality and efficiency.

Nursing literature offers little research on the topic of case management results, although some research has been documented. For example, in one study addressing cost effectiveness of case management in preventive services, Buescher, Roth, Williams, and Goforth (1991) found that for each dollar spent for maternity care coordination services among Medicaid women, $2.02 was saved in costs of infant medical care beginning within 60 days of birth (p. 1625). Buescher et al. (1991) estimated that Medicaid saved more than $2 million in North Carolina during 1988 and 1989, when only 31 percent of eligible pregnant women on Medicaid received case management.

Studies measuring the effectiveness of case management in community mental health settings revealed that community mental health clients receiving case management used more community services than those not receiving case management (Bigelow and Young, 1991; Borland, McRae, and Lycan, 1989; Franklin, Solvitz, Mason, Clemons, and Miller, 1987; Goering, Wasylenki, Farkas, Lancee, and Ballantyne, 1988; McRae, Higgens, Lycan, and Sherman, 1990). This would indicate an improvement in client quality of life, which would consequently lead to fewer hospitalizations. Another study suggested that case management improves adherence to agreed-upon service plans and medication regimens among adults with severe psychiatric disabilities

(Bush, Langford, Rosen, and Gott, 1980).

In studies of hospitalized patients in acute care settings, case management appears to be cost effective. Results from a case management program at New England Medical Center Hospitals with ischemic stroke and adult leukemia patients suggest that case management decreases the average length of stay and, consequently, overall costs related to the patient (Zander, 1988). The literature, then indicates that the greatest economic contribution case managed care can make to a hospital is cost savings through reduced lengths of stays.

Case Management and The Technological Challenge

While changing to some degree, case management is still largely managed through a manual, labor-intensive process. In other words, case management as a viable form of coordinating care across the continuum has continued to grow without much help from information technology. Today, nurse case managers use existing systems for assistance with documentation, order management and, in some cases, patient education.

The reason information technology has been limited to these functions is that most information technology in use today is episodic-oriented or transaction-based (i.e., one order here, one charge there). If information technology is to meet all the needs of a comprehensive case management program, certain advancements will be required, including a *common nursing language, a longitudinal electronic patient record (serving as a common data base), intuitive (i.e., easy) technology and a pervasive information network*. Information technology is moving rapidly in these areas, and some predict that many of these breakthroughs will be available within the next 5 to 10 years.

As the profession of nursing becomes more involved in the development and management of these emerging technologies, more and more researchers, too, have become involved in the science of nursing informatics, which has been defined as follows: "The combination of computer science, information science and nursing science designed to assist in the management and processing of nursing data, information and knowledge to support the practice of nursing and the delivery of nursing care." (Graves and Ozbolt, 1993, p. 407).

Clinical nursing informatics has also been described as dealing with theories and processes of clinical reasoning and the management of uncertainty in clinical nursing practice (Lange, 1993).

The Nursing Barrier: Lack of a Common Language

Probably the single most pronounced barrier to effective case management software is the lack of a common nursing language or nursing minimum data set. Nursing is the primary focal point for most clinical documentation, yet the profession as a whole has yet to come to an agreement about a universal nursing minimum data set. Computers work in absolutes, so "X" must always mean "X," and "Y" must always mean "Y"; otherwise the computer cannot "compute." However, the profession of nursing seems to be in a constant state of argument about what "X" or "Y" means precisely, whether that argument is across units, across organizations or across academic research centers.

According to Graves and Ozbolt (1993),

It is the absence of codified data that has inhibited the inclusion of nursing information in the *various discharge abstract databases* on which health policy decisions are increasingly based. Only the clinician knows practice well enough to understand how clinical problems are represented, described, and solved. Only the clinician schooled in informatics knows how to represent clinical problems in a computer system so that computer support of diagnosis, treatment and evaluation of treatment follows the natural flow of practice. (pp. 411, 416)

The adoption of a nursing minimum data set is probably the most important step in the advancement of nursing technology and, in particular, nursing case management technology. Case managers must be able to access data bases regarding patient status, physician orders, nursing diagnoses and other patient information across institutions to be able to effectively manage patient care and education across the continuum.

Longitudinal Electronic Patient Records

Despite the rapid advancements in technology during the last two decades, today's patient records continue to be predominantly paper-based. Patient records remain primarily the domain of nursing and would serve as a key means of communicating patient status and needs in a case-managed environment.

Since the early 1990s, the Institute of Medicine (IOM) has been advocating that computer-based-patient records be established by the year 2000. Such computerized patient records would have a unique potential to improve the care of both individual patients and populations and, concurrently, reduce waste through continuous quality improvement (Simpson, 1991, p. 22).

Currently, the IOM and its various committees are developing standards for a computerized patient record that would support users through availability of complete and accurate data, practitioner reminders and alerts, clinical decision support systems, links to bodies of medical knowledge, and other aids (Simpson, 1991, p. 22). This vision would move patient records and information technology in use today from episodic management of events to providing a fluid, continuously updated, longitudinal account of patient care. The goal of the IOM is to have electronic patient records available by the end of the decade.

Clearly, a longitudinal account of care or patient record would assist the nursing case manager in significant ways. It would be the difference between piecing together limited "snapshots" of care episodes over a limited period of time, and watching a moving film of the patient's status over long periods of time and over the continuum of care throughout various institutions and, perhaps in the future, over the continuum of a patient's life.

Intuitive, Easy-to-use Systems

If future systems are to be effectively used at all levels of nursing practice, particularly in "the field" for case managers, they must be flexible, fast, intuitive and extremely easy-to-use. Technology cannot require that nurses spend days or weeks in training to master fundamental principles of its use. In the 1970's when the first information systems were introduced, three to four weeks were required to orient nurses to the technology. In the early 1990's, however, that time frame has dropped to a matter of hours (four to eight) in brief training sessions. Time spent on learning new technology will continue to drop, with the goal that future systems will be so intuitive, (i.e., easy to use), they would require *no* formal computer-training.

Technology will also play an increased role from the patient's point of view. Just as banking customers have become accustomed to using automated teller machines for basic banking transactions, it is predicted that within the next 10 years, health care patients will also be asked to "input" or report basic health statuses into patient-oriented computing systems. Patients would also have the option to "research" symptoms and disease states via networked computer systems, as well as communicate with practitioners, case managers and even other patients via an electronic bulletin board facility.

Because increased patient participation in using technology is expected within the next decade, information systems will have to be extraordinarily simple and easy-to-use. they will likely feature colorful graphic icons and touch screens or a mouse for easy navigation. Graphics and color will be employed to help users understand and interpret information, in summarized or highlighted form. Such information systems might also feature voice or sound alarms to remind patients and/or care givers about upcoming medical visits or schedules for taking medications or changing dressings. In all cases, nurse case managers would serve as the key focal points for advancing patient-oriented technology and networks.

A Pervasive Information Network

For technology to assist case management in profound ways, great advancements need to be made in connectivity and accessibility. This will occur at a point when society is able to support a pervasive information network.

A pervasive technology is one that is more noticeable by its absence than its presence, in just the way that automobiles, televisions and telephones are today (Simpson, 1994). Within the last few decades, most citizens of North America have become habituated to finding a telephone or television in most hotel rooms—yet in the future, they may find computers are "standard" too. Similarly, most patient rooms in hospitals today feature telephones and televisions; in the future, personal computers will also become standard.

It is important to keep in mind that only persons born before a technology is developed think of it as a "technology"—to others who are accustomed to it, it is merely part of the environment. For example, children in today's society do not consider the telephone or the television as "technology"—each is merely part of life—i.e., a technology that has become all-pervasive. In the future, computers will enjoy that same level of acceptance and "universality."

Medical applications in technology will never become pervasive because they require specialized training by a relatively small fraction of the population. An information network will become pervasive, however, linking patients, practitioners, case managers and institutions across town and across the country.

The development of a national information network was (and still is) a top priority. Commonly known as the "electronic superhighway," this network would allow nurse case managers to take nursing practice beyond the walls of the institution and into individual patient homes. In such a future, most homes would come equipped with a personal computer (just as most homes today come equipped with stoves and microwave ovens). Most apartment homes would provide computing network access, just as most provide cable access (indeed the cable access would serve as both cable and computer access as televisions evolve into featuring both interactive power and computing power). (Elmer-Dewitt, 1993). Some futurists also predict a time when there will be a "computer company," just as there is a telephone company today in each American community to serve the needs of its citizens. (Indeed they may be one and the same company because most computer networks are accessed via telephone networks.) Citizens would call the "computer company" to have their networks turned on, just they do now with other types of utility companies. In other words, it is predicted that there will be an " information utility" similar to today's telephone, gas or electric utility.

In a future in which computers are as ubiquitous as telephones and television sets, case-managed care across the continuum would become easier to implement and manage. Indeed, one can see the effectiveness of computer networks for group-managed care in early trials. Researchers at the Frances Payne Bolton School of Nursing at Case Western Reserve University studied the efficacy of computer networks to link AIDS patients with nurses and with each other, as well as linking Alzheimer's patient caregivers with nurses and with each other.

In the AIDS patients study, patients were supplied with computer terminals and modems and given 24-hour access to a central computer network. Using existing technology, patients were able to access a communications module which included a bulletin board through which they could "converse" with each other and with nurses; a decision support module which helped patients make daily living and self-care decisions; and an information module, a database filled with encyclopedic data about the disease (Simpson, 1994).

The "experiment" in linking patients with a case manager via a network was an unqualified success. Thirty-one of the AIDS participants in the study generated more than 10,000 accesses during the six-month test period. The typical user accessed the network 125 times, for an average of four to five times a week. Researchers found that patients enthusiastically "posted" encouraging messages on the bulletin board and freely shared ideas for self-care and managing the formal health system with other "networked" patients. From the nursing perspective, nurse managers also found it easier to disseminate information to patients and to reinforce patient education.

Clearly, early studies show that case-managed care with the help of computer networks will have a great impact on the quality of individual care. Through networked computers, nurses could have daily "contact" with patients for follow-up consultations, questions about medications, steps for patient follow-through, and so on, all without ever leaving the hospital or institution. Voice or sound computer-generated reminders or alarms could also be used to remind patients or family members about everything from taking insulin shots, to changing their dressings regularly and correctly, to keeping their appointment for their latest check-up. In return, the patient could report to the case manager unusual symptoms or ask questions over the same network.

The advent of an "information utility" featuring computer network access by a majority of the patient population is still perhaps about a decade away. In order for the electronic superhighway to be viable, however, the proper infrastructure must be in place. Networks must be plentiful, cheap and easy to access. Patients must have easy access to computers and modems or interactive televisions. And systems must be extraordinarily user-friendly so patients will feel comfortable in using the technology on a daily or frequent basis. Despite these challenges, it is clear that this is the direction in which information technology is moving. A global or universal network by its very definition requires an open, standards-based technology, whereby vendors do not limit access by proprietary technology and designated users can access the technology via the same standards, no matter what "make" or "model" they are using.

Summary

Case-managed care is clearly an evolutionary process. Today, leading nursing case management groups are proving that it is a viable and effective way to manage patients in a complex environment while improving quality, enhancing access and reducing overall costs. Current models of case management are primarily managed via a manual process. Yet the future of information technology—with an electronic patient record, universal network access and common databases—shows tremendous potential in fulfilling the true promise of case management for both nurses and patients.

References

Bigelow, D. A., and Young, D. J. (1991). Effectiveness of a case management program. *Community Mental Health Journal, 27*(2), 115-223.

Borland, A., McRae, J., and Lycan, C. (1989). Outcomes of five years of continuous intensive case management. *Hospital Community Psychiatry, 40*(4), 369-376.

Buescher, P. A., Roth, M. S., Williams, D., and Goforth, C. M. (1991). An evaluation of the impact of maternity care coordination on Medicaid birth outcomes in North Carolina. *American Journal of Pubic Health, 18*(12), 1625-1629.

Bush, C. T., Langford, M. W., Rosen, P., and Gott, W. (1990). Operation outreach: Intensive management for severely psychiatrically disabled adults. *Hospital Community Psychiatry, 41*(6), 647-649.

Elmer-Dewitt, P. (1993, April 12). Take a trip into the future on the electronic superhighway. *Time,* 50-55.

Erkel, E. (1993, January). The impact of case management in preventive services. *The Administration of Nursing Administration, 23*(1), 27-31.

Ethridge, R. A. (1991, July). Nursing HMO: Carondelet St. Mary's experience. *Nursing Management, 22*(7), 22-26.

Franklin, J. L., Solovitz, B., Mason, M., Clemons, J. R., and Miller, G. E. (1987). An evaluation of case management. *American Journal of Public Health, 77*(6), 674-678.

Goering, P. N., Wasylenki, D. A., Farkas, M., Lancee, W. J., and Ballantyne, R. (1988). What difference does case management make? *Hospital Community Psychiatry, 39*(3), 272-276.

Graves, J. R., and Ozbolt, J. G. (1993). Clinical Nursing Informatics—Developing Tools for Knowledge Workers. *Nursing Clinics of North America, 28*(2), 407-417.

Lamb, F. (1992). Conceptual and methodological issues in nurse case management research. *Advance Nursing Science, 15*(2), 16-24.

Lange, L. (1993, December). Clinical Informatics. Letter to the Division of Nursing.

McRae, J., Higgens, M., Lycan, C., and Sherman, W. (1990). What happens to patients after five years of intensive case management stops? *Hospital Community Psychiatry, 41*(2), 175-180.

Simpson, R. L. (1991, October). Computer-Based Patient Records. Part I: The Institute of Medicine's Vision. *Nursing Management,* 22-23.

Simpson, R. L. (1994). Computer networks show great promise in supporting AIDS patients. *Nursing Administration Quarter, 18*(2), 92-95.

Zander, K. (1988). Nurse case management: Strategic management of cost and quality outcomes. *Journal of Nursing Administration, 18*(5), 23-30.

Information Systems to Measure the Cost/Quality of Patient-Centered Outcomes

Alexis A. Wilson, MPH, RN
President, Wilson and Associates
Outcome Concept Systems
Gig Harbor, Washington

Introduction

In the current environment of health care reform, cost-containment, and renewed enthusiasm for quality assurance (QA), there is an accelerating effort to integrate information systems that will measure both the cost and quality of patient outcomes. While many software vendors, consultants, and would-be quality gurus often claim that they have all of the answers for health care information, measurement, and accountability problems, nurse managers should know some basic tenets to enable them to understand and select information systems. In addition, a thorough understanding of what patient outcomes are, how to factor in costs, as well as some of the differences between various information systems, is critical to the selection, use, and long-term utility of information systems to measure the cost and quality of outcome information.

Most nurse managers have little or no preparation for the information requirements to document, nor can they measure the impact of such services on patients' health status (patient outcomes). While nursing informatics is beginning to be a part of our professional language, few practitioners are comfortable using the required computer technology. Although it is not essential for nurse managers and administrators to immerse themselves in computer science and programming courses, a familiarity with basic computer language and how manual data systems feed into automated systems can make the difference between effective and ineffective information processing.

To date, very few systems are able to measure patient outcomes, let alone cost and quality; however, this situation is about to change as the 1990s usher in an era of health care reform, cost containment, a resurgence of attention to the concept of patient value, and new consumer attitudes.

This chapter begins with a discussion on information system technology and then reviews some basic information about computers as a part of overall information system development. The second section reviews patient outcome measurement theory and current trends in QA. Finally, two automated information systems currently available in home health care are introduced as examples of the possible use of information systems to measure cost/quality of patient outcomes. While most examples stem from the author's area of expertise in the home health care setting, the information presented is applicable throughout the health care continuum.

Information System Technology

Information system technology is rapidly becoming a major component of the health care industry. The complexity in automating health care documentation is that it is an extremely information-intensive industry. Computerized information systems are believed to result in an increase in the RN's productivity and to improve use of the RN's skills while providing appropriate documentation of nursing's contributions to the outcomes of care (Barry and Gibbons, 1990). The health care industry, in its efforts to seek ways to control costs, increase worker productivity and job satisfaction, improve service levels, decision making, and cash flow, and improve the quality of information to support quality of care and outcomes, has turned to computer assistance. Multiple studies are under development or in progress to examine the use of the computer, staff and the patient in relation to all of the above. The nursing profession faces a big challenge if it is to assume a leadership position to answer the financial, public policy and consumer questions about its own value relative to the outcomes of care received. If it does not, others will, which inadvertently will also define a significant portion of future nursing practice.

While Ball, O'Desky, and Douglas (1991) point out the tools which already exist in computer technology and promise to change the process of health care, such as voice activation, graphics, visualization, bar code technology, and specialized data bases, they apply caution in the area of outcome studies because outcomes cannot be studied unless inputs are well defined and carefully controlled.

Understanding Computers

A basic mistake often made by administrators and managers in a position to influence computer purchasing or design decision is the lack of understanding about exactly which tasks they want the computer to accomplish. Horror stories are often heard about the creation of information monsters within hospitals or other health settings, generally because someone in a decision-making position was sold (by an ambitious vendor, or management information system [MIS] specialist) a system that was quite incompatible with the information needs, or capability of the organization, much less the computer skills of individual staff members. Although many managers may be reluctant to admit it, they are often intimidated by computer professionals. This situation may lead them directly to a poor purchase, or to depend upon the sole expertise of the MIS department; in this process, they may overlook perhaps the practical components (and nursing input) for successful overall organizational implementation. Couple this with the already difficult concept of patient outcome measurement, the cost of nursing and multidisciplinary services, and the decision tree itself becomes impossible to articulate. By far, the best approach is to keep the process simple: break it down into manageable components. The key to the development and integration of a successful patient outcome measurement system is to gain insight into each component of information that needs to be captured, and to know what type of computer and software is needed to accomplish and maintain the task at hand.

For a typical large health care organization, the initial decision to go forward with an automated information system was probably made during the 1960s. Most likely, the architecture of the system was based on a large mainframe, supporting a network of terminals that were used to interact with a variety of data bases maintained on large disk drives. The primary applications of these systems were often financial, with ancillary systems created to support the financial systems. As information systems moved into the 1970s (Ball et al., 1991), many of the ancillary departments in hospitals, such as laboratory or radiology, justified the purchase of minicomputers for their departments. Since the mainframe and minicomputers were probably purchased from different manufacturers, the communication between the information systems was, and often still remains, a very difficult task.

To identify individual system needs, especially before tackling costs and patient outcomes, basic components of all information systems, at least in concept, must be mastered. This does not require advanced study; what is important is that the manager has a genuine interest in understanding the automated information needs of the organization or nursing department. The language of computers is not all that difficult; in fact, it is important to remember that computers are, by design, without content. They are only as intelligent as the person designing their software and supplying the computer with pieces of information (data). In other words, the old adage "garbage in-garbage out" is an accurate statement.

The first step in contemplating the purchase of computer technology is to evaluate the organization's current needs in a computer system. Once decision makers understand whether their organization's needs are multi-use (data base management, word processing, or so forth) versus single-use, how often it will be used, what type of work will be done with it, how powerful the needs are, whether employees need color (or just want it), whether the system needs to be portable or not, the next step is to match a computer system with those needs. Needs should be ranked by priority—what is absolutely necessary and what can be lived without. Remember that most computers are expandable, so that even if a model does not fit an organization's needs exactly, there will be an add-on component available.

Using Computerized Data Bases

Data collection can be an expensive and time-consuming process. Many hospitals have extremely large data bases, but they may not have the specificity of information to select the information desired in relation to cost, quality, or outcomes. Temple (1990) considers the problems and risks of using large data sets for outcome assessment, especially to assess effectiveness or to compare treatments. Essentially this interpretation is steeped in research theory, but it narrows down to the fact that data bases are retrospective and unblinded, and do not minimize a variety of kinds of bias especially patient selection bias and analyst bias. Kovner (1989), on the other hand, suggests that utilizing data collected and compiled into data bases for regulatory agencies, for patient care, for third-party payers, and for management, might be useful for nursing research and/or QA. Hegyvary (1991) states that measures which reflect outcomes are not comparable across institutional systems, and that the basic incompatibility among data bases and data systems points out the need for the nursing profession to achieve consensus on data elements to reflect nursing interventions.

Two well-recognized data bases that collect patient information based on nursing diagnosis are: (1) the North American Nursing Diagnosis Association (NANDA) (1989), and (2) The Classification Scheme for Client Problems in Community Health Nursing from the Visiting Nurse Association (VNA) of Omaha (1986). Currently, however, nursing diagnosis data cannot be aggregated across settings until the same nursing diagnosis classification scheme is agreed upon. Werley, Devine, Zorn, Ryan, and Westra (1991) encourage implementation of The Nursing Minimum Data Set to standardize the collection of essential nursing data, and suggest coding both the NANDA and Omaha systems to allow data collection from more settings. At basic issue here is the fact that no single classification system is widely used or universally accepted. The nursing profession must use caution in its insistence on the use of a nursing diagnosis-based classification system as the only mechanism to "give credit to" the profession's unique contribution, lest it lose sight of the proverbial forest for the trees.

The Center for Health Policy Research (CHPR) is a multidisciplinary health policy research organization which is developing an outcome measurement data collection instrument that is more oriented toward patient functional status than nursing diagnosis. The Health Care Financing Administration (HCFA) funded a five-year CHPR project beginning in 1988, to develop and test outcome-based measures, or indicators of quality, for

Medicare home health services. The measures that are developed may be considered for incorporation into Medicare's home health QA programs. CHPR's Study Paper 6 (Shaughnessy, 1991) documents progress in the development of a consolidated set of outcome measures, and the possibility of recommending a uniform data system for home health care. The measures developed may eventually be used by the Medicare Program, and if used, they will be tested as part of the empirical phase of the project. The project has outlined a specific array of outcome measures that can be evaluated to assess the quality of care provided for specific patient conditions.

Quality Assurance and Patient Outcomes

Before an effective information system to measure patient outcomes can be implemented, an understanding of the concepts of patient outcome-oriented information is necessary. The most basic concept about patient outcome measurement is to first have an understanding of what a patient outcome is. Typically, nursing is extremely focused on the process of nursing care rather than the outcome of the patient in relation to health status, knowledge, behavior, mental status, activities of daily living (ADLs), and overall satisfaction with services. If no method is in place to capture the outcomes of care in the current documentation, then no computer system is going to magically capture the outcomes of care on a computer screen. Furthermore, if no mechanism is in place to quantify the costs of nursing, or other ancillary services, there will be no primary basis of comparison for the cost of services once patient outcomes are achieved.

Quality Assurance Programs

Traditional programs of quality assurance are changing their focus to quality improvement (QI). QI often includes total quality management (TQM) and continuous quality improvement (CQI), which are concepts borrowed from industry and adapted to health care management. TQM and CQI have a broader focus than traditional QA programs in health care, providing a tighter link between organizational service, finance, management, and other components. Out of these concepts is arising a new "buzzword" in health care called outcomes management (OM). Conrad (1991) points out that where the emphasis of modern TQM is on "doing things right" the first time, OM is equally concerned with "doing the right thing." Therefore, ideally, the two concepts will be integrally related to focus on enhancing the health status of the populations served by health care organizations. Conrad further cites the challenge for organizational leadership to support information networks and interactive clinical-managerial structures that will produce, monitor, and act systematically on outcome information diffused rapidly throughout the institution. Donabedian (1993) outlines the differences and the similarities of the traditional health care model of quality with the adapted industrial model. He points out what can be learned, but concludes that adopting an oversimplified definition of quality could deflect attention from clinical effectiveness to the efficiency of supportive activities.

OM places emphasis on the word "management," and not measurement. Nash and Markson (1991) emphasize that OM will never be adequately summarized in a single statistic or quality score, and that the field involves more than the massive collection of data. While it is difficult to rationalize patient outcome measurement away from the actual patient outcomes documented (most likely through a statistic or quality score), it is apparent that this focus is geared to synthesizing and integrating the perspectives of researchers, payers, executives, and clinicians. Nash and Markson provide a comprehensive view of the perspectives of OM, from researchers, to regulatory agencies and clinical guidelines, to purchasers. In summary, they conclude that OM should be thought of as part of a tripod designed to support improved quality of care, that moves beyond the structure, process, and outcome evaluation established by Donabedian (1985). Citing a theory developed by Ellwood (1988), that an effective health outcomes management strategy could bring order to the health care system, the other legs of the tripod are a commitment to TQM and a willingness to abide by clinical guidelines. Jones (1993) builds on this theory at the macro-level across hospitals and at the micro-level with epidemiologic approaches. She concludes with a call for the need to design computer systems to track nursing interventions, costs, and outcomes attributable to nursing actions, and development of a minimum nursing data set.

Williamson (1988) proposed a philosophic approach for the systematic management of the quality of health care in the 1960s, which he called Health Accounting. With an emphasis on outcomes, yet recognizing Donabedian's structure, process, and outcome triad, Williamson suggested an initial focus on unacceptable outcomes or health problems with a deductive problem-solving inquiry to identify "correctable determinants." This is one of the earliest models of a problem-based approach to QA. Williamson also recognizes that the focus of QA activities cannot be restricted to available data sets such as medical records, and he stresses the principle that QA must start with individual and organizational values. In other words, the success of QA, QI, TQM, CQI, and/or OM is directly related to the internal motivation of the individual organization and persons involved.

One concept of OM has been designed by The New England Medical Center Hospital's Center for Nursing Case Management that examines relationships between tasks and outcomes, nursing case management by Diagnosis Related Grouping (DRG), physician collaboration, and managed care maps along timelines, critical paths, and variance analysis (Maturen and Zander, 1993). Maturen and Zander define case management as "a clinical system that focuses on the accountability of an identified individual or group for coordinating a patient's care; insuring and facilitating the achievement of quality, clinical and cost outcomes . . . ." DiJerome (1992) describes computerizing both the interdisciplinary team plan of care and critical pathways to develop standardized care plans in an inpatient setting. The critical pathway prioritizes, summarizes, and places time limits on all of the activities on the care plan. Desired patient outcomes are selected according to nursing diagnoses and printed out on a case management plan. Outcomes selected are goals that need to be met before discharge can occur, and are determined with consideration to the patient's health care needs and DRG length of stay limitations. Each goal has a time limit designed to keep the patient outcomes on track. Intermediate goals also give direction to nurses and other team members for choosing appropriate interventions. A critical path form serves as a worksheet to monitor the progress of the interventions and the patient's response to care. Rather than measuring the actual results of care, this method manages care outcomes by prospectively "mapping" the process of care to drive practitioner interventions through standardized care plans. Costs could be calculated in terms of days or visits. With this type of OM, discharge practices need to be closely monitored with analysis of variances.

Cuddeback (1993) appears to support this concept of quality and OM, noting that payers now want clinical data with much more detail. The payers of the past who received bills for services after care was provided, now want to confirm, in advance, the appropriateness of care. In information system development, he suggests building into the process of care, steps to make the system more attractive to purchasers.

Edison and Esmond (1991) identify the information requirements for assessing quality of care and outcomes as predominantly satisfaction from the perspective of the patient, the perceived value of care from the perspective of payers, and for providers, the relationship between the cost of care and the effectiveness of the care delivered. A model for outcome quality assessment is described to structure a methodology to assist in analyzing the care provided to groups of similar patients, with a second component to develop clinical profiles to quantify expectations for resource use and the quality of care delivery. The goal of the model, which was designed for physicians, is to effectively plan and price services to reduce uncertainty and reduce costs by eliminating inappropriate medical services.

OM, then, is closely linked with traditional QA to confirm quality in the process of care which can lead to more positive patient outcomes. The major difference between OM, TQM, and CQI and traditional QA is an expanded view that includes business, financial, and overall management components of a health care system, and this also includes a renewed interest in process of care documentation and monitoring systems. Outcome measurement, on the other hand, is the study of the relationship between patient care processes and outcomes to quantify cost effectiveness and to classify changes in patient health status.

Patient Outcome Classification

Lang and Marek (1990) provide an overview of efforts to classify patient outcomes, including a strong historical focus on the identification and use of outcomes within the nursing profession. The discussion reinforces the need for the inclusion of nursing data in the development of national data bases, the effectiveness of nursing care on patient outcomes, and entering nursing interventions into the reimbursement system. In the article, Lang and Marek also describe a pilot classification of outcomes, in an attempt to classify existing outcomes as found in the nursing literature. Marek (1993) has continued to build on this work in Nursing Sensitive Outcomes, which provides a comprehensive review of the past and present use of outcome measures in the evaluation of nursing care, examples of research, and a framework for outcomes research for nursing. This work identifies the need for consensus about the relationship of outcomes to process and structure variables, and the necessity of consensus about the naming of the variables among nurses in practice, research, and in organized nursing. Delaney (1992) reinforces the need for nursing management to use a minimum data set to capture nursing interventions and nurse-sensitive outcomes, which is discussed elsewhere in this book. A review of outcome measures in home care with a practice focus (Rinke and Wilson, 1987) provides a broad resource for developing outcome-oriented QA measures by: (1) an historical overview; (2) examples of promulgated standards by professional organizations; (3) examples of programmatic standards for community-based services; (4) a medical diagnosis approach; (5) exploration of other discipline specific approaches; and (6) functional status approaches. Rinke (1987) also edits an anthology on home care research to provide a reference to the classic and current literature addressing outcomes in home care.

A basic decision for nurse managers to make is to choose the perspective from which the organization, or department, views health problems, stated goals, and actual outcomes achieved. As health care becomes more competitive, effective communication of information about care quality, costs and associated outcomes is paramount. The medical and nursing diagnosis perspectives are the most common classifications used to view patient problems. Systems designed to communicate the effects of care in relation to nursing diagnoses, however, still need to be interpreted to the larger health care community, to payers and to consumers of the care received. Conversely, systems which depend on only medical diagnosis do not interpret the impact of nursing interventions on patient care.

Rinke (1988) devised a clear classification of outcomes incorporating the medical, nursing, and functional status perspectives for the home health care setting that can also be applied to outcome measurement within institutions. Rinke's analysis of the dimensions of the concept, complexity, and variety of outcome statements suggests a framework that can be used to start to define and measure individual and aggregate health care outcomes. By first defining the individual components of a patient outcome statement, that is, who is going to achieve the outcome, what is the outcome to be achieved, and when, or the timeframe in which the outcome is to be accomplished, the organization can identify outcome statements in relation to patient health problems. Rinke's work, while well within the purview of nursing, provides a departure from the classification of patient outcomes within the perspective of medical or nursing diagnoses, and into a categorization of physical, behavioral, psychosocial, knowledge, and functional outcomes. This concept is effective when considering the need to communicate the outcomes of care in a language understood by other disciplines in health care, payers, and patients.

Several trends become apparent as a result of this review. First of all, in the nursing domain, the field of home care appears to be the most fully developed in the outcome measurement arena. This is due primarily to the fact that nursing is the predominant service in home care, and home care agencies have traditionally chosen nurses as the Chief Executive Officers. Secondly, since nursing has been the major factor in home care, and costs are traditionally viewed on a cost per home visit basis, it is somewhat easier to attribute many agency costs to nursing interventions. Outcome measures that are widely published in the medical and hospital realm frequently pay little attention to nursing as a factor, but do recognize the multiple input and cost centers that factor into the overall outcomes achieved. The HCFA, the Joint Commission of Accreditation of Healthcare Organizations, as well as, to some extent, NLN's Community Health Accreditation Program have also had an effect on the development of information systems to measure the outcomes of patient care, from both perspectives of cost and quality. Costs are becoming a greater factor in the equation as the emphasis on health reform and shrinking dollars becomes a reality. To be truly accurate in the outcome, cost and quality equation, factors including ADLs, case mix and caseload variations, and patient acuity will also need to be considered.

Patient Acuity/Intensity

Patient acuity/intensity of care can be defined and measured in many ways. Home care agencies and nursing departments will often design acuity systems to factor in the level of care required for different patients, which may have the same or similar diagnoses. Intensity systems try to address the issues of why one patient may consume more care resources than another. Ideally, acuity measures will be factored into an information system to examine the costs of care and the outcomes achieved. Few are published, however, and even fewer are standardized between health care settings or institutions. Another important issue is reliability and validity of the data collected. According to Pallas and Giovannetti (1993), obtaining patient specific intensity data is a prerequisite for the evaluation of efficacy (and costs) of nursing care. Pallas suggests that intensity methods which place patients into categories of care (e.g., Medicus) may be more valid over time than systems that are based on task and time approaches (e.g., GRASP), although task and time approaches may seem more meaningful to the nurses that use them. Giovannetti recognizes that while establishment of reliability and validity in the practice setting can be time-consuming and expensive, attention to these issues will greatly influence the quality of the data retrieved. Once established, a still greater commitment for staff and administration will be required to monitor the systems in place.

The Easley-Storfjell Caseload/Workload Analysis (Allen, Easley, and Storfjell, 1986) is a classification system to rate patients according to the time required and complexity of care delivery. The information is graphed to help nurses and managers plan patient care in a cost-effective fashion, based on more information than the technical care and medical diagnosis would provide. The system allows for a testing process to monitor the accuracy of assessment, interrater reliability, and validity. To assess computerization potential, the system was compared to guidelines for workload measurement, developed by a MIS project, to ensure that the necessary components for effective information management were available in major systems being utilized around the country. The Easley-Storfjell Instrument provides a mechanism for home care agencies to project and evaluate staffing needs and determine nursing costs, based on a method that encompasses the comprehensive demand on nursing resources in a home care agency. Coupled with a system to reliably measure patient outcomes, this system, or an adaptation of it, could yield promising results.

Products to Measure Outcomes in Relation to Cost and Quality

Visiting Nurse Association of Eastern Montgomery County (MD)

The Visiting Nurse Association of Eastern Montgomery County began an outcome-based information system in 1985 for these stated purposes: (1) to accommodate envisioned changes in the home care reimbursement system, and (2) to support its belief that nursing diagnoses, rather than medical diagnoses, influence the level and amount of services home care patients require. This association is interested in identifying costs and determining rehabilitation potential within nursing diagnoses.

Harris (1994) builds on the methodological research in nursing relative to patient classification systems, to utilize a tool developed by Daubert (1979) called the Rehabilitation Potential Patient Classification System (RPPCS). Daubert's method offers five client categories to describe the characteristics of patients, with sub-objectives assigned to each category. Actual functioning of the patient at discharge, according to the RPPCS, is compared with the classification of the patient on admission to determine if the patient achieved the outcome objectives of the admission classification. The RPPCS categories include recovery, self-care, rehabilitation, maintenance, and terminal care. Harris combines RPPCS with classification systems including Major Disease Category (MDC), Nursing Diagnosis (ND), and International Classification of Diseases or ICD-9 codes. A variety of outcome data are generated through VNA's computer system, including total charge per case, as well as per case by discipline, average length of stay (LOS), and average number of visits by case and discipline, RPPCS, ND, and MDC. To determine the dollar value of the care provided, the staff indicates the percentage of total time spent on each nursing diagnosis, along with the start and stop dates for each diagnosis. The charge for services is calculated by dividing the percentage of time spent on each diagnosis by the total case number. Each diagnosis may only be a percentage of the total charge for care, depending on the number of NDS identified for that patient (see Table 1). At any time, this system can print out three years of cumulative data to document the charge for care by ND, to identify ND within the RPPCS and MDC, to identify the average LOS, and average number of visits per case by ND (see Tables 2 and 3). The correct identification of the RPPCS and ND for each patient is included as one aspect of VNA's QI program, and builds in several checkpoints to ensure accuracy. Clinical outcomes are included from all disciplines. Nursing or therapy managers assure that the outcome data for therapy are consistent with

Table 1.

Most Expensive Nursing Diagnoses, June 30, 1993

Nursing Diagnoses	Charge	Visits	Cases
Impaired skin integrity	$1,049	18	2,239
Potential for impaired skin integrity	676	21	34
Ineffective breathing pattern	663	12	1,611
Altered tissue perfusion	656	13	177
Altered urinary elimination pattern	623	15	580
Pain	549	12	677
Knowledge deficit	535	7	2,877
Ineffective coping (individual)	426	10	55

Reprinted from Handbook of Home Health Care Administration by M. Harris, 1994, Rockville, MD: Aspen Publishers.

Table 2.

Outcomes by RPPCS 6/30/93

Category	Number of Patients	Total Visits	Charge by RPPCS	Average Visits	Average LOS
Recovery	616	3,251	$ 491	5	11
Skilled Care	23	170	$ 748	7	15
Rehabilitation	2,591	63,548	$2,442	25	32
Maintenance	46	1,908	$4,694	41	54
Terminal	266	5,096	$2,068	19	22

Reprinted from Handbook of Home Health Care Administration by M. Harris, 1994, Rockville, MD: Aspen Publishers.

Table 3.

Three-Year Cumulative Discharge Data for Ten Major Disease Categories (MDC) Summary Data—June 30, 1993

Major Disease Category	Number of Cases	Median Length of Stay	Average Number of Visits	Average $ Charge Per Case
Circulatory	970	34	24	2,554
Neoplasm	498	24	14	2,211
Respiratory	419	34	20	2,211
Digestive	156	28	20	2,102
Musculoskeletal	143	27	33	3,412
Perinatal	140	10	5	439
Endocrine	136	33	27	2,604
Skin/Subcutaneous	123	41	44	4,497
Genito-urinary	64	22	13	1,416
Nervous	53	31	35	3,833
Overall Total*	3,595	29	22	2,321

*Overall totals include all MDCs, not only the 10 shown.

Reprinted from Handbook of Home Health Care Administration by M. Harris, 1994, Rockville, MD: Aspen Publishers.

the nursing outcomes and goal attainment documented on the agency's problem-oriented medical record system.

Harris emphasizes the need to concentrate on measurement of clinical outcomes of care to meet certification and accreditation standards. She also documents the need for agency administrators to have the ability to associate costs and charges of care by other methods than the traditional per visit basis. The system developed at the VNA of Eastern Montgomery County (MD) can assist agencies in determining what changes need to be made to continue to provide quality home care services through examination of the clinical and financial outcome information it provides.

Outcome Concept Systems

Wilson (1992) developed Outcome Concept Systems (OCS) as a method to integrate patient outcome measurement from the functional status perspective, and to communicate the cost and outcomes of services provided in a common language of care that is not dependent on either the medical or nursing diagnosis. Building on the work of Wilson and Rinke (1988), the system captures patient-oriented, quantifiable outcome statements that enable home care agencies to measure patient changes between admission and discharge. The operational definition of OCS is the documentation and interpretation of patient information at admission to and discharge from home care services, with analysis in the following five dimensions: Health Status (physical condition of the patient); Knowledge Function (what a patient or caregiver needs to know to assume responsibility for care); Skill Function (what a patient or caregiver needs to do to assume responsibility for care); Psychosocial Function (what social/emotional supports are necessary to assume responsibility for care); and Activities of Daily Living (what change can be documented in patients' toileting, ambulation, dressing, feeding, transferring, and bathing). To measure the patient information specified, Wilson has developed Patient Functional Assessment Tools to classify patients in the domains of health status, knowledge, skill and psychosocial function, and operationalized them into a nursing care plan, utilizing a health systems assessment and planning approach at the VNA of Hudson Valley, NY (Wilson, Hartnett, and Ferrari, 1992). To measure ADLs, an existing model was integrated that captures the categories of independence, partial dependence and dependence (Christensen, 1987).

OCS has developed a software program to accompany the documentation system to enable agencies to analyze and view the impact of services on patient outcomes through a variety of reports and graphs, either by individual patient, or by specified groups of patients. In addition, a cost option permits users to include dollar and visit data on graphs and/or reports (see Tables 4, 5, and 6). Costs, integrated with the outcomes of care, can assist in demonstrating the expenses associated with the outcomes achieved, as well as the value of services provided in a changing health care environment (Wilson, 1993). Costs and visits may be viewed by totals, averages, and/or by individual disciplines providing service. Costs can be further broken down to include the average and total cost per case, or the average and total costs per actual recipient of care.

In the training manuals provided to OCS users, emphasis is made on the importance of establishing interrater reliability of the items used for measurement. Written instructions and often on-site training are provided to the staff to establish interrater reliability (80% consensus at a minimum) before implementing the measurement items in the field. In addition, ongoing interrater reliability is assessed by joint visits to 10% of the patients admitted. OCS is utilized in both internal QA and external marketing efforts of the agency. Internally, outcomes may be tracked according to case manager and as a part of agency utilization review. Externally, the agency can demonstrate the effects of service to

Table 4.
Change in Ability to Administer Insulin Injections Between Admission and Discharge for Diabetic Patients

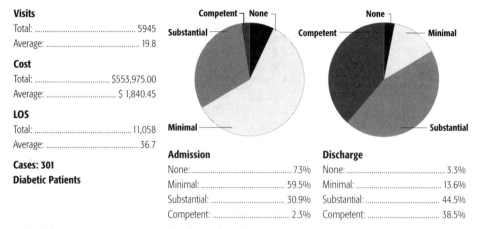

Skill Function
Ability to administer insulin

Visits
Total: 5945
Average: 19.8

Cost
Total: $553,975.00
Average: .... $ 1,840.45

LOS
Total: 11,058
Average: 36.7

Cases: 301
Diabetic Patients

Admission		Discharge	
None:	7.3%	None:	3.3%
Minimal:	59.5%	Minimal:	13.6%
Substantial:	30.9%	Substantial:	44.5%
Competent:	2.3%	Competent:	38.5%

Reprinted from Outcome Concept Systems by Wilson and Associates, 1993, Gig Harbor, WA: Author.

Table 5.
Change in Activities of Daily Living (ADLs): Bathing, Transferring, and Ambulation with Average Cost per Case

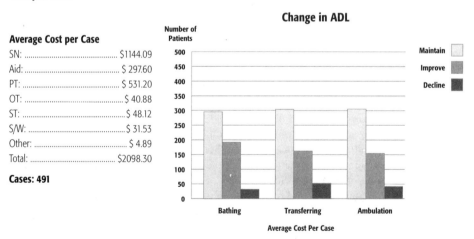

Change in ADL

Average Cost per Case
SN: $1144.09
Aid: .... $ 297.60
PT: .... $ 531.20
OT: .... $ 40.88
ST: .... $ 48.12
S/W: .... $ 31.53
Other: .... $ 4.89
Total: $2098.30

Cases: 491

Reprinted from Outcome Concept Systems by Wilson and Associates, 1993, Gig Harbor, WA: Author.

Table 6.
Sample Cost Analysis of 526 Patients

**Outcome Concept Systems
Cost Analysis**

Date: 09/02/1993
Sample Rate Record Discipline Rates   Total Cases: 526

Providers	Total Visits	Average Visits per Case	Rates	Total Cost	Average Cost per Case	Service Recipients	Average Visits per Recipient	Average Cost per Recipient
S/N	5823	11.1	105.00	611,415.00	1,162.39	516	11.3	1,184.91
Aides	2606	5.0	65.00	169,390.00	322.03	141	18.5	1,201.35
P/T's	3004	5.7	90.00	270,360.00	513.99	281	10.7	962.14
O/T's	225	0.4	90.00	20,250.00	38.50	33	6.8	613.64
S/T's	233	0.4	105.00	24,465.00	46.51	21	11.1	1,165.00
S/W's	131	0.2	120.00	15,720.00	29.89	44	3.0	357.27
Others	109	0.2	25.00	2,725.00	5.18	64	1.7	42.58
	12,131	23.1		1,114,325.00	2,118.49			
	Total LOS 24,120	Average LOS 45.9						

Reprinted from Outcome Concept Systems by Wilson and Associates, 1993, Gig Harbor, WA: Author.

referral groups, physicians, and the community at large. From a research and public policy perspective, the system has potential to provide reliable information about patient outcomes with multiple independent variables (demographics, nursing or medical diagnosis, discharge disposition, health problem, knowledge deficits, referral sources, visit numbers, and so forth), including the costs to provide the care.

Summary

Much work remains to be done on multiple issues in the development of information systems designed to measure the cost and quality of patient outcomes. A basic issue inherent in this entire discussion is the fact that many systems currently in use are undocumented in the current literature, or hidden behind unyielding superiors. Furthermore, while one system may measure outcomes, it often does not look at costs. Hospital departments or home care agencies almost never agree on a method to capture information in a uniform fashion. Many excellent documentation methodologies are available in manual form, but have little likelihood of computerization for lack of time or resources. Interdisciplinary efforts to look at outcomes, cost and quality are gaining momentum, but are not yet fully developed. The question of perspective will be a continuing issue for nursing, as well as the use of standardized nursing data to communicate the outcomes and costs of care.

Simplicity is probably the most important issue to keep in mind when developing or purchasing a system to examine outcomes and cost. Certainly no one will gain from an elaborate research system that is improperly used, or worse yet, not used at all. If a third party comes in to collect the data from clinical records, or patient interview, the critical point of practitioner/patient contact will be lost. Conversely, if the staff has not invested in the patient outcome measurement process, and it becomes cumbersome, little will be gained from it. If the systems we design cannot work within the framework of medical, nursing and any other kind of classification, we will continue to maintain multiple data bases that are unable to communicate.

Quite possibly, before consensus is reached among professionals, institutions, researchers and the like, the federal government could mandate a method to document outcome and patient quality issues, and tie it to prospective reimbursement, managed care, and/or continued participation in the Medicare program. Unfortunately, this will not make many happy, but it will provide a forced consensus on measurement issues, data sets, and how much the whole package should cost. On the other hand, if left to market forces, as in a managed competitive environment, the organizations that can demonstrate a cohesive method, and data to demonstrate acceptable patient outcomes for a cost-sensitive price, will likely remain standing after the tidal wave of health reform and a managed care environment passes over the health care industry.

References

Allen, C. E., Easley, C. E., and Storfjell, J. I. (1986). Cost management through caseload/workload analysis. In F. A. Shaffer (Ed.), Patients & Purse Strings. Patient Classification and Cost Management (pp. 331-346). New York: National League for Nursing.

Ball, M. J., O'Desky, R. I., and Douglas, J. V. (1991). Status and progress of hospital information systems (HIS). International Journal of Biomedical Computers, 29, 161-168.

Barry, C. T., and Gibbons, L. K. (1990). Information systems technology: Barriers and challenges to implementation. Journal of Nursing Administration, 20(2), 40-42.

Christensen, M. L. (1987). Development and use of functional client outcome measures. In L. T. Rinke and A. A. Wilson (Eds.), Outcome Measures in Home Care—Volume II: Service (pp. 249-254). New York: National League for Nursing.

Conrad, D. A. (1991). Editorial. Frontiers of Health Services Management, 8(2), 1-2.

Cuddeback, J. K. (1993). Computers for clinical practice and education in radiology. Radiographics, 13, 445-456.

Daubert, E. A. (1979). Patient classification systems and outcome criteria. Nursing Outlook, 27, 450-454.

Delaney, C. (1992). Standardized nursing language for health care information systems. Journal of Medical Systems, 16(4), 145-159.

DiJerome, L. (1992). The nursing case management computerized system: Meeting the challenge of health care delivery through technology. Computers in Nursing, 10(6), 250-258.

Donabedian, A. (1985). The epidemiology of quality. Inquiry, 22, 292.

Donabedian, A. (1993, January-March). Continuity and change in the quest for quality. Clinical Performance and Quality Health Care, 1, 9-16.

Edison, S., and Esmond, T. (1991). Information requirements for assessing quality of care. Topics in Health Care Financing, 18(2), 75-80.

Ellwood, P. (1988). Outcomes management: A technology of patient experience (Shattuck lecture). New England Journal of Medicine, 318, 1549-1556.

Harris, M. (1994). Clinical and financial outcomes of patient care. In Handbook of Home Health Care Administration. Rockville, MD: Aspen Publishers.

Hegyvary, S. T. (1991). Issues in outcomes research. Journal of Nursing Quality Assurance, 5(2), 1-6.

Jones, K. R. (1993). Outcomes analysis: Methods and issues. Nursing Economics, 11(3), 145-151.

Kovner, C. (1989). Using computerized databases for nursing research and quality assurance. Computers in Nursing, 7(5), 228-231.

Lang, N. M., and Marek, K. D. (1990). The classification of patient outcomes. Journal of Professional Nursing, 6(3), 158-163.

Marek, K. D. (1993). Nursing sensitive outcomes. Papers from the Nursing Minimum Data Set Conference. Edmonton, Alberta: Canadian Nurses Association.

Maturen, V. L., and Zander, K. (1993). Outcomes management in a prospective pay system. Caring, 12(6), 46-53.

Nash, D. B., and Markson, L. E. (1991). Managing outcomes: The perspective of the players. Frontiers of Health Services Management, 8(2), 3-45.

North American Nursing Diagnosis Association. (1989). Taxonomy 1—Revised 1989: With Official Diagnostic Categories. St. Louis: Author.

Pallas, L. O., and Giovannetti, P. (1993). Papers from the Nursing Minimum Data Set Conference (pp. 70-72). Edmonton, Alberta: Canadian Nurses Association.

Rinke, L. T. (Ed.). (1987). Outcome Measures in Home Care: Volume I—Research. New York: National League for Nursing.

Rinke, L. T. (1988). Outcome Standards in Home Health: State of the Art (pp. 40-45). New York: National League for Nursing.

Rinke, L. T., and Wilson, A. A. (Eds.). (1987). Outcome Measures in Home Care: Outcome II Service. New York: National League for Nursing.

Shaughnessy, P. W. (1991). A Study to Develop Outcome-Based Quality Measures for Home Health Services Study Paper 6 (Part of a report series funded by the Health Care Financing Administration, Department of Health and Human Services Contract No. 500-88-0054.) Denver: Center for Health Policy Research.

Temple, R. (1990). Problems in the use of large data sets to assess effectiveness. International Journal of Technology Assessment in Health Care, 6, 211-219.

Visiting Nurse Association of Omaha. (1986). Client Management Information System for Community Health Nursing Agencies (NTIS No. HRP-0907023). Rockville, MD: Dept. of Health and Human Services, Division of Nursing.

Werley, H. H., Devine, E. C., Zorn, C. R., Ryan, J. W., and Westra, B. L. (1991). The nursing minimum data set: Abstraction tool for standardized, comparable, essential data. American Journal of Public Health, 81(4), 421-426.

Williamson, J. W. (1988). Future policy directions for quality assurance: Lessons from the health accounting experience. Inquiry, 25, 67-77.

Wilson, A. A. (1992). Outcome Concept Systems: A Guide to the Measurement of Outcomes in Home Care. Harrison, NY: Wilson & Associates.

Wilson, A. A. (1993). The cost and quality of patient outcomes: A look at managed competition. Nursing Administration Quarterly, 17(4), 11-16.

Wilson, A. A., Hartnett, M., and Ferrari, P. (1992). Outcome measurement from the functional status perspective. Home HealthCare Nurse, 10(3), 32-46.

Wilson, A. A., and Rinke, L. T. (1988). DRGs and the measurement of quality in home care. Nursing Clinics of North America, 23(3), 569-578.

Using the Computer to Measure Outcomes of Nursing Care

Mary S. Tilbury, EdD, RN, CNAA
Assistant Professor
Department of Education, Administration, Health Policy and Informatics
School of Nursing
University of Maryland at Baltimore

Introduction

Nursing literature is replete with calls for the evaluation of nursing practice effectiveness (del Bueno, 1993; Hegyvary, 1991; Hinshaw, 1992; McCormick, 1992). While the profession was first urged to focus on this topic some 20 years ago (Block, 1975), the current health care environment demands that this area of research receive priority consideration.

Factors such as runaway health care costs, consumer dissatisfaction and significant numbers of individuals with inadequate or no health insurance coverage, represent only a few of the forces shaping the powerful health care reform movement now underway. The nursing profession is faced with significant change and challenge as this transition unfolds; but most of all nursing is faced with significant opportunities generated by a reform movement that must not be ignored. How the profession responds to this challenge will in large measure shape nursing practice in the foreseeable future (Strickland, 1992).

This chapter explores why nursing should focus on outcome measurement; examines the current status of nursing's readiness to conduct effectiveness evaluation; addresses attendant outcome evaluation issues; details what must be done to enhance the profession's contribution in outcome measurement, and identifies how professionals in nursing informatics can contribute to this effectiveness agenda.

The Need for Outcome Measurement

Diminished economic resources and consumer concerns regarding the high cost of health care are increasingly advancing efforts to develop programs and examine factors related to the cost, benefits and outcomes of care. The responses of leaders and organizations in the health care arena are both comprehensive and varied. For instance, Medicare-related Peer Review Organizations (PRO's) are developing resources to document and share information on electronically generated geographic patterns and outcomes of care. Generally, this represents a major departure from the PRO's former focus which featured a manual review of hospital-specific records designed to make judgments and take action on questions primarily related to resource utilization, treatment regimes and care outcomes (McPhillips, 1992).

The Agency for Health Care Policy and Research (AHCPR), established under the auspices of the U.S. Public Health Service in 1989, is centered on medical treatment effectiveness research and the development of multidisciplinary clinical practice guidelines. In addition, AHCPR is concerned with the evolution of data bases that can adequately support the evaluation of patient outcomes. Finally, in addressing its oversight responsibilities, the Joint Commission on the Accreditation of Healthcare Organizations, developed its Agenda for Change, which reflected increased emphasis on quality management and evaluation. As exhibited by the programs and practices of the public and private bodies cited above, significant resources are now allocated toward finding the answers to fundamental questions concerning not only what is effective treatment, but what is cost-effective treatment. These steps speak directly to a changing landscape and the newly re-ordered national priorities of quality care, responsible economics and sound management of the health care system.

The health care system, and those providers participating as major players, are challenged to demonstrate that they make a difference, articulate how they make a difference in patient outcomes, and specify the fiscal resources necessary to achieve specified outcomes. These structures will support the purpose of outcome evaluation—to test the effectiveness of services provided by professionals, institutions and networks of managed care.

How effectiveness research questions are answered will impact heavily on the future of nursing as a profession. At best, the promise of practice expansion, increased nursing knowledge, the effective utilization of economic resources, enhanced influence in public policy decision-making, as well as the improved health status of millions of Americans is possible. An inadequate response will leave a void which inevitably will be filled by others. It is the profession's choice and a vital one. Without the findings yielded by outcome evaluation, nursing is not positioned to gain in status by responding to society's changing expectations.

Nursing's Readiness to Conduct Outcome Research

Ozbolt (1992) asserts that:

> . . . the prime requirement for effectiveness research is utterly lacking in nursing: valid, reliable, useful data from multiple sites structured in data bases that allow easy, preferably automated, entry from clinical records and ready access for whatever analyses the investigators may choose to perform. (p. 211)

Furthermore, she argues that the profession's failure to identify and agree upon data elements for inclusion in information systems, as opposed to prejudice or denial of inclusion requests, is primarily responsible for this set of circumstances (Ozbolt, 1992). Major aspects of this apparent dilemma are reviewed.

Advances in information management and computer technology have significant implications for the collection, retrieval and analysis of nursing practice information. For the better part of 35 years, Werley has called for the profession to standardize essential nursing data (Werley, Devine, Zorn, Ryan, and Westra, 1991). The utilization of such essential elements of nursing care would allow for the development of a nursing information data base across regions, populations and settings. Furthermore, Werley says, "if nurses are to describe, compare and assess their practice, they must be able to communicate with each other using comparable data" (Werley et al., 1991).

The work of Werley and her associates has yielded a list of 16 data elements. Of these 16, only six are not currently included in the Uniform Hospital Discharge Data Set: a unique record number for the patient, an individual number for the registered nurse provider, nursing diagnosis, nursing intervention, nursing outcome and nursing intensity (Werley, 1991). The collection of the information related to the first two items is primarily a matter of policy; however, it is the last four items that present significant challenges to the profession. Nursing must name what it does.

McCormick asserts that information systems must be developed that document client nursing care needs (McCormick, 1991). The attainment of this objective is entirely dependent on the development, evaluation and acceptance of a diagnostic taxonomy. As

Block argued some 20 years ago (Block, 1975), it is essential that a common set of problems be developed so that expectations regarding the response of the patient to nursing actions/interventions can be established. In other words, the relationship between diagnoses, interventions and outcomes begins with establishing patient need, continues with the identification and implementation of interventions, and ends with the evaluation of patient response. The nursing process must remain intact if the measurement of nursing outcomes is achieved.

The most comprehensive work in this area remains that of the North American Nursing Diagnosis Association. While far from attainment, the apparent goal of this group is the development of a complete set of nursing diagnoses. How the work of other groups and individuals, such as the Omaha Visiting Nurses' Association community health nursing practice project will be addressed, remains to be seen.

In addition to nursing diagnosis developmental issues, significant questions related to the validity and reliability of assessment criteria must also be addressed. As Ozbolt points out, " . . . nursing is far from possessing a valid and reliable assessment guide for establishing the presence, absence or degree of a comprehensive set of nursing diagnoses" (Ozbolt, 1992, p. 212).

The development and testing of a taxonomy of nursing interventions is substantially complete. The primary work in this area has been done by Bulechek and McCloskey (1989). Similar projects have also been reported by Grobe (1990) and the Omaha Visiting Nurses Association (Martin and Scheet, 1992). A more comprehensive discussion of standardizing nursing language can be obtained in an earlier chapter. Suffice it to say, nursing intervention language problems have made rapid progress over the last few years. Although much work, including that of national nursing data base inclusion, remains to be done, nursing can point with pride to this effort.

The definition, classification and categorization of nursing outcomes remains largely unresolved. Conceptually, scholars agree that outcomes are the end result of treatment or intervention (Hegyvary, 1991; Lang and Marek, 1990; Strickland, 1992). In the Nursing Minimum Data Set, nursing outcome is defined as "resolution status of the nursing diagnosis[es]" (Werley and Lang, 1988).

The definition and measurement of service outcomes has not been a common activity. Indeed, Ingersoll, Hoffart and Schultz (1990) report a total of 113 nursing outcome studies were conducted from 1980 through 1989. This is primarily related to the difficulty in defining and measuring both the processes of care and the evaluation of the results of that care.

Certainly there is a high degree of familiarity with more traditional outcome measurements such as morbidity, mortality and disability or the more recent classification of the 5 D's—death, disease, disability, discomfort and dissatisfaction. More positively stated indicators of outcomes, such as states of health in the physiological, physical and emotional domains are increasingly seen, as are measures related to the ever-increasing emphasis being placed on consumer satisfaction. Thus, the definition of outcomes is not as simple as it might first appear. Various numbers and types of outcomes clearly apply to individual clinical situations (Hegyvary, 1991). "Thus, development of language and measurement standards for outcomes of nursing care lags behind development of such standards for diagnoses and interventions" (Ozbolt, 1992, p. 213).

Information related to the level of nursing intensity presents similar problems. Although patient classification systems are familiar tools commonly utilized in patient care settings to measure the amount of nursing care required, they are not standardized and may yield differing measurement outcomes from unit to unit, even when the same tool is utilized organizationally. Furthermore, the classification tool is rarely linked to the actual plan of care, and when utilized as a means of evaluating the cost of patient care, obvious problems regarding validity and reliability surface. While the Nursing Minimum Data Set includes initial efforts to standardize assessment and classification methods, the need for further development and investigation in this area is extensive.

In summary, although much progress has been made in determining and developing the basis for nursing's readiness to conduct effectiveness research, there is much work that remains. Questions regarding validity, reliability and utility must be answered and concerns related to comprehensiveness and standardization will require continuing effort.

Outcome Evaluation Issues

Although we have the technology to conduct meaningful effectiveness research and have initiated attempts to formulate the development of a comprehensive nursing data base, other theoretical and practical issues hamper professional consensus and hence progress. Hegyvary (1991) suggests that issues such as the level of analysis, timing and attribution in outcome research warrant examination.

Outcome evaluation involving individual situations, group orientations, specific localities or the public as a whole will require varying methodological approaches and measurement approaches. The purpose of the inquiry must be carefully considered in any evaluation of outcomes.

A second issue, timing, refers to the identification of the timeframe in which a specific outcome can be expected to occur. When examining the relationship between patient teaching and compliance, for example, it is clear that different outcomes may be expected over time. Patient compliance may be high during the immediate period following instruction, but deteriorate over time. Thus, investigators may elect to look at immediate results or outcomes related to survival. Studies which include repeated measures seem particularly desirable in addressing the relationship between time and outcomes.

The attribution issue affects all studies and outcome evaluation. As Hegyvary (1991) points out, most effectiveness evaluation has been focused on immediate responses to physician interventions. The consideration of structural variables, such as staffing ratios or governance practices, are rarely considered. By the same token, nursing studies which deny the influence of other disciplines on patient outcomes are flawed.

The term *nursing outcomes* should rarely if ever be used. The focus of outcomes is not the provider but the recipient of care. Future studies using a multivariate analytical approach will enable us to determine the levels of variance explained by nursing, medicine, organizational, demographic, environmental, and numerous other variables. (Hegyvary, 1991)

McCormick (1992) argues that the impact of nursing interventions in treatment effectiveness studies does not receive the scientific attention that it warrants. She suggests that there are many areas of inquiry that should be embraced by the nursing research community, including patient preference research, treatment compliance investigations, patient versus treatment outcome studies and cost/quality comparisons related to different systems and providers, among others. Additional areas of inquiry are also reviewed by del Bueno (1993). The domain of effectiveness research is indeed rich.

Data Base Development

The effectiveness of nursing practice requires measurement at multiple levels. There can be no question, however, that the most powerful evaluation of nursing's contribution comes through the utilization of large data bases to conduct outcome research. Breaux

(1992) cites three major sources of large data bases for nursing effectiveness research: federal and/or public sources, Veteran's Administration tapes, and those data bases held by private concerns, such as insurance companies, or organizations such as the American Hospital Association.

Three major systems are fundamental in any attempt to conduct outcome research. Two of these are derived from the federal arena, specifically the Health Care Financing Administration (HCFA), the Medicare Claims File and the Uniform Clinical Data Set (UCDS), currently under development within HCFA. The third source of information are the registries, such as the tumor registry, that include clinical elements characteristic of their focus.

The HCFA data bases, which are primarily related to service utilization, costs and reimbursement for Medicare and Medicaid, represent the largest health care data base in the world. The National Claims History DataBase, a relatively new HCFA information source, will be used to monitor services and influence policy decision-making. Of particular interest is the development of the UCDS.

The UCDS will enable PRO's, HCFA and researchers to analyze the effectiveness of medical interventions. We will use the data set to find out what really works well, what has marginal value, and what simply does not work. (McPhillips, 1992, p. 195)

The UCDS is based on several years of Professional Review Organization experience and has been tested in several states across the nation including Alabama, Colorado, Connecticut, Iowa, Utah and Wisconsin. Currently one thousand clinically relevant data elements are abstracted from each case under review (C. Wark, HCFA, personal communication, September 1993). These elements are then exposed to automated quality screens, which if positive, will refer the case for additional analysis by the PRO. Although the system has generated controversy and has yet to undergo reliability and validity testing, the data base does contain elements that may be helpful to nurse researchers—functional status, patient education and specialty referrals.

Those issues cited above, as relevant to the NMDS, certainly apply to health care data bases. The need for comprehensive and comparable data, both within and across geographical sectors and divisions of information systems is critical. Currently, one of the problems in using major data bases is the informatics expertise and time required to access and analyze the data. Of a more critical concern is the lack of nursing data elements being routinely included in these systems. While the existence and formulation of large and potentially meaningful information systems for outcome research are available, the work of nursing in these systems is for the most part invisible. Thus, none of these data bases includes data elements that can be systematically used to measure nursing outcomes. In the future, however, when these challenges have been successfully addressed, systems that will facilitate research and evaluation, through the utilization of data that is rich in nursing content will emerge (McPhillips, 1992, p. 195).

Recommendations and Implications for Informatics

Nursing's effectiveness agenda will challenge the profession well into the 21st century. To adequately address the multiple demands generated by this significant opportunity, the nursing profession must develop strategies and allocate the resources necessary to achieve this ambitious goal. The efforts generated on behalf of measuring nursing's effectiveness in patient outcomes must be at all levels within the health care system, particularly for those in leadership positions.

It is imperative that nurses with expertise in informatics be included in decision-making regarding the planning, development and implementation of clinical information systems. This would include activities that are agency-specific, such as the selection of automated charting or documentation systems, or at the national level where policy decisions shape the ability of nursing to contribute to the evaluation of patient outcomes. It is particularly imperative that nursing administrators and informatics specialists work together to see that the Nursing Minimum Data Set, or elements thereof, are included in information systems whenever possible.

Informatics specialists will also play a vital role in establishing meaningful working relationships with vendors, so that they are educated in the importance of including the NMDS in their products. Indeed, these nursing specialists will play a major role in the development of future systems.

Individual and collective efforts must continue to work for the inclusion of nursing nomenclature in health care information systems. This is particularly important in relation to specialty organizations and for those organizations that speak for nursing at the national level.

Finally, it is essential that the development of informatics specialization in nursing continue. This will facilitate the development of teams composed of clinicians, administrators, researchers and informatics specialists who can adequately address the outcome effectiveness for nursing and appreciate the power and versatility of the computer in measuring the outcomes of patient care.

Summary

The evaluation of patient care outcomes is of paramount importance, not only to the nursing community, but to all those who strive to meet the needs of individuals and families seeking services in the health care system. With diminishing economic resources, the goal becomes one of offering the highest quality care at the lowest possible cost. A principle means of achieving this goal is to fully utilize the skills and competencies of each health care provider. Outcome research promises to be a powerful tool in supporting the expanding role of nurses in health care.

The effectiveness research agenda cannot move forward in a meaningful manner until the work of nursing is catalogued, categorized, classified, routinely collected and systematically evaluated for its contribution to the care of patients. As long as the work of nursing remains essentially invisible in health care data bases, the ability of the profession to influence future policy decisions is severely restricted. Through the development of informatics expertise, cooperation and collaboration within the discipline and outside the discipline, and the appropriate utilization of resources, nursing's future is assured.

References

Block, D. (1975). Evaluation of nursing care in terms of process and outcome: Issues in research and quality assurance. *Nursing Research, 24*(4), 256-263.

Breaux, K. (1992). Database Sources for Research in Quality of Care and Utilization of Health Services. *Houston Center for Quality of Care and Utilization Studies.* Veterans Affairs Medical Center, Houston, TX, Document Report. HCACUS: TR 92-01, April 1, 1992.

Bulechek, G., and McCloskey, J.C. (1989). Nursing interventions: Treatments for potential diagnoses. In E. M. Carroll-Johnson (Ed.), *Proceedings of the Eighth Conference NANDA* (pp. 23-30). Philadelphia: J. B. Lippincott.

del Bueno, D. J. (1993). Outcome evaluation: Frustration or fertile field? *Journal of Nursing Administration, 23*(7/8), 12-13, 19.

Grobe, S. J. (1990). Nursing intervention lexicon and taxonomy study: Language and classification methods. *Advances in Nursing Science, 13*(2), 22-23.

Hegyvary, L. J. (1991). Issues in outcome research. *Journal of Nursing Quality Assurance, 5*(2), 1-6.

Hinshaw, A. L. (1992). Welcome: Patient Outcomes Research Conference. In *Patient Outcomes Research: Examining the Effectiveness of Nursing Practice.* (NIH Publication Na. 93-3411, pp. 9-10). Washington, DC: U.S. Department of Health and Human Services, Public Health Services, National Institutes of Health.

Ingersoll, G. L., Hoffart, N., and Schultz, A. W. (1990). Health services research in nursing: Current status and future dissections. *Nursing Economics, 8*(4), 229-238.

Lang, N. M., and Marek, K. D. (1990). The classification of patient outcomes. *Journal of Nursing, 6*(3), 158-163.

Martin, R., and Scheet, N. (1992). *The Omaha System: Applications for Community Health Nursing.* Philadelphia: W. B. Saunders Co.

McCormick, K. A. (1991). Future data needs for quality of care monitoring, DRG considerations, reimbursement and outcome measurement. *Image, 23*(1), 29-32.

McCormick, K. A. (1992). Areas of outcome research in nursing. *Journal of Professional Nursing, 8*(2), 71.

McPhillips, R. (1992). National and regional data bases: The big picture. In *Patient Outcomes Research: Examining the Effectiveness of Nursing Practice* (NIH Publication Na. 93-3411, pp. 191-199). Washington, DC: U.S. Department of Health and Human Services, National Institutes of Health.

Ozbolt, J. G. (1992). Strategies for Building Nursing Data Bases for Effectiveness Research. In *Patient Outcomes Research: Examining the Effectiveness of Nursing Practice* (NIH Publication Na. 93-3411, p. 210-218). Washington, DC: U.S. Department of Health and Human Services, Public Health Services, National Institutes of Health.

Strickland, O. L. (1992). Measures and Instruments. In *Patient Outcomes Research: Examining the Effectiveness of Nursing Practice* (NIH Publication Na. 93-3411, pp. 145-153). Washington, DC: U.S. Department of Health and Human Services, Public Health Service, National Institutes of Health.

Werley, H. H., Devine, E. C., Zorn, C. R., Ryan, P., and Westra, B. L. (1991). The nursing minimum data set: Abstraction tool for standardized, comparable, essential data. *American Journal of Public Health, 81*(4), 441-446.

Werley, H. H., and Lang, N. M. (Eds.). (1988). *Identification of the Nursing Minimum Data Set.* New York: Springer Publishing Co.

Electronic Networking for Nurses

Susan M. Sparks, PhD, RN, FAAN
Research Education Specialist
National Library of Medicine
Educational TechnoLogy Branch
Lister Hill Center

Introduction

Electronic networking for information access is becoming increasingly crucial to nursing. The technology infrastructure currently in use can be considered somewhat undeveloped in terms of ease of use, functionality, and available resources. Much research and development activity is on-going and the quantity and quality of resources are expanding rapidly.

Electronic networks link computers of various kinds and sizes, ranging from mainframes to laptops. Computers connected to a given network share certain common specifications, called "protocols," that allow such systems to "talk" to each other. Individual computers, which send and receive messages on a network, are called "nodes." A node may serve one person or thousands. Nodes are managed by systems operators (truncated to "sys-ops").

Even within one network there is considerable disorganization, so much so that in very large systems, such as Internet, it is difficult to know the exact number of nodes and users. Also, some networks have allowed individual nodes to tailor commands and features to suit their "local" needs. For the would-be-user, this means that commands at one node may not function at all or may function differently at another node.

The two major international electronic networks of high relevance to nurses are: Internet and FidoNet. Other networks, such as BITNET, which is international, and FITNET, a private network linking nurses in the United States and Canada, are also valuable to nurses. In addition to facilitating electronic mail (e-mail), each of these networks offer specific resources useful to the nursing profession.

Internet, which is managed by the National Science Foundation, is the world's largest international computer network. This network alone is estimated to have about 160,000 nodes and to be attaching additional nodes at the rate of about 60 nodes a month. Developed in the late 1970s, Internet was known then as the Advanced Research Projects Agency Network, with the purpose of linking major mainframe computers. Internet is currently composed of computers of various sizes, including mainframe computers. Membership in Internet is institutional and consists primarily of academic and research organizations.

FidoNet consists of about 18,000 nodes worldwide. This network began in the early 1980s as a result of the efforts of two computer hobbyists attempting to automate communication with each other via computers and modems. FidoNet is considered a network of "amateur volunteers" in that participation is not primarily a function of the users' professional position. Node sys-ops themselves own the computer and communication resources, giving access and service to participants via their computers and modems at no charge.

Initiated in 1986, BITNET, an acronym for Because It's Time NETwork consists of about 3,000 nodes linking academic, research, and some government and commercial organizations. BITNET is available in many countries; however, there are some notable exceptions (e.g., Australia, New Zealand). BITNET is managed by EDUCOM, a nonprofit organization of universities.

FITNET, the private network of the Fuld Institute for Technology in Nursing Education Network, consists of a single computer located in Athens, Ohio. It serves several hundred members of the Fuld Institute for Technology in Nursing Education Consortium who access the system via computers and modems using two 800 (toll-free) datalines.

E-mail may generally be exchanged between participants on Internet, FidoNet, and BITNET whether or not they are on the same wide area network. System dependent modification of an electronic address is usually all that is required to exchange e-mail across networks. Due to individual network differences and incompatibilities, however, exchange of e-mail between different networks cannot always be guaranteed. FITNET participants may exchange private mail messages only with others on FITNET.

While e-mail can usually be exchanged from one wide area network to another, there are other forms of electronic communication that may not be available between different wide area networks. These include interactive communications, file transfers, and telnet sessions.

Interactive communications, consisting of one message line at a time in realtime, can take place between two participants when both are online on Internet. This feature is also available between some BITNET nodes. "Online chats," interactive realtime communications, can take place between a FidoNet sys-op and any participant who is online. FITNET has the capability of placing any combination of two participants and a sys-op into an online chat mode.

File transfer service, if available, can only take place between participants on the same wide area network. Therefore, an Internet participant can only transfer a file with another Internet user.

A telnet session, in which a host computer on a network provides a communication session for a participant, can take place only when the participant and the host computer both share the same network. Therefore, only participants on Internet can access Internet host computers.

On Internet

As of February 1994, The Internet "electronic landscape" includes only a handful of very powerful resources of significance to nursing. This number is expected to increase dramatically over time.

Major resources currently available on Internet include access to the National Library of Medicine MEDLARS family of data bases. Internet access also allows telnet sessions to E.T.Net, a computer conferencing system operated by the National Library of Medicine; to Sigma Theta Tau International's Virginia Henderson International Nursing Library; to ALF, the Agricultural Library Forum, which carries information vital to rural health and rural nurse midwives; and to FDA, the network of the Food and Drug Administration. Community-supported electronic networks, FREENETS, are available in several areas via Internet.

MEDLARS

MEDLARS (MEDical Literature Analysis and Retrieval System) is the computerized system of data bases and data banks offered by the National Library of Medicine. This family of more than 40 data bases includes those well-known and used by nurses such as MEDLINE (MEDlars onLINE), AIDSLINE (AIDS information onLINE), and AVLINE

(AudioVisuals onLINE), which are accessed via GRATEFUL MED. Three of the newer data bases, with which nurses may be somewhat less familiar, are ALERT, HSTAR, and HSTAT. ALERT is a full-text data base announcing the immediate cessation of NIH-supported clinical trials for reasons such as proven efficacy or harm to subjects. HSTAR (Health Services/Technology Assessment Research) provides access to the published literature of health services research. HSTAT (Health Services/Technology Assessment Text) is free and provides electronic practice guidelines and other documents useful in health care decision making. While there is a charge for use of most of the MEDLARS data bases, currently there is no charge to use AIDSLINE, AIDSDRUGS (Substances being tested in AIDS-related Clinical trials), AIDSTRIALS (AIDS Clinical TRIALS), and DIRLINE (Directory of Information Resources onLINE and HSTAT. For additional information, call or write:

MEDLARS Management Section
National Library of Medicine
8600 Rockville Pike
Bethesda, MD 20894
(800) 638-8480 (voice)
(301) 496-6193 (voice)

Virginia Henderson International Nursing Library

A telnet session to the Virginia Henderson International Nursing Library of the Sigma Theta Tau International Honor Society of Nursing furnishes access to the online Directory of Nurse Researchers and to abstracts of recent scientific sessions. The process of adding to the directory and the abstracts is continuously ongoing. Plans are under way for various interactive resources and services; for instance, in the future, dial-in access will be available to those with a computer and modem. For more information, contact:

Virginia Henderson International Nursing Library
Sigma Theta Tau International Honor Society of Nursing
550 West North Street
Indianapolis, IN 46202
(317) 634-8171 (voice)

For an additional subscription, users may access Sigma Theta Tau International's Online Journal of Synthesized Nursing Knowledge, the first electronic serial in nursing of any kind. It is also possible to subscribe to the online journals of other vendors. For more information, contact Sigma Theta Tau International.

Food and Drug Administration

A telnet session to the Food and Drug Administration (FDA) gives read-only access to information on the following topics: News releases; Enforcement Report (weekly recall list); Drug and Device Product Approvals List; Medical Devices and Radiological Health News; FDA Medical Bulletin; Special section on AIDS information; FDA Consumer Magazine, index and selected articles; FDA Federal Register summaries (available by subject or date); answers arising from questions in news stories; Congressional testimony by FDA officials; speeches by FDA officials; Veterinary Medicine News; Centers for Devices and Radiological Health Bulletins; upcoming FDA meetings; and Import Alerts. FDA may be accessed via Internet or dial-in, including toll-free datalines. Use is free-of-charge. For more information about the FDA Electronic BBS, contact:

FDA Press Office
5600 Fishers Lane
Rockville, MD 20857
(301) 443-3285 (voice)

FREENETS

FREENETS are community-access electronic networks that allow sharing of discussion and information about topics and issues of importance to the community. Access is free and management of the various components of each is usually performed by volunteers. Cleveland was the first community to have such a resource. Now, there are private conferences on the Cleveland Free-Net, initiated by Patricia F. Brennan, PhD, RN, who pioneered the use of electronic networking for support of persons with AIDS and caregivers of Alzheimer's patients. At this writing, there are 21 additional communities with Freenets and many others are considering the development of such a resource. Currently the Denver Free-Net has the most extensive health/nursing related resources. For more information, contact:

> School of Nursing
> University of Colorado
> 4200 East Ninth Avenue
> Denver, CO 80262
> (303) 270-8665 (voice)

Newsgroups

Internet also offers "newsgroups." These are subject-matter, interactive message areas, or electronic bulletin boards, where participants exchange messages about "news" on a specific subject of interest. Although there are hundreds of internationally available newsgroups and variable numbers of regionally and locally available newsgroups on a myriad of topics, currently there are no nursing-relevant newsgroups. But, following instructions available in "newsgroup administration" (one of the newsgroups), users could easily and rapidly be created. There is no charge for participating in newsgroups, but entering newsgroups is an active process. A potential user must seek out particular newsgroups to join in order to access their "news" service. Participants are "transparent"; i.e., not seen, in a newsgroup unless they post a message.

LISTPROCs

LISTPROCs (list processors) are electronic mailing lists. They are virtual interest groups that exchange communications by all members of the list by e-mail. The current LISTPROC of greatest interest to nurses is the Nursing Informatics List owned by Gordon Larrivee, MS, RN, CNS. Participation in a LISTPROC is considered a passive process. Once registered to a LISTPROC, members receive all mail sent to the list. There is no charge for participating in a LISTPROC. Since registration to any list is managed by its host computer, specific steps must be followed to allow the registrations to be performed automatically. Since LISTPROC communications are e-mail, participants on BITNET and FidoNet can, with minor modifications of the electronic address, subscribe to and participate in Internet LISTPROCs. For more information about the Nursing Informatics LISTPROC, contact:

> Gordon Larrivee, MS, RN, CNS
> larrivee@umassmed.ummed.edu

Future Internet Resources for Nursing

Many nursing organizations are actively involved in initiating electronic resources to be accessed on Internet. The National League for Nursing is designing a resource for organizational and membership use. For more information, contact:

> National League for Nursing
> 350 Hudson Street
> New York, NY 10014

(212) 989-9393 (voice)

The American Journal of Nursing Company (AJN), a wholly owned nonprofit subsidiary of the not-for-profit American Nurses Association, is mounting AJN-Net, which will be initiated as a dial-in resource via computer and modem, later to be available on the Internet. AJN-Net, which is supported by a grant from the Division of Nursing, Health Resources and Services Administration, U.S. Public Health Service, will provide continuing education opportunities, expert consultation, and unique programming, with a special emphasis on AIDS information. For more information about AJN-Net, contact:

Director, Interactive Technologies
American Journal of Nursing Company
555 West 57th Street
New York, NY 10019-2961
(212) 582-8820, ext. 541 (voice)
(800) CALL AJN, ext. 541 (voice)
For more information about Internet, contact:
National Science Foundation
Computer and Information Science and Engineering
1800 G Street, NW
Washington, DC 20550
NSF Network Service Center
nnsc@nnsc.nsf.net

The best source of information about Internet access and use is usually available through a potential user's local institutional computer center administration or staff. While Internet nodes must share certain common protocols to communicate, there are many features that are specified locally. Registering for an Internet account, learning the commands required, and learning the options available are best done on a local basis.

On FidoNet

FidoNet nodes are plentiful, but not ubiquitous, in the United States. In addition, there is at least one health-related node in each of the following countries: Australia, Canada, Germany, Hong Kong, Italy, Netherlands, Spain, and the United Kingdom. Each FidoNet node carries subject matter discussions of the sys-op's choice. This person is the one who owns the computer and gives free "service" to his or her participants. While there are nodes that specialize in nursing, health-related, and medical topics, many more FidoNet nodes do not carry health-related discussions.

FidoNet subject matter discussion areas are called "echos." All messages in one echo are batched and exchanged with all nodes that carry that echo at a regional level. They are further batched and exchanged with counterpart nodes at national and international levels. Thus, all messages in an echo are exchanged with each other at a low-use time, usually during the night. It may take one night to exchange messages within an echo within a region, and a couple of nights to exchange messages within an echo with another country. As messages are exchanged and copied, they "reverberate" or echo throughout the system. Over a period of just a few days, each node of an echo posts all messages within that echo from around the world.

One particularly pertinent echo is the International Nurses' Net which is carried by many nodes in the United States and also in Canada, the Netherlands, and the United Kingdom. Some of the subjects that have been discussed recently on the International Nurses' Net echo are: Joint Commission for the Accreditation of Healthcare Organizations standards and site visits, nursing diagnosis, shift work, availability of software, pro-

Table 1.
Approximate Names of FidoNet Health-Related Echos

AIDS/ARC National Discussion

Alcoholism and Drug Abuse National Echo–Recovery (AA & Al-Anon)

Alzheimer's Disease

Anesthesia Discussion Echo

Blinktalk

Carcinoma

(Child Abuse Echo)–Please

Chronic Fatigue Syndrome

Chronic Pain

Cerebral Palsy

Diabetes National Discussion

Disabled Interests National Echo

European Disabled Users Echo

Fire/EMS National Echo

Grand Parents

Grand Rounds National Medical Discussion

Health Physics Echo

Hearing Disabilities Echo–Deaf Users Echo

Holistic Health National Forum

Incest

International Nurses' Network

Multiple Sclerosis

Organ Transplant Echo

Overeaters Anonymous Echo

Problem Child

Physicians Only National Conference

Psychiatry/Psychology Echo–National Psychiatry Echo

Rare Disease

Social Services National Echo

Spinal Injury National Echo–Spinal Cord Injured

Spouse & Child Abuse Echo

Stress Management Echo

Stroke

Survivor

Traumatic Head Injury & CerebroVascular Accident National Discussion

Visual Disabilities

Radiology Echo

Table 2. Nurse Managed FidoNet Nodes

Node Name	Location	Dataline	Nurse Manager
Nurse Corner	Orlando, FL	(407) 299-4762	Nurse Manager
PC Nurse	New Castle, DE	(302) 335-3088	Nurse Manager
SON*NET	Austin, TX	(512) 471-7584	Nurse Manager
The Nurses Station	South Shore, KY	(606) 932-9597	Nurse Manager
Trilogy	Laurel, MD	(301) 880-0965	Nurse Manager

gramming languages, IV certification, and breast implant information.

Many health-related echos actually consist of electronic support groups (ESGs). These are generally medical diagnosis-named echos where patients and clients and sometimes, nurses, physicians, and other health professionals share information, opinions, solutions, problems, dreams, and fears. Since local sys-ops are able to name echos on the screens, such as the Main Menu, that they create, the names of the ESGs may vary somewhat from node to node. Table 1 lists the approximate names of the current health-related echos.

Table 2 lists nurse-managed FidoNet nodes, their locations, and their datalines. For more information about FidoNet, contact one of the nurse sys-ops or:

Ed Del Grosso, MD. Black Bag Medical BBS List.

Black Bag BBS (150/140) (302) 994-3772 (dataline)

CIS 71565,1532

Genie: E. DELGROSSO

Internet: delgross@apache.dtcc.edu

On BITNET

The most significant electronic resources currently on BITNET designed specifically for nurses are LISTSERVs. "LISTSERV" is the acronym for "list server." These are the BITNET equivalent of Internet LISTPROCs.

Since listserv communications are e-mail, participants on Internet and FidoNet can, with minor modifications of the electronic address, subscribe to and participate in BITNET listservs. At this time there is no specific LISTSERV specifically of special interest to nurses.

To learn more about BITNET, contact the local institutional computer center administration or staff. Like Internet, BITNET nodes vary from site to site.

EDUCOM
BITNET Network Information Center
1112 16th Street NW, Suite 600
Washington, DC 20036
(202) 872-4200 (voice)

On FITNET

Participation in FITNET provides access to a bulletin board where messages are posted about technology in nursing education in general, about specific interactive technologies available to members of the FITNE consortium, and about technology-based problems and solutions. There are also Special Forums for discussion of software, of matters related to instructional development, for information about conferences, and for sharing news and abstracts of research.

For more information about FITNET, contact:

FITNET
Fuld Institute for Technology in Nursing Education
28 Station Street
Athens, OH 45701
(614) 592-2511 (voice)

Participation in networking, once one knows which network(s) to access, is relatively simple. Many users already involved in networking are pleased to help neophytes find their way to the information and the form of electronic communication desired. Help is usually available online.

To make good use of networking to support and fulfill your goals, you need only use the networks; in this way you enhance the network by your direct participation in the process. The more informed the participants, the better the networking. Letting the network participants know what subjects you are interested in, need assistance with, can offer assistance with, are essential to tailoring communications to meet your networking and information needs. Please come and share the future of nursing electronically by joining and participating in one of the networks and resources described here!

New Electronic Health Care Community: The Denver Free-Net

Diane J. Skiba, PhD, RN
Associate Professor and Director of Informatics
Center for Nursing Research
University of Colorado Health Sciences Center

Drew T. Mirque, BA
Project Administrator
University of Colorado Health Sciences Center

Introduction

The current crisis in U.S. health care has precipitated a critical analysis of the costs and delivery of health care to citizens. Such publications as *Healthy People 2000* (Department of Health and Human Services, 1991), *Healthy America: Practitioners for 2005* (Shugars, O'Neil, and Bader, 1991), and *Healthy People in a Healthy World: The Belmont Vision for Health Care in America* (Institute for Alternative Futures, 1992) have advanced specific ideas of what changes are needed in the health care arena. One such document is *Nursing's Agenda for Health Care Reform* (American Nurses Association, 1991), which provides a blueprint for the restructuring of the health care system. The authors of this document advocate the principles of equal access to health care, a balance between health promotion/prevention and illness services, and a consumer focus: The Agenda is described as "a plan that encourages health care consumers' participation and promotes nursing care as the link between the consumer and the health care system" (Reifsnider, 1992, p. 65). *Nursing's Agenda* demands a new approach to health care delivery—taking health care to the consumer who will be an increasingly informed participant in decisions affecting his/her care (National League for Nursing [NLN], 1992). This demand will create new opportunities for health care to be delivered in a variety of new settings, such as the workplace or school-based clinics. According to the National League for Nursing publication, *An Agenda for Nursing Education Reform*, (1992), hospitals and other institutions will no longer be the dominant influence; the consumer will assume that position.

Within this context of change, many opportunities arise for nurses to explore the use of information systems in the health care delivery system. The purpose of this chapter is to examine the use of electronic networks as an option for health care delivery. This chapter specifically explores the use of electronic networks with a consumer-based focus. It contains three sections: The first section presents the challenge—providing consumers with access to health care information as one component to facilitate their active participation in health care decisions. The second section highlights the opportunities to meet this challenge that are currently available in the areas of information systems and health-oriented telecommunications. A review of electronic network usage in nursing care delivery provides additional support for a consumer-based system. The final section describes a community computing project in Colorado designed to empower consumers to become active participants in maintaining a healthy community.

The Challenge

Providing access to high-quality, cost-effective care that is consumer-oriented is not a simple task. Access to health care incorporates two key areas: health care for the more than 37 million who cannot find ready access (Shugars et al., 1991) and access to health care information that has normally been under the purview of the health care professional. Information about quality and a focus on the measurement of health outcomes are concerns for both the consumer and the health care provider. The cost of health care must also be examined as it places limits on the capacity to respond to the issues of access and quality (Shugars et al., 1991). Consumer-oriented health care also requires major changes in the value systems of individuals and health care professionals. *Healthy People in a Healthy World* (Institute for Alternative Futures, 1992) advocates that our health care system be based upon a social contract, a conscious exchange of rights and responsibilities between individuals and their communities. Health rights allow all consumers to participate in a universal health care system in which society must recognize this equal participation and seek to reduce inequalities in access to health care. According to this vision, "society, through publicly set priorities, defines and limits certain medical care choices . . . [and] individuals have the right to make appropriate choices." To make those choices, consumers need access to comprehensive information. These rights also imply greater individual responsibility for personal health habits, the health of one's family, community and the environment, as well as the viability of the health care system itself. According to the authors of *Healthy People in a Healthy World,* consumers must make informed choices and appropriate use, and above all, maintain reasonable expectations of the health care delivery system.

Given these new assumptions of health care, consumer models and the consumer/provider relationship must be examined. According to Gustafson, Bosworth, Hawkins, Boberg, and Bricker (1992), "effective health care delivery increasingly involves a partnership between providers and consumers in which effective treatment depends upon a well-informed consumer who can make difficult health care decisions" (p. 161). Access to health care information and support for optimal treatment decisions are often barriers for consumers to make informed health care choices. Information pertinent to make choices about personal health behaviors, health care providers and therapies must be provided to consumers. Health promotion and prevention materials must be emphasized. Consumers need information about wellness programs, exercise, nutrition and self-care therapies to promote active involvement in health maintenance (Shugars et al., 1991).

To achieve these health care goals, individuals must understand the relationship between lifestyle behaviors and their medical consequences. To promote this understanding, individuals must have readily accessible health care information. This information needs to be accessible at the time a health care decision is being made. According to McDonald and Blum (1992), 95% of all first-line health decisions are made at home or in the workplace by the person and family or friends. Additionally, most individuals wait too long to handle health care problems, resulting in longer, more complex and costly care (McDonald and Blum, 1992). Many health care policy authors (Grundner and Garrett, 1986; Melmed and Fisher, 1991; Olson, Jones, and Bezold, 1992) believe that taking effective self-care and health promotion into the home is of critical value in resolving the health care crisis.

To date, most printed information, as well as computerized information systems, remains in the service of health care professionals (Melmed and Fisher, 1991). Information systems are designed to address such issues as staffing, scheduling, budgeting, strategic planning, administrative operations, clinical care, ancillary care and research. All have in common the need for the health care professional to access, process and manage information to provide high-quality, cost-effective health care. The missing component is the patient's access and management of information required to be an active participant in the health care process.

The recent work of the Computer-based Patient Record focuses on computer uses for health care professionals. Even the White House Task Force on Healthcare Reform's (Workgroup in Information Systems) development of Community Health Management Information Systems (CHMIS), based on the computerized patient record, focuses on linking key parties in the health care delivery system. According to Scott (1993), under CHMIS, key parties (physicians, nurses, other health care professionals, hospitals, nursing facilities, home health care agencies, clinical laboratories, pharmacies, payers, state health departments, employers and health insurance purchasing cooperatives) will have access to pertinent clinical and administrative data. The CHMIS concept, pioneered by the Hartford Foundation, should create more efficient claims and financial settlement transactions, as well as provide an unobtrusive system designed to meet the community's shared data needs. The CHMIS will also provide the community with information on costs and effectiveness of health care plans and provide data for community-wide wellness studies and health outcomes research. Although the consumer appears to be missing in this health network concept, several authors (Gabler, 1993; Simpson, 1993; Wakerly, 1993) reported that patients will be phased into these networks toward the end of the 1990s. Gabler projects that development of health information networks will come in stages, and that it is not until stage 4 (Value-added enhancements) and stage 5 (Open architecture utility) that consumers will be an integral part of the network.

The Opportunity

Gustafson et al. (1992) stated that if consumers are to participate actively in health care decision-making, barriers such as access to health information, need for confidentiality, limited financial resources and support for understanding complex medical problems must be overcome. According to Gustafson et al., "a computer-based support system can reduce these barriers by the provision of information and support that is convenient, comprehensive, timely, non-threatening, anonymous and controlled by the user" (p. 161). The marriage of computer and communication technologies in the last decade has promoted the use of information networks. Simpson (1993) has predicted that health information networks will become pervasive in society and their use will allow health care professionals to take health care "beyond the walls of an institution." Nurses will be able to use information systems to communicate with and monitor patients at home. Nurses in this scenario could have daily contact with their patients for follow up on medications, questions and a host of reminders for health promotion and prevention. In addition, patients could communicate with their health care providers and inform them of any unusual symptoms or concerns. Simpson projects that information *systems* will become information *utilities* in the future similar to the telephone or electric utility services. The constant blurring among technologies such as video phones, cable television and computer systems with communications facilities will make this information utility a possibility in the near future.

The National Information Infrastructure (NII) or the Information Superhighway proposed by the Clinton and Gore administration illustrates the administration's plans for an enhanced national communications environment (Ishida and Landweber, 1993). Video conferencing, access to libraries and information repositories, multimedia entertainment options and support for health care consultations are just some of the services projected to be available to homes, schools and institutions via the NII. The concomitant promotion of NII is viewed as one potential solution to many of the social, economic, health and education issues facing our nation. General interest magazines abound with articles on the "information superhighway" with promises of interactive multimedia services available in your home (Elmer-Dewitt, 1993). A recent draft of a Public Interest Communication Policy Agenda (Center for Civic Networking, 1993) supports the notion that the NII is a key to a revitalized American economy and civic culture. Examples of this revitalization include opportunities for local economic growth; improved delivery of government services; reduction of health care costs through prevention; early detection of disease and streamlining health care administration; equalization of children's educational opportunities; and reduction of pollution, road maintenance and child care costs via telecommuting.

In recent years the health care community has produced several documents advocating use of a telecommunications infrastructure to provide health, education and civic applications in the home. Melmed and Fisher (1991) provided numerous examples of communication and information applications that could be available to the public and provide considerable benefits to society. Examples included interactive health care consultation systems, interactive systems with access to governmental and civic information, electronic systems to improve the political process and educational applications such as job training, literacy and English as a second language training. A similar report by Olson et al. (1992) highlighted interactive multimedia systems with specific health care consultation and educational examples. A recent study by the Environmental Science and Policy Institute (McDonald and Blum, 1992) stated that a telecommunication infrastructure could provide health care to the poorest and most disaffected segments of the population. Health-oriented telecommunications could save hundreds of billions of dollars over the next two decades. According to this report, the proposed interactive network could provide: access to patient electronic medical records, integration of clinical data bases and preventive care, self-care medical advice and other health care information to consumers. These documents provide support for the continued development and implementation of network systems for the community.

Health Care Delivery Via Electronic Networks

The possibility of provision of health care via electronic networks have been examined by several researchers in nursing and medicine. For many years, several electronic bulletin boards (BBSs) have provided information and communication resources for health care professionals. Electronic support groups were initiated by many BBSs within the last five years (Sparks, 1992). Electronic support groups were available according to specific diseases (HIV+/AIDS, Diabetes, mental health, alcoholism). The electronic support groups provided 24-hour service in which consumers could selectively participate in discussions about their health problems. This non-face-to-face communication provided a non-threatening environment in which to ask questions, share feelings and communicate with others who experienced similar consequences of their specific diseases/health problems. One such network is the Nurse Corner in which several electronic support groups have been flourishing for years. The Nurse Corner's philosophy, according to Sparks, "is to help participants manage situations as independently as possible, yet know when and how to get help when needed" (p. 62). The Nurse Corner participants also have access to a knowledge-based, decision-support system that provides information and management options for several different health care problems. Besides Nurse's Corner, several other BBSs such as NurseLink (Skiba and Warren, 1991), SON-NET, and Nightingale carry these electronic support groups for their users. These discussion groups were shared nationally and internationally across the FidoNet network that supports several thousand BBSs.

An examination of electronic BBSs and their uses by the disabled was investigated by Hassett, Lowder, and Rutan (1992). Their study surveyed current users of BBSs and electronic support groups relating to physical disabilities. A total of 26 users responded to the survey that provided information about the usage and benefits of an electronic network. The majority of the users connected to the networks from home and used the network on a daily basis. Communication, information, fun and support were the primary reasons listed in descending order for the use of the networks. Few participants used the network for employment purposes. Hassett et al. (1992) concluded these results demonstrated the feasibility of using electronic networks for the provision of information, services, assistance and support for the disabled population and their caretakers.

Two extensive studies examined the use of an electronic network in the provision of care for both Persons Living with Aids (PLWAs) (Brennan, Ripich, and Moore, 1991) and caretakers of Alzheimer's Disease (AD) patients (Brennan, Moore, and Smyth, 1991). In both studies, Brennan and her colleagues investigated the use of an electronic network, ComputerLink, to bring support services into the homes of patients or caretakers. The first study was a pilot study to investigate the use of a computerized network to provide services for PLWAs. The ComputerLink system provided three basic services: an electronic encyclopedia, a decision-support system and a communication pathway. The electronic encyclopedia was designed to meet the patient's informational needs and served as a clearinghouse for factual information about AIDS, clinical care and local community services (Brennan, Ripich, and Moore, 1991). The decision-support tool was tailored to meet the problem-solving needs of patients and used a decision-modeling tool based upon multi-attribute utility theory. The communication pathway functioned as a social and professional contact to decrease patients' social isolation needs. This pathway allowed patients to talk with their health care provider, each other and other members of the electronic community served by the Cleveland Free-Net system. Within the communication pathway, patients could access the question and answer (Q & A's) section to read and post anonymous questions that would be answered by the project nurse.

The first segment of the pilot study focused on the introduction and use of this computer-mediated communication system. Each patient was given a computer system complete with a modem and instructions on how to connect to the Cleveland Free-Net, a free electronic community system available 24 hours per day. The Cleveland Free-Net served as the core computer network for this project. The system provides text-based community resources, electronic mail (e-mail) services, and interactive communication opportunities. In this phase, 15 patients used the Free-Net system most often for e-mail services. Mail was used as a means to communicate with the nurse project director as well as to others on the system. Patients also explored such areas as the Public Kiosk (an open discussion forum) and clinical data bases on the Free-Net.

The second study phase focused on the use of ComputerLink and its sequestered AIDS services area. According to patient self-reports, all nine patients used the decision-support system at least once and used the electronic encyclopedia to review at least eight different sections. The communication pathway was used most often by patients. Communication usage included both private mail between patients and with their nurse, as well as public communication via the discussion groups and Q & A sections. Brennan, Ripich, and Moore (1991) concluded that a computer network was feasible to maintain social contact and to provide self-care information.

In the case of caretakers of AD patients, ComputerLink provided three services for the caretaker. The first service facilitated communication between the caretaker and the nurse, as well as discussions among the caretakers themselves. This communication pathway was conceived as a "support group without walls" (Brennan, 1992). The second service was an information resource that included an AD electronic encyclopedia and numerous patient educational materials. The third service was a decision support tool similar to the one provided for the PLWAs in the previous study.

The study demonstrated the feasibility of using a computerized network for the delivery of health care services to caretakers of AD patients. Caretakers (N = 47) accessed the system 3,888 times in the course of one year. Caretakers averaged 84 connections to the system with an average encounter lasting 12 minutes. The most widely used service was the communication pathway, followed by access to information resources. Caretakers accessed the private mail function, discussion groups, and the Question and Answer section as a part of the communication pathway. Information resources were accessed over 500 times by caretakers. The least used service was the decision support tool that was accessed over 100 times. Brennan (1992) concluded that ComputerLink promotes peer collaboration around complex health care problems and prepares individuals to better participate in health care decision-making.

Parietti and Atav (1993) reported on the use of a computerized network to provide nursing consultation, case management, social support and information resources for HIV+/PLWAs in rural upstate New York. The BBS system, AIDSNET, is operated by the School of Nursing at the State University of New York in Binghampton. The system is available 24 hours per day, 7 days a week at no cost for registered users. These registered users can read and send electronic messages, read and receive information from national AIDS networks, read health education presentations and communicate with a nurse consultant. The nurse consultant is a master's prepared nurse currently employed in a primary care clinic for AIDS patients. The system has an average of 30 users and receives 177 calls per month. According to Parietti and Atav, AIDSNET demonstrates the potential of improving the home health care of rural, isolated patients by providing a crucial link to a primary care nurse.

Another system, designed by the University of Wisconsin, is the Comprehensive Health Enhancement Support System (CHESS). The system was developed for users to: anonymously communicate with each other and health care providers, access information in a variety of formats, assess their health risks and decide how to regain control over their lives (Gustafson et al., 1992). CHESS currently contains five specific content areas: breast cancer, AIDS/HIV Infection, Sexual Assault, Substance Abuse, and Academic Crisis.

The CHESS system offers nine distinct services: Q & A (compilation of common questions in each topic area); Instant Library (data base of articles, brochures and pamphlets); Getting Help/Support (information about how to get help and support); Personal Stories (stories written by people who are living and coping with their health crises); Expert Mail (area to ask experts anonymous questions); Discussion Group (area to anonymously discuss topics with others); Decision Aid (tools to facilitate decision-making using multi-attribute utility models for both specific health care and generic decisions); Action Plan (tools to help users analyze their plans to implement their health care decisions based upon a change theory framework); and Assessment (a risk factors assessment tool). The authors anticipated CHESS would affect three major outcomes: health status (by making informed decisions, a better physical and emotional health status should be achieved), improved health behavior (tools like the decision and action analyses plus social support should facilitate the maintenance of healthy behaviors) and cost-effective service utilization (providing support for consumers to be effective users of health care services).

The CHESS system was pilot-tested in homes of patients with breast cancer and AIDS/HIV infection with positive outcomes related to appeal, usefulness and usability. Ten women with breast cancer used CHESS services 546 times during a 50-day pilot and 11 men with AIDS/HIV infection used the services 581 times during a 34-day pilot. The average amount of time was approximately 20 minutes/subject/day. The Communication and Information & Referral Services were the most frequently used services. As in Brennan, Ripich, and Moore's (1991) study, the decision support tools were used with less frequency. Many participants reported positive emotional outcomes of using CHESS. A more controlled evaluation of health status and outcomes is planned with the AIDS/ HIV infection population. An additional evaluation of CHESS usage in community sites is planned.

Early research findings have demonstrated the feasibility of electronic networks as health care delivery mechanisms. Several networks were successfully implemented in rural, urban and academic medical settings providing health care services for caretakers of AD patients, PLWA/HIV+ patients, breast cancer patients and the disabled population. Communication with peer groups and their health care providers was the most widely used service followed by access to information and referral resources. The benefits of decision support tools were yet to be realized within the medium of computer-mediated communication systems. Users reported both positive emotional support and other beneficial outcomes of electronic networks as health care delivery systems.

Nursing and Electronic Communities

Clearly the new health care reform demands, as well as the opportunities provided by electronic networks, will facilitate changes in the role nurses will play in the restructured health care delivery system. Nurses will function as patient care managers, i.e.,

> Someone who combines the roles of patient advocate, knowledgeable advisor, triage officer and channel of access to the system and someone who helps the patient and the family choose wisely when they face the knowledge gap between them and the health care professional while dealing with the anxiety usually associated with actual or potential illness and disability. (NLN, 1992)

Nurses are now in the position to explore all the possibilities that might promote consumer participation. Electronic networks provide one opportunity to facilitate consumer involvement.

To further this idea, let us examine one Electronic Health Care Community established within a new electronic community called the Denver Free-Net. To begin this exploration, the Denver Free-Net will be described and several examples provided of the health care building within our electronic community. The Denver Free-Net's Electronic Health Care Community embraces the concepts promoted by the work of Brennan (1992) and Gustafson et al. (1992), yet is placed within the context of a healthy community framework. According to the World Health Organization ("Colorado Trust," 1992), a healthy community is defined as "one that includes a clean, safe, high quality physical environment and a sustainable ecosystem; provision of basic needs; an optimum level of appropriate, high quality, accessible public health and sick care services; and a diverse, vital and innovative economy."

Denver Free-Net is best described as a community computing system available to anyone who has access to a computer equipped with a modem and telecommunication software. Users may connect through the phone lines or remotely log in to the system via the Internet, a globe-spanning network of networks. It is a menu-driven system allowing users to choose the number of the item they wish to view and then press the return key.

Denver Free-Net employs the features one would find on most bulletin board systems found all over the world; that is, users can read text and leave messages for other users and/or moderators. In addition to text-reading and e-mail, Denver Free-Net includes other valuable features. These include among others, file transfer, real-time chat, effective data base search tools, and the ability to participate in an on-going discussion.

The system allows users to access and read any type or format of document. The document can be presented in narrative form. Elementary data base search tools are used on Denver Free-Net to develop many support tools in the health care arena. The combination of the above features allows users of Denver Free-Net to effectively communicate with other professionals, access critical health care information, and play an important part in promoting and improving their own health care and the well-being of others.

The menus are organized and laid out on the model of a typical community. Users are presented with a main menu of "buildings," such as the Health Care Building, a Schoolhouse, Post Office, and so forth. The buildings contain all the information found on Denver Free-Net. Information on sending e-mail can be found in the Post Office where users can learn how to transfer files between their computers and Denver Free-Net in the Communication Center. The Administration Building will house all the information related to the operation of the Denver Free-Net. From the Main menu, all the information is designed to branch out from the main building. The user can envision the structure to represent a family tree diagram. Within the Health Care Building are numerous submenus which correlate to major health care topics: The Cancer Center, Consumer Health Tips, Online Publications for the Practitioner, and so forth.

As mentioned previously, one of the more valuable features on Denver Free-Net is the ability to develop and utilize data bases. Data bases can be searched by the users applying a variety of methods through keywords or a combination of keywords. A functional data base online allows users to search the Denver metro area for support groups on a particular condition or topic.

<<< The Support Groups Center–From A to Z >>>
(go support)

1 About the Support Groups Center
2 Support Groups Index
3 Search and Display Supp9ort Group Information

(h)elp, (m)ain, (p)revious, e(x)it DFN.

Your Choice = = >

One can search the data base by topic or condition; another search may involve the topic and the zip code desired; still another may be topic and location, such as a general town or geographic area. After entering the criteria, the user will receive a list of support groups conforming to the search criteria. Upon choosing the particular group by number, complete information about that group may be read on-line or downloaded to the user's computer to be read and utilized at a later time. This service is particularly helpful for both the consumer and health care professional; applicable support groups are provided by a wide range of interested parties.

The following screen highlights what users would see upon completing their search for a support group. The group was displayed after searching for the keywords of "AIDS" and "teens." Information displayed is what would be deemed of most value to both consumer and health care provider.

```
=============== Freenet Support Groups ===============
              Support Group Type is: AIDS
```
                  Colorado Aids Project (CAP)
Support & referral services offered for HIV+ & AIDS-diagnosed persons.
Services include hospital visitation, emergency financial assistance, food
bank, housing, transportation, legal referrals, support groups.
Contact: Phone: 837-0166 V/TDD:
            information line 830-AIDS
            (830-2437) V/TDD

            Colorado Aids Project (CAP)
            P.O. Box 18529
            Denver, CO 80218

            Meeting Information
            P.O. Box 18529

```
================================================
```
Type a Number to view a record, 'r' to repeat list, 'n' for a new query, or
'q' to quit ->

The user may continue with a search, repeat the list to identify more resources or quit the program.

On-line data bases are crucial in the drive to give health care providers essential tools in providing high-quality care in an efficient manner as well as providing consumers with the information necessary in promoting and improving their own health. However, on-line data bases are not the only tools Denver Free-Net can provide. Access to the Internet is another important resource which allows all users a connection to critical information found at other computer sites. Denver Free-Net connects its users to the Internet in a variety of ways, allowing them access to the infinite variety of resources found throughout the Internet. One method of bringing Internet to Denver Free-Net is by setting up Usenet newsfeeds. Usenet is a combination of worldwide discussion groups on an equally infinite variety of topics. One such newsgroup on Denver Free-Net is the HIV/AIDS Discussion newsgroup. The discussion is contributed to and developed by leading HIV authorities and includes the daily summary report generated by the Center for Disease Control. Consumers and health care professionals alike find this an invaluable resource. Usenet newsgroups can be found in all areas of Denver Free-Net's Health Care Building, as well as throughout the other buildings. Once connected to the desired group, the user chooses the item of interest, based on the subject heading. A sample Usenet newsgroup session follows:

The user is presented with a list of available health care Usenet newsgroups.

```
=== MGNR v2.3 ===================== [normal mode] ===
          (mod)       1 sci.med.aids
          (unmod)     2 sci.med.dentistry
          (unmod)     3 sci.med.nutrition
          (unmod)     4 sci.med.occupational
          (unmod)     5 sci.med.pharmacy
          (unmod)     6 sci.med.physics
          (unmod)     7 sci.med.telemedicin


          'p': Parent dir 'm': Main dir 'q': Exit MGNR 'h':  Help

          Enter command:
```

Users may choose the "sci.med.aids" newsgroup and participate in that group by posting messages, reading critical reports, or downloading or transferring the messages to their work directory on Denver Free-Net. The user would see a menu similar to the following:

First message is #4115, last message is #4327

4115. CDC Summary 08/12/93
4116. Re: Response to UML inquiry
4117. Re: Condoms
4118. Immigration ban
4119. Re: (10436) CDC Summary 7/26/93
4120. direct immunomagnetic quantification of CD4 and CD8
4121. VAMC NEWSLETTER
4122. Re: Response to UML inquiry
4123. Response to UML inquiry
4124. Exactly what is a T-cell count
4125. Re: Response to UML inquiry
4126. CDC Summary 08/13/93
4127. Re: Response to UML inquiry

---

c = Contribute a new message
n = Read next unread message
s = Read next unread message with same subject
h = Help, list of additional commands
q = Quit

Enter command:

The ability to set up newsgroups has provided Denver Free-Net with the opportunity to connect consumers to a variety of health care professionals. Users may enter a local newsgroup dedicated to School Health or Adolescent Health. They may leave a question for the moderator of the particular group and expect to receive an answer in a timely manner. Newsgroups can be moderated or chaired; unmoderated, so anyone may post a question or message; or the group may be anonymous, allowing users to ask questions without having their user ID identified. This anonymous variation has been found to be helpful in areas such as School Health and HIV/AIDS.

E-mail is an effective and essential method of communication on the Denver Free-Net. Registered users have access to a very powerful tool. Various editors, which allow the user to compose and format documents and messages, are available. Users may also choose to compose off-line and upload their text. This option is important for those who do much of their editing and composing at off times and do not have the luxury of accessing Free-Net during the workday. The e-mail function allows users to send messages and files to other users on the system or to any user who has an e-mail account on the Internet.

Users can always take advantage of the extensive on-line help section. These help files accommodate everyone from the least experienced user to the advanced system user. The help files cover every feature found on Denver Free-Net, ensuring that users can always immediately address any uncertainty they may encounter on the system.

The many features of Denver Free-Net provide a comprehensive and practical resource for both the health care provider and consumer. There is a wealth of consumer-oriented information available. The information is readily accessible and easy to retrieve. Consumers can also communicate with health care providers in the question and answer forums. The consumer may also participate in worldwide discussions about health care topics. The health care professional has the same privileges as the consumer. In addition, there is the option for the health care professional to become an information provider and present information resources to the public. What has been presented about the resources available represents only a fraction of what exists and can exist on the system. The Denver Free-Net is a community resource built within a health community context with a health care consumer focus.

Summary

The world of health care reform is providing numerous challenges to the health care professions. One challenge is to provide an accessible cost-effective, consumer-oriented health care delivery system. This challenge builds upon the assumption that consumers and health care professionals will enter into a social contract in which there are certain rights and responsibilities. The world of computer-mediated communications and community health information systems provide numerous opportunities for nurses to create new health care delivery systems. Electronic health care communities have been studied in the nursing arena and represent a viable delivery mechanism to provide nursing care and support for patients in the community. The Electronic Health Care Community affords both the consumer and the nurse new methods of communication and fosters new patient/provider relationships. Most importantly, the use and development of this Electronic Health Care Community truly allows the nurse to become a patient care manager in this restructured health care environment.

References

American Nurses Association. (1991). *Nursing's Agenda for Health Care Reform*. Kansas City, MO: Author.

Brennan, P. (1992). Computer networks promote caregiving collaboration: The ComputerLink Project. In M. Frisse (Ed.), *Proceedings of the Sixteenth Symposium of Computer Applications in Medical Care*. New York: McGraw-Hill Book Co.

Brennan, P., Moore, S., and Smyth, K. (1991). ComputerLink: Electronic support for the home caregiver. *Advances in Nursing Science, 13*(4), 14-27.

Brennan, P., Ripich, S., and Moore, S. (1991). The use of home-based computers to support persons living with AIDS/ARC. *Journal of Community Health Nursing, 8*(1), 3-14.

Center for Civic Networking. (1993, July). *A Vision of Change: Civic Promise of the National Information Infrastructure*. Cambridge, MA: Author.

Colorado Trust unveils strategic study. (1992). *The Colorado Trust Quarterly*.

Department of Health and Human Services. (1991). *Healthy People 2000: National Health Promotion and Disease Prevention Objectives* (DHHS Publication No. PHS 91-50212). Washington, DC: U.S. Government Printing Office.

Elmer-Dewitt, P. (1993, April 12). Take a trip into the future on the electronic superhighway. *TIME*, 50-55.

Gabler, J. (1993, March). Shared information boosts competition in networks. *Computers in Healthcare*, 20-23, 25-26.

Grundner, T. M., and Garrett, R. (1986). Interactive Medical Telecomputing: An Alternative Approach to Community Health Education. *New England Journal of Medicine, 15*, 982-985.

Gustafson, D., Bosworth, K., Hawkins, R., Boberg, E., and Bricker, E. (1992). CHESS: A computer-based system for providing information, referrals, decision support and social support to people facing medical and other health-related crisis. In M. Frisse (Ed.), *Proceedings of the Sixteenth Symposium of Computer Applications in Medical Care* (pp. 161-165). New York: McGraw-Hill Book Co.

Hassett, M., Lowder, C., and Rutan, D. (1992). Use of computer network bulletin board systems by disabled persons. In M. Frisse (Ed.), *Proceedings of the Sixteenth Symposium of Computer Applications in Medical Care* (pp. 151-155). New York: McGraw-Hill Book Co.

Institute for Alternative Futures. (1992). *Healthy People in a Healthy World: The Belmont Vision for Health Care in America.* Alexandria, VA: Author.

Ishida, H., and Landweber, L. (1993). Internetworking: An introduction. *Communications of the Association of Computing Machinery, 36*(8), 28-29.

McDonald, M. D., and Blum, H. L. (1992). *Health in the Information Age: The Emergence of Health-oriented Telecommunication Applications.* Berkeley, CA: University of California.

Melmed, A., and Fisher, F. (1991). *Towards a National Information Infrastructure: Implications for Selected Social Sectors and Education.* New York: New York University.

National League for Nursing. (1992, October). *An Agenda for Nursing Education Reform.* New York: Author.

Olson, R., Jones, M., and Bezold, C. (1992). *21st Century Learning and Health Care in the Home: Creating a National Telecommunications Network.* Washington, DC: Institute for Alternative Futures and The Consumer Interest Research Institute.

Parietti, E., and Atav, A. (1993). AIDSNET. *Connections, 2*(1), 2.

Reifsnider, E. (1992). Restructuring the American Health Care System: An analysis of Nursing's Agenda for Health Care Reform. *Nurse Practitioner, 17*(5), 65, 69-70, 72, 75.

Scott, J. (1993, July). Community health MIS. *Computers in Healthcare,* 22-23, 25, 28.

Shugars, D., O'Neil, E., and Bader, J. (1991) *Healthy America: Practitioners for 2005, An Agenda for Action for U.S. Health Professional Schools.* Durham, NC: Pew Health Profession Commission.

Simpson, R. (1993). Case-managed care in tomorrow's information network. *Nursing Management, 24*(7), 14-16.

Skiba, D., and Warren, C. (1991). The impact of an electronic bulletin board to disseminate educational and research information to nursing colleagues. In E. Hovenga, K. Hannah, K. McCormick, and J. Ronald (Eds.), *Nursing Informatics '91: Proceedings of the Fourth International Conference on Nursing Use of Computers and Information Science, 42,* 704-709. Berlin: Springer-Verlag.

Sparks, S. (1992). Exploring electronic support groups. *American Journal of Nursing, 92*(12), 62-65.

Wakerly, R. (1993, March). Open systems drive health information networks. *Computers in Healthcare, 30,* 32-33, 35.

Quality Improvement via Clinical Information Systems

Carol A. Romano, PhD, RN, FAAN
Director, Clinical Systems and Quality Improvement
National Institutes of Health Clinical Center

Introduction

Modern health care institutions are experiencing a major transformation in their managerial efforts to improve quality of care. Currently, the movement from traditional quality assurance programs to initiatives focused on continuous improvement to the quality of care is changing institutional methods of managing health care.

The Quality Paradigm

Berwick (1989) discusses two theories of quality that describe the climate in which health care is delivered. The first theory suggests that quality is achieved through inspection, and thresholds for acceptability are established. This theory, commonly referred to as "The Bad Apple Theory," asserts that hazards and deficiencies in health care are caused by poor intentions. The theory implies that the cause is staff members who do not care enough to do their best, or what they know is right. This Bad Apple Theory can be contrasted with the Theory of Continuous Quality Improvement. From this alternative perspective, improvements in quality care are said to depend on understanding and revising the systems and processes within an organization. Theorists of this alternative persuasion assert that every process produces information from which the process can be improved (Deming, 1982). The focus of this approach, however, is on continuous improvement throughout the organization as a result of a constant effort to reduce waste, rework, and complexity. Historically, quality assurance programs in the United States have focused on the Bad Apple Theory. Contemporary quality programs are beginning to incorporate the theory of continuous improvement; in contrast, quality assessment initiatives focus on the objectives of productivity and improvement in quality through refinement and revisions to systems of work, systems of information and systems of communication. The fact that quality can never be assured is acknowledged. The objective, instead, is to assess the level of quality that exists, and then to direct initiatives to improve the existing quality.

Quality Principles

The new quality paradigm embraces several key management principles (Appel, 1991) usually referred to as Total Quality Management or Continuous Quality Improvement (CQI). These principles suggest that first, quality improvement requires the direct involvement and commitment of top *clinical and managerial leaders*. Next, an organization must define quality in terms of meeting the needs and *expectations of customers*. Third, quality improvement must occur through *examination* and continuous improvement *of the key processes and systems* through which health care and services are delivered to customers. Fourth, to be skilled in providing quality, an organization must become skilled in *information gathering and use*. And finally, CQI principles assert that employees must be educated, empowered, and supported to pursue *quality through teamwork.* These principles support the belief that for a system to be improved, the system itself must first be assessed and understood. The reduction of variance in the performance of work routines or in the processes of delivering, as well as in communicating care and service, is also required so that quality can be consistent and predictable.

Role of Clinical Information Systems

A computerized clinical information system is defined as an automated information processing system that is designed to support the operations, management, and decision functions related to delivering or administering clinical care or services. Such a system has the capability to collect, transmit, process, store, retrieve and distribute information. From the perspective of CQI, a computerized information system to support the practice of medicine and nursing can be viewed both as a vehicle for improving the communication and information systems within an organization and as a mechanism through which other organizational processes and systems of work can be improved. Improvement can be accomplished by decreasing the variance or inconsistency in handling information and thereby eliminating the redundancy of information that is sent, received and archived. The computerized information system can also extract specific data for the systematic assessment of quality. In this manner, the system can support the principles of CQI through the provision of educational information regarding the quality standards for specific clinical functions. Further, a computer information system has the potential to trigger collaboration in problem solving related to the use and management of patient information. Finally, this technological innovation can be used to communicate support for CQI initiatives from the top management level throughout the organization.

Several clinical applications for a specific Hospital Information System (HIS) were developed for a 500-bed teaching-research hospital. For the past 18 years, the Clinical Center of the National Institutes of Health has implemented, evaluated and maintained an integrated hospital-wide computerized information system for clinical care. This system is used to write and process medical orders, to report clinical test results, and to record nursing notes and plans of care (Romano, 1984). Most importantly, the system provides an electronic patient record. In the ongoing development of the system, specific information management innovations were made in the area of advance directives, blood administration, patient allergy identification, infection control, medication administration, communication of continuing care needs, and nursing assessments in inpatient and ambulatory care settings. Each application is presented below from the perspective of the defined need for the improvement, a description of the applications, and the response of the health professional. The evaluation of each application was done through organizational meetings, focus groups, and/or internal surveys.

Clinical Applications

Advance Directives

An advance directive is defined as a written document that specifies, in advance, a person's preferences concerning medical treatment. This treatment includes use of life-sustaining technologies and management of the advance of a medical condition or cognitive impairment that may render the person incapable of making health care decisions at a future time. In 1991, health care legislation required that the existence of such a directive for any patient be assessed upon each patient's admission. In addition, a patient's request for more information about advance directives needs to be assessed and accommodated

(Dimond, 1992). To address this need, the HIS was designed to prompt an admission clerk to solicit and record this information during the admission process. The information provided becomes a part of the permanent electronic patient record. Advance directive information is incorporated into the computerized nursing admission note to reflect standards of practice regarding the nursing responsibility in this area. The technology facilitates the collection, recording, and processing of consistent and complete information. The admission note with its added request for further information was also designed to trigger a written request for a bioethics consultation to the Hospital Office of Ethics.

The status and type of advance directive for each patient is programmed to print on specified patient documents like the Kardex or medical care plan. The on-line retrieval of the information during and after discharge is also available to prompt a review of this information by the caregiver on subsequent patient admissions. Organizational feedback from physicians and nurses regarding this application has been favorable. Implementation of the legislation and the resulting hospital policy was facilitated, and medical and nursing responsibility was clarified throughout the computerized system.

Blood Administration

The need to comply with standards for prescribing irradiated blood components, to streamline the medical ordering of blood, to clarify nursing certification requirements for blood administration, and to simplify the reporting and recording of adverse blood transfusion reactions were identified as improvement opportunities. In response, several revisions were made to the clinical information system. First, criteria for use of irradiated blood components were established in policy and incorporated as a requirement into the physician's computer pathways for ordering blood. All blood ordering was performed directly by the physician via the HIS. Second, the process for ordering blood component(s) on the computer was designed to differentiate between two specific medical orders: (1) a request to prepare blood from the Transfusion Medicine Department, and (2) the administration instructions to the nurse for rate and volume. Third, this information was organized to print as a separate category of medical orders on the patient's plan of care (Kardex). Fourth, nurse certification requirements for blood administration were automatically programmed to print on nursing care plan documents, along with the standards of practice and standing medical orders for managing a potential transfusion reaction.

In the event of an adverse transfusion reaction, the HIS also was programmed to facilitate documentation of this patient event in the patient record, as well as to report the required regulatory information to the Transfusion Medicine staff. The nursing and medical standards for symptom identification and management were also programmed into the documentation pathways. The HIS eliminated duplication of effort by allowing the nursing documentation to simultaneously trigger the report of this information to the Blood Bank for follow up. All required specimen collection requisitions were also programmed to automatically print out in the nursing area when an adverse blood reaction was reported. An internal evaluation indicated that the medical and nursing response to this application was favorable. The computer application eliminated extra clerical work, forced consistency in the processes related to blood component administration, facilitated compliance with standards of care, and streamlined information management.

Patient Allergy Identification

The need to provide consistent and updated medical and nursing assessments regarding a patient's sensitivity/allergy to medications, foods, or other products across patient encounters in the inpatient and ambulatory care setting was identified as a quality improvement opportunity. In response, the HIS was designed to prompt physicians and nurses to conduct a standardized assessment of a patient's allergies/sensitivities on each encounter.

This information includes identification of the allergy/sensitivity, the source of information, the history and the supporting data or manifestations. This information is recorded and stored on-line so that a review of information on each subsequent patient encounter is possible. This ensures that the information is available when patients are seen for follow up in the ambulatory care clinic.

In addition, patient allergy information also prints on key patient documents, including the nursing plan of care. The process for physician ordering of any medication or diet in the HIS is also designed to prompt the prescriber with information regarding a patient's allergy history. The information is also available on-line to pharmacists and dieticians. Customer response to this application was evaluated internally and found to be positive. The inconsistency between nursing and medical assessment of allergies was eliminated; the availability of information on inpatients as well as outpatients provides continuity of information and hence continuity of care; and the accessibility of the information to other departments (i.e., nutrition and pharmacy) is available.

Infection Control

A mechanism to provide mandatory education regarding Universal Precautions to all physicians was needed. In addition, the need to communicate a patient's infectious status to hospital escort personnel when nurses requested patient transportation services was identified. The HIS was used as the vehicle to provide improvements in both these areas. First, educational content related to Universal Precautions was identified and programmed into the HIS so that physicians or nurses can access the information at their convenience. An interactive on-line evaluation of learning was also designed so that a self-assessment is conducted by the physician and feedback on incorrect responses is provided. Upon completion of the on-line training session, a written verification prints to confirm compliance with the requirement for the annual review of Universal Precautions information. This verification is sent to the medical credentialing office. Organizational feedback from physicians has been positive as the logistics and paperwork of annual continuing education are simplified.

To address the lack of communication of a patient's infectious status to hospital escort personnel, standards for gown/gloves/mask use for the transport of specific types of patient was clarified with Nursing, Hospital Epidemiology and Patient Escort Service. An HIS application was then designed to provide nursing with a mechanism to send an electronic request for service to the patient escort staff. The request was designed to include the patient's isolation status as well as precaution information related to contagious diseases. This information is used by the patient escort service to ensure that only employees with specific disease immunities would be assigned to certain patient care situations. The HIS also provides a means to clarify requests for service so that the patient transportation time and the patient appointment time are differentiated. This clarification helps to facilitate planning and the timely escort of patients. An internal interdisciplinary evaluation was very favorable, as employees felt that their safety needs, as well as the patient's, were being addressed. Customer satisfaction was clearly achieved.

Medication Administration

The need to decrease medication errors and to provide consistent planning for emergency drug administration were identified as targeted areas for improvement. To improve the medication administration process, the HIS was used to reformat the documents that communicate a patient's current medication orders to nursing. Medications were categorized to print on the care plan documents according to the type of administration schedule. The printout was designed to subgroup medications into: (a) those with a scheduled time for administration; (b) medications to be given on request [prn]; and (c) medications to be given according to a conditional schedule (i.e., on call). Because of the volume and complexity of medications for some patients, this reorganization allows the nurse to more easily review, verify and synthesize information, and to plan to meet patient requirements. An internal survey indicated that the response has been very favorable.

The HIS was also used to provide more accurate and timely information on emergency drug dosages. Standard medication dosages and rates are used for adults in an emergency situation. However, for children, medication management in an emergency situation is contingent on the weight of these pediatric patients. To support more accurate medication administration, the recording of a pediatric patient's weight on admission was designed to automatically activate a computerized printout of emergency medication dosages specific for that patient's weight. A written document is always ready to use in the event of an emergent patient clinical situation. This application eliminates the need for complex calculations during an emergency. It also allows for the availability of this information at all times at the patient's bedside. The information can always be updated if the patient's weight changes.

Continuity of Care

To enhance patient education, discharge instructions need to be legibly written, explained, and given to the patient and family. To support the continuity of care, these instructions must be recorded in the patient's clinical record. In addition, all verbal interactions that occur between provider and patient must be recorded. The need to avoid duplication of effort and inconsistency in recording discharge instructions in the patient record, as well as in a document given to the patient upon discharge, was identified. The capacity to record patient telephone encounters with the nurse after the patient is discharged also needed to be accommodated. To address these improvement opportunities, the computerized HIS was programmed to communicate to the nurse the standards of practice for patient discharge instruction. In addition, the ability to record this information in the electronic patient record was developed to generate a printout for the patient upon discharge. The information in both documents was produced with one entry by a nurse. The patient document, however, was re-formatted for easy readability. The information was designed to stay on-line 60 days after a patient's discharge so that retrieval of the information is available for easy reference and follow up if needed.

To accommodate documentation of telephone encounters between patient visits, content on the HIS was developed to allow the nurse to enter an assessment, planned interventions and patient outcomes resulting from any telephone interaction. This information is also kept on-line for 60 days and then automatically printed on a permanent patient record document and filed. A patient's name is never removed from the on-line information system; thus, the ability to access the patient's record and to record information on-line is always available.

All patient information for inpatient and outpatient encounters is integrated into one electronic patient record. Access to patient information across care settings has been very well received. The fragmentation found with separate inpatient and outpatient charts is eliminated, and accessibility to information from a prior patient encounter is available to physicians and nurses so that continuity of care can be provided.

Nursing Documentation

The need to improve consistency in patient assessments related to mental status, substance abuse, and pain/discomfort was identified by clinical nurses. The potential outcome to be achieved was an increase in the reliability of patient data collection in these areas and the ability to compare and evaluate patient responses and outcomes over time.

To accomplish this, standards of practice were developed for assessment in each of these areas. Where possible, valid assessment instruments such as the Folstein Mini Mental Status were incorporated into the visual displays of the HIS. In a research environment, this eliminated duplication of data entered into the patient record and the research data base. Information from the HIS can be extracted for analysis. In addition, on-line graphic capabilities for the trending of quantitative information is available as the HIS operates using multipurpose personal computers and graphics software.

Administrative Perspective

Administrative support for the involvement of customers in assessing quality of care is critical to the identification of areas for improvement. Customer involvement is also essential to help develop, implement, and evaluate clinical information systems if these systems are to be used successfully. Structures such as committees, task forces, or focus groups need to be constructed to include individuals who directly use clinical information to support patient care decisions. These users or customers of information are best suited to articulate what an information system should be designed to do and what constitutes a successful application. The structures and the tasks need to be carefully managed. The review, critique, testing prototypes of new innovations, and provision of feedback regarding the effectiveness and consequences of specific applications require skillful planning and leadership. The applications described above could not have been developed and implemented without these elements.

Summary

The development and implementation of the new paradigm of CQI was demonstrated through a description of the application of a hospital-wide computerized system, with an extensive nursing component. Evolving concepts of quality assessment, quality assurance, and quality improvement as they relate to use of information systems were reviewed. Specific clinical computer applications in relation to the defined need for improvement, the description of the application, and the health professional's response to the implemented innovation were detailed.

References

Appel, F. (1991). From quality assurance to quality improvement: The Joint Commission and the new quality paradigm. *Journal of Quality Assurance, 13*(5), 26-29.

Berwick, D. (1989). Continuous improvement as an ideal in health care. *New England Journal of Medicine, 320*(1), 53-56.

Deming, W. E. (1982). *Quality, Productivity, and Competitive Position.* Cambridge, MA: Massachusetts Institute of Technology, Center for Advanced Engineering Study.

Dimond, E. P. (1992). Oncology nurses' role in patient advance directives. *Oncology Nursing Forum, 19*(6), 891-896.

Romano, C. (1984). A computerized approach to discharge care planning. *Nursing Outlook, 32*(1), 23-25.

Strategies and Support for Managing Administrative Information

Integration of Managed Care with Information Systems 200

Maximizing Technology for Cost-Effective Staff Education
and Training 216

The Value of Bedside Computer Systems in Restructuring
Nursing Care 222

Communication Technologies for Nurse Executives 230

Nurse-Designed Voice-Activated Computer Systems for
Nursing Documentation 239

Automated Systems for Staffing, Scheduling, and Resource
Management 245

Integration of Managed Care with Information Systems

Bonita Ann Pilon, DSN, RN, CNAA
Assistant Professor and Director of Nursing Administration Program
Vanderbilt University
School of Nursing

Maria Hill, MS, RN
Senior Consultant
The Center for Case Management
South Natick, Massachusetts

Introduction

The current movement toward health care reform is a reality that is changing the nature of health care rendered by professionals in all delivery systems. The viability of the corporate American hospital as it now functions is threatened by the revelation of great system inefficiencies and fragmentation of care. In the new health care environment, the industry must respond to the demands clearly identified by national and local business alliances, managed care companies, federal and state governments, and patients and families, if it is to deliver quality care at reasonable cost. Health care systems or networks that focus on organization of care across the health continuum are now under development. In an effort to better understand and evaluate care management, the leaders in the health care industry must demonstrate a commitment to advances in information technology, team management of patient case types across the continuum of care, and refinement of advanced critical thinking skills.

According to Zander (1993), "The much-bemoaned inefficiency and fragmentation in health care is mirrored and perpetuated by existing information systems" (p. 34). These information systems fail to integrate data housed in the cost accounting, medical records, quality assurance, utilization/appropriateness review and acuity measurement programs within hospital systems. In addition, these systems fail to capture and report data, in real time, across geographic locations as the patient transitions back into the community. Computerization of the sophisticated tools and processes developed to coordinate care within health care systems has never been more essential. The integration of data bases contained within information systems must shift from isolated host/character-based systems to distributed, interconnected data management systems serving multiple clients, multiple providers and multiple media (Spitzer, 1993). In the near future these systems should be integrated using the CareMap® tool as the core of the electronic medical record.

Care Designed For Systems Improvement

The CareMap® and Case Management Systems, as well as the need to computerize the existing paper tools required to concurrently manage and retrospectively review patient outcomes achieved and cost of care delivered, are described in this chapter. The first section describes the tools and goals of CareMaps® and Case Management systems. The following section describes the successful application of information technology to support such systems as well as directions for the future. The chapter concludes with a discussion of some barriers to product development.

CareMap® and Case Management Systems are pragmatic and flexible systems designed to span the care continuum with a focus on cost and quality care outcomes. These systems were devised at the New England Medical Center in 1985 in response to: (1) implementation of diagnostic-related groups (DRGs) as a basis for reimbursement by the federal government; (2) the lack of integration of professional care plans into one working record/document of care; (3) the advancement of nursing knowledge without concomitant expansion of skills and roles; and (4) the introduction and integration of the Sociotechnical Systems approach to work redesign at the Medical Center (Zander, 1992). These systems have evolved over the past nine years; the current foci include identifying patient and family needs by case type, determining the timeframes necessary to achieve quality patient outcomes, reducing length of stay and inappropriate use of resources, and clarifying the appropriate environment, providers, and timeliness of interventions across the health care continuum. The systems mimic the production process of patient care, thus reflecting the core business of health care. Computerization of CareMaps® and case management tools would, therefore, allow concurrent management of resources, serve as both a document and record of care, and would have the potential to interface with multidisciplinary documentation and acuity/severity systems, cost accounting systems and operations management systems.

The CareMap® System

This system is designed to provide continuity of the plan of care and consists of four key components: (1) CareMap® tool; (2) variance analysis system with integration into the Continuous Quality Improvement (CQI) or quality management structure; (3) communication processes including change of shift report, discharge planning conferences, discussions with utilization review staff and patient care conferences; and (4) collaborative group practices which are designed to meet quarterly to perform case reviews and to review variance data, patient educational materials, and standing orders.

A CareMap® tool consists of a traditional critical pathway, a patient problem/issues list, benchmark goals demonstrating the clinical progression to end outcomes for each problem/issue identified, and a variance record designed to capture chronological deviations from the norm (Center for Case Management, 1992b). The CareMap® is created for a specific case type (designated by DRG, ICD-9 code, procedure or condition) by a team of professional staff members. Team members include representatives of the professional staff routinely providing care to patients and families in the case type selected. For example, the team comprised to develop a CareMap® for patients undergoing open-heart surgery may include representatives from cardiovascular surgery; anesthesiology; respiratory therapy; nurses from the operating room, recovery, intensive care, telemetry and home care; cardiac rehabilitation; social work; discharge planning; utilization review; dietary; pharmacy; and quality management.

Prior to a CareMap® session, team members may identify current patterns of care for the case type through chart review, evaluation of standards of care and practice, a comparison of clinical practice guidelines published by professional organizations, an analysis of institutional policies and procedures, review of physician orders, and results of discussions with patients and families regarding their perception of care received. Team members may also review patient bills to become aware of charges incurred for equipment, procedures and care rendered.

During a CareMap® session the team identifies key problems/issues experienced by a majority (75%) of patients presenting to this case type and the appropriate clinical outcome for each problem/issue. In addition, intermediate goals which build toward the clinical outcomes are identified and listed for each problem/issue for appropriate time intervals or phases of clinical progression. The team then builds the interventions and tasks into the body of the CareMap® tool driven by the outcomes to be achieved. The use of this tool, however, challenges the traditional aspects of care delivery. The group embarks on a process of clinical inquiry, questioning: What resources are used to deliver care? Are the tests obtained, value-added? With which outcomes are these interventions affiliated? What can be changed to positively impact the quality of care? When does the teachable moment occur for patients and families, and are we capitalizing on this moment? And, is discharge planning occurring prior to admission? Following discussion and principled negotiation, tasks, interventions, intermediate goals and outcomes are entered into the appropriate cells of the template. Through this evaluative effort the group is moving from current to best practice. The tool is then tested on several patients admitted to the case type for accuracy of the clinical information identified, ease of access to the tool as a multidisciplinary plan of care and ease of use as a record of care. Appropriate changes are made to the tool and then it is retested. Following this evaluation period, policies and guidelines are established for CareMap® use and the tool is used with every patient admitted to the case type.

At Montclair Baptist Medical Center in Birmingham, Alabama, the staff used the tool shown in Figure 1 to manage the care of patients undergoing open-heart surgery.

The staff implements the tool on patient admission to the cardiac surgery service and individualizes it for issues such as a secondary active diagnosis or specific patient clinical or emotional needs. Once individualized, health care team members involved in the patient's care use the document to manage the care delivered and outcomes to be achieved during the five-day acute care length of stay.

For patients undergoing this procedure, key problems and associated outcomes identified include risk for decreased cardiac output or altered hemodynamics post-surgery. The intermediate goal to be achieved is maintenance of hemodynamic parameters within the normal limits 12 hours after arrival in the intensive care unit. Parameters monitored include the cardiac index, systemic venous resistance, left atrial and pulmonary artery pressures, systolic blood pressure, and cardiac rhythm.

Another problem is the risk of decreased mobility after surgery. Progressive ambulatory programs have been demonstrated to enhance efficient recovery. The intermediate goals include: dangling at the bedside 24-hours post-operative; ambulate with assistance to the bathroom and sit in a chair for meals on post-op day two; ambulate the length of the hallway with assistance and sit in chair for one hour (three times) on post-op day three; independent ambulation for increasing time periods and sitting up in a chair for one hour (four times) on post-op day four. Through creation of key benchmarks demonstrating the patient's clinical progression, care can be well-managed.

Goals and outcomes are shared with patients and families via an educational tool given to the patient and family upon patient admission to the hospital (see Figure 2).

This intervention has been demonstrated to greatly improve patient and family satisfaction (P. Midyette, personal communication, November 29, 1993).

In institutions or agencies using CareMaps®, nurses typically micro-manage patient care, as these nurses spend the most time in provision of direct care. As micro-managers, nurses coordinate team efforts to meet identified intermediate goals and outcomes at the appropriate times (Zander, 1992). Each team member, however, is responsible for documenting information on the CareMap® tool which has incorporated and replaced in many

Figure 1.
CABG CareMap® (Montclair Baptist Medical Center, Birmingham, Alabama)

✝ MONTCLAIR
BAPTIST MEDICAL CENTER

Coordinated CareMap®
CASE TYPE–OPEN HEART SURGERY
DRG 106, 107—CABG W, W/O CATH
DRG 104, 105—VALVE W & W/O CATH

(Addressograph)

SURGEON: _____ AGE: _____ PRE-OP WEIGHT: _____

TYPE OF SURGERY: _____ OTHER DIAGNOSIS: _____

CONSULTING PHYSICIANS: _____ PULMONARY DISEASE: YES _____ NO _____

_____ DIABETES: YES _____ NO _____

ALLERGIES: _____ RENAL DISEASE: YES _____ NO _____

NAME/RELATIONSHIP: _____ FAMILY PHONE NUMBERS: (___) _____

NAME/RELATIONSHIP: _____ FAMILY PHONE NUMBERS: (___) _____

NAME/RELATIONSHIP: _____ FAMILY PHONE NUMBERS: (___) _____

	1900-0700			0700-1900	
DATE	SIGNATURE	INITIAL	DATE	SIGNATURE	INITIAL

Signature/Date/Initial each shift indicating plan of care reviewed.

Coordinated CareMap® - **OPEN HEART SURGERY (CABG and VALVE)**   M-93-5455 Rev. 12/7/93 P

(continued)

Figure 1. *(continued)*

CABG CareMap® (Montclair Baptist Medical Center, Birmingham, Alabama)

✝ **MONTCLAIR**
BAPTIST MEDICAL CENTER

Coordinated CareMap®

OPEN HEART SURGERY — CABG & VALVE

Key: Highlight Completed Tasks And Goals, Circle Variances
and Focus. Date and Highlight Variances Once Completed.

(Addressograph)

	PRE-OP DATE DATE/INITIAL _____	DAY OF SURGERY (*ACTUAL P.O.D.:* _____) DATE/INITIAL _____	P.O.D. 1 (*ACTUAL P.O.D.:* _____) DATE/INITIAL _____	P.O.D. 2 (*ACTUAL P.O.D.:* _____) DATE/INITIAL _____
CARDIOVASCULAR High risk for decreased cardiac output or altered hemodynamics post-surgery		OUTCOME: **GOAL:** Hemodynamic parameters within normal limits for patient within 16 hours after arrival in OHICU (CI, SVR, LA, PAP, BP) NSR with rare ectopy.		
Vital Signs **ECG Monitor** **Invasive Monitoring**	Vital Signs QID	Vital Signs every 30 minutes Continuous ECG monitoring RA LA ART PA Pacing wires present	Vital Signs every 2 hours Telemetry D/C RA, D/C LA, D/C ART, D/C PA - - - - - - - - - - - - - - - -	Vital Signs every 4 hours - - - - - - - - - - - - - - - -
PULMONARY High risk for respiratory insufficiency, retained secretions, and inadequate oxygenation.		**GOAL:** Extubated and with normal breathing patters within 16 hrs after arrival in OHICU. AGBs per protocol Suction PRN Extubated@ Nasal O2@ **GOAL:** Oriented x3, normal thought process	**GOAL:** Clear airway and adequate oxygenation Decrease nasal O2 by 2 liters May use O2 PRN Incentive spirometry + CPT q 2° while awake, cough and deep breathe q 2°	**GOAL:** Off nasal O2 with minimal resp. effort. SaO2 > 90 D/C nasal O2 I/S q 2-4° w.a. Cough and deep breathe q 4°
ELIMINATION **GASTROINTESTINAL** **NUTRITION** High risk for altered bowel function and nutrition	NPO after midnight	NGT — Gravity NPO until extubated, then ice chips	D/C NGT **GOAL:** BS present, abd flat Ice chips to clear liquids then progress as tolerated to full liquid then Phase I AHA diet or _____ ADA	**GOAL:** Absence of N and V - - - - - - - - - - - - - - - -
PSYCHO-SOCIAL/ **SPIRITUAL** Coping difficulties related to surgery and recommended lifestyle change	1. Assess support system and need to verbalize. 2. Consider allowing time to listen. 3. Consult Pastoral Care	1. Assess response to recommended treatment and allow time to listen. 2. Answer or seek answers to patient/family questions. 3. Pastoral Care. - - - - - - - - - - - - - - - -	- - - - - - - - - - - - - - - -	**GOAL:** Pt/Family will verbalize concerns to nurse - - - - - - - - - - - - - - - -
ALTERED FLUID BALANCE High risk for hypovolemia		**GOAL:** Normal LAP/PAD and U/O > 20 cc/hr, CTD < 200/hr I & O hourly - - - - - - - - - - - - - Pre-Op Weight: _____ lbs. Foley Catheter - - - - - - - - - - - Chest tubes **GOAL:** CTD < 200/shift	I & O q 2 hr. - - - - - - - - - - Dialy weights - bedtime	**GOAL:** Normal bladder function I & O q shift - - - - - - - - - - - - - - - - D/C foley D/C chest tube
ACTIVITY High risk for decreased mobility	Up ad lib	Passive ROM Complete bedrest Turn q 2 hr. if stable ➤HOB 20 **GOAL:** Absence of motor deficits	Dangle with assistance Transfer Move to: _____ - - - - - - - - - - - - - - - - Feeds self	**GOAL:** Ambulate w/ assist. ambulate to bath-room. Up in chair for meals. Head of bed as desired. ➤FOB. - - - - - - - - - - - - - - - - Bath w/assistance
INTEGUMENTARY High risk for impaired skin integrity/wound healing and infection	Chin to toe prep Hibiclens bath	All incisions covered: Chest, leg, RA/LA sites, chest tubes, peripheral IV, triple lumen.	**GOAL:** Incisions dry and intact Incisions covered: RA/LA, wires, chest tubes, chest. Leg incisions open to air. Incision care BID. Triple lumen remains	Clean chest incision when tubes out. Gauze dressing if needed. Incision care BID Triple lumen dressing care
PAIN		**GOAL:** Pain controlled with IV pain meds.		**GOAL:** Pain controlled with po pain meds.
KNOWLEDGE DEFICIT of expected progression of care in hospital and at home	**GOAL:** Verbalizes and understands surgery prep, I/S, immediate post-op expectations. Film _____ ,Booklet, _____ Patient CareMap® _____	Reinforce I/S, weaning, extubation, coughing and deep breathing, equipment. Topics reinforced Verbalized understanding	Teaching/Understands 1. Progression of activity 2. Routine care, Meds, Equipment 3. Begin D/C instructions w/ family 4. Evaluate D/C needs.	Reinforce teaching: Activity 02, medications, diet. Review plan of care Verbalizes understanding
LAB WORK/TESTS	EKG, CBC TYPE/CROSS S-27 HCT/HGB U/A PT/PTT	HCT/HGB } K+ } On Admit CXR ACT BS if diabetic	HGB/HCT } K + } at 0500	HGB/HCT } K + } at 0500 CXR after tubes out Pt. if valve
CONSULTATION		Evaluate need for discharge planning	Consult Cardiac Rehab	

Coordinated CareMap®- **OPEN HEART SURGERY - CABG & VALVE**

M-93 5455 Rev. 12/13/93 P

Figure 1. *(continued)*
CABG CareMap® (Montclair Baptist Medical Center, Birmingham, Alabama)

✝ MONTCLAIR
BAPTIST MEDICAL CENTER

Coordinated CareMap®
CABG
Expected discharge 106, 107 - POD 5

(Addressograph)

P.O.D. 3 *(ACTUAL P.O.D.: ____)* DATE/INITIAL _____	P.O.D. 4 *(ACTUAL P.O.D.: _____)* DATE/INITIAL _____	P.O.D. 5 *(ACTUAL P.O.D.: _____)* DATE/INITIAL _____	P.O.D. 6 *(ACTUAL P.O.D.: _____)* DATE/INITIAL _____	P.O.D. 7 *(ACTUAL P.O.D.: ____)* DATE/INITIAL _____
Vital Signs QID Telemetry Pacing wires present	D/C telemetry 2 hrs after wires removed **GOAL:** Normal sinus rhythm with occasional to no PVCs/PACs D/C wires if rhythm stable for previous 24 hrs.	·+·+·+·+·+·+·+·+·+·+·		
I/S q 4° while awake Cough and deep breathe q 4°	I/S QID QID	**GOAL:** Lungs clear to ausculation and by CXR ·+·+·+·+·+·+·+·+·+·+· ·+·+·+·+·+·+·+·+·+·+·		
Assess need for PRN laxative **GOAL:** Tolerates diet > 50% no N and V Phase I AHA diet or _____ ADA diet	Bowel movement **GOAL:** Resume normal pre-op bowel pattern ·+·+·+·+·+·+·+·+·+·+·	·+·+·+·+·+·+·+·+·+·+·		
1. Assess response to recommended treatment and allow time to listen. 2. Answer or seek answers to patient/family questions. 3. Pastoral Care.	·+·+·+·+·+·+·+·+·+·+· ·+·+·+·+·+·+·+·+·+·+·	**GOAL:** Pt. complaint with plan of care. ·+·+·+·+·+·+·+·+·+·+· ·+·+·+·+·+·+·+·+·+·+·		
Daily weights	**GOAL:** Post-Op weight = pre-op weight. Hct > 21 Daily weights	Weight _____ lbs.		
Walk length of hall w/ assist. TID 1 2 3 up in chair 1 hr. TID. HOB as desired. Increase FOB Feeds self Performs own personal care	**GOAL:** Independent ambulation. Increase ambulation time QID 1 2 3 4 up in chair 1 hr. QID 1 2 3 4 ·+·+·+·+·+·+·+·+·+·+· ·+·+·+·+·+·+·+·+·+·+· Shower if wires out	Expected discharge date ___ 1 2 3 4 (Walk QID) ·+·+·+·+·+·+·+·+·+·+· ·+·+·+·)) ·+·+·+·+·+·+ Shower		
GOAL: Temp. <101. Invasive line sites w/o redness or purulent drainage. All incisions open to air Incision care BID Triple lumen remains	D/C triple lumen 2 hr. after wires removed. All incisions open to air ·+·+·+·+·+·+·+·+· ·+·+·	**GOAL:** No inflammation or purulent drainage from incisions. Temp. < 100°F. D/C incision care.		
Pain meds prn	·+·+·+·+·+·+·+·+·+·+·	·+·+·+·+·+·+·+·+·+·+·		
Reinforce instructions on activity, telemetry, diet, meds, I/S Verbalizes understanding	Receives instructions for: Diet _____ Stress _____ Cardiac Rehab//Home Activity _____ Receives Booklet _____	**GOAL:** Understands discharge instructions verbalizes understanding medication supplements provided Discharge _____		
Resume home diabetic regimen	CBC } S-6 } at 2100 ECG } CXR } in PM	**GOAL:** CBC, S-6 WNL		
	Cardiac Rehab Evaluation Home Walk Instructions	·+·+·+·+·+·+·+·+·+·+·		

Coordinated CareMap®-OPEN HEART SURGERY-CABG   M-93-5455 Rev. 12/13/93 P

(continued)

Figure 1. *(continued)*
CABG CareMap® (Montclair Baptist Medical Center, Birmingham, Alabama)

✝ MONTCLAIR
BAPTIST MEDICAL CENTER

Coordinated CareMap®
OPEN HEART SURGERY - VALVE
Expected Discharge - POD 7

(Addressograph)

P.O.D. 3 *(ACTUAL P.O.D.: ____)* DATE/INITIAL ____	P.O.D.4 *(ACTUAL P.O.D.: _____)* DATE/INITIAL _____	P.O.D. 5 *(ACTUAL P.O.D.: _____)* DATE/INITIAL _____	P.O.D. 6 *(ACTUAL P.O.D.: _____)* DATE/INITIAL _____	P.O.D. 7 *(ACTUAL P.O.D.: ____)* DATE/INITIAL ____
Vital Signs QID Telemetry Pacing wires present	Vital Signs QID D/C telemetry 2 hrs after wires removed **GOAL:** Normal sinus rhythm with occasional to no PVC/ PACs, or controlled A-Fib D/C wires if rhythm stable for previous 2 hrs.	· · · · · · · · · · · · · ›	· · · · · · · · · · · ›	· · · · · · · · · ›
			GOAL: Lungs clear to ausculation and by CXR	
I/S q 2-4° while awake Turn, cough and deep breathe q 4°	· · · · · · · · · · · · · › · · · · · · · · · · · · · ›	I/S QID QID	· · · · · · · · · · · › · · · · · · · · · · · ›	· · · · · · · · · › · · · · · · · · · ›
Assess need for PRN laxative **GOAL:** Tolerates diet > 50% no N and V	Bowel movement		**GOAL:** Resume normal pre-op bowel pattern	
Phase I AHA diet or _____ ADA diet	· · · · · · · · · · · · · ›	· · · · · · · · · · · ›	· · · · · · · · · · · ›	· · · · · · · · · ›
			GOAL: Pt. complaint w/Plan of Care	
1. Assess response to treatment and allow time to listen. 2. Answer or seek answers to patient/family questions.	· · · · · · · · · · · · · › · · · · · · · · · · · · · ›	· · · · · · · · · · · › · · · · · · · · · · · ›	· · · · · · · · · · · › · · · · · · · · · · · ›	· · · · · · · · · › · · · · · · · · · ›
		GOAL: Post-Op weight ⊜ pre-op weight. Lab work normal		
Daily weights	· · · · · · · · · · · · · ›	· · · · · · · · · · · ›	Weight _____ lbs.	
		GOAL: Independent ambulation.	Expected dischrg. Date ____	Discharge
Walk length of hall w/ assist. TID 1 2 3 up in chair 1 hr. TID. Feed self	Walk in hall w/assist. QID 1 2 3 up in chair 1 hr. TID.	Increase ambulation time QID 1 2 3 4 Chair 1 HR QID 1 2 3 4	Chair HR QID 1 2 3 4	Walk QID 1 2 3 4 Chair 1 HR QID 1 2 3 4
Performs own personal care	· · · · · · · · · · · · · › Shower if wires out	· · · · · · · · · · · › Shower if wires out	· · · · · · · · · · · › Shower	· · · · · · · · · › Shower
GOAL: Temp. <101. Invasive line sites w/o redness or purulent drainage. All incisions open to air Incision care BID Triple lumen remains	All incisions open to air D/C Triple Lumen	D/C incision care	**GOAL:** No inflammation or purulent drainage from incisions. Temp < 100°F.	
Pain meds prn	· · · · · · · · · · · · · ›	· · · · · · · · · · · ›	· · · · · · · · · · · ›	· · · · · · · · · ›
Reinforce teaching on activity, telemetry, VS, diet, Coumadin, I/S	· · · · · · · · · · · · · ›	Receives instructions for: Diet ____ Stress _____ Cardiac Rehab _____ Coumadin _____	Verbalized understanding: Diet ____ Stress _____ Cardiac Rehab _____ Coumadin _____	**GOAL:** Understands discharge instructions Reinforce discharge instructions
Verbalizes understanding	Verbalizes understanding	Receives Booklet _____	Receives Booklet _____	Medication supplements Discharge _____
Resume home diabetic regimen Regimen	CBC⎫ S-6 ⎬ at 2100 ECG ⎫ CXR ⎭ in PM	**GOAL:** CBC, S-6 WNL **GOAL:** Pt. regulated for INR 2.5-3.5		
Daily PT	Daily PT	Daily PT	Daily PT	Daily PT
	Cardiac Rehab Home Walk Inst.			

Coordinated CareMap®-**OPEN HEART SURGERY-VALVE**

M-93-5455 Rev. 12/13/93 P

Figure 2.
Patient CareMap® (Montclair Baptist Medical Center, Birmingham, Alabama)

OPEN HEART SURGERY PLAN OF CARE

✝ MONTCLAIR
BAPTIST MEDICAL CENTER

The following is a brief day-by-day outline of what you can expect after open heart surgery. This is only a guideline and may vary with each individual. A Case Coordinator will oversee your progress and is available to answer your questions or assist you should any problems arise.

UNIT	DAY OF SURGERY	Day 1 After Surgery	Day 2 After Surgery	Day 3 After Surgery	Day 4 After Surgery	Day 5-7 After Surgery
	OPEN HEART INTENSIVE CARE	Open Heart ICU Stepdown	Open Heart ICU Stepdown	Open Heart Progressive Care	OHPC	OHPC ➡➡➡ HOME
Lines and Tubes	1. **Endotracheal** (breathing tube) connected to ventilator. Will be weaned off ventilator within 12 hrs. after surgery.	Nasal Oxygen	Oxygen discontinued			Criteria for discharge: 1. Lab work normal 2. Weight equal to pre-op weight 3. Lungs clear 4. Temperature < 100°F 5. No inflamma-tion at incision site 6. Understands discharge instructions 7. Walking in halls
	2. Chest tubes (drain blood from around heart)	·······→	Chest tubes out			
	3. Nasogastric (NG) Tube (drains stomach)	NG tube out				
	4. Foley catheter (drains bladder)	·······→	Foley catheter out			
	5. Arterial line (measures blood pressure)	Arterial, PA, LA, RA lines out				
	6. Pulmonary Artery, Right Atrial, Left Atrial Lines (measures pressures in the heart)					
	7. Intravenous catheters (1 or 2 in neck veins and arm - for IV fluids)	IV in arm out Keep IV in neck	·······→	·······→	IV in neck out	
	8. Pacing wires (for regulating heart rhythm with pacemaker if needed)	·······→	·······→	·······→	Pacing wires out if heart rhythm stable	
	9. Heart Monitor	·······→	·······→	·······→	Heart Monitor off	
Activity	Bedrest	Sit on side of bed Weigh every night Feed Self	Walk with assistance to bathroom Up in chair for meals	Walk length of hall with assistance 3 times today Sit in chair for meals	May shower Walk independently in hall at least 4 times a day until discharge	Continue walking in halls Move around frequently in room
Diet	Can have ice chips when breathing tube is out	Clear liquids, then diet as tolerated	Low-fat diet	Low-fat diet Laxative if needed	Need to have BM today	
Incisions	Chest incision Leg incision	Chest incisions covered Leg incisions uncovered	Clear dressing over chest incision when CT out		All incisions uncovered	
Lab Tests	Blood work Chest X-Ray				CXR ECG Blood Work	
Teaching	Pain medication every 3 hours if **requested until discharge**	Cardiac Rehab	·······→	·······→	Diet & Stress Classes	Reinforce discharge instructions includ-ing medications

· OPEN HEART SURGERY PLAN OF CARE   M-92-5414 Rev. 8/92 P

institutions the traditional nursing kardex, the independent care plans for each discipline, the standards of care and practice, utilization management criteria, quality assessment monitors and shift by shift documentation. Incorporation of the tool into the documentation system has reduced redundant documentation, promoted assumption of individual responsibility for tasks and outcomes on a shift-by-shift basis, and improved outcome and variance tracking. In institutions where daily use of CareMaps® is truly multidisciplinary, each discipline is responsible for initialing appropriate interventions, intermediate goals, and outcomes achieved. In addition, each team member must identify, record on the variance-tracking sheet and act on variances in a timely fashion.

Variance Analysis

Variances occur when a deviation from the norm or the unexpected occurs. Variance can be positive, when a patient progresses ahead of schedule, or negative, when a patient does not progress as identified on the CareMap®. This may occur when interventions are not completed, and/or the patient does not meet the expected intermediate goals, outcomes or identified length of stay.

The three variance categories are: (1) Patient/Family, (2) Clinician, and (3) System (Center for Case Management, 1992c). Patient/Family variances occur when a patient's clinical condition changes or length of stay and resources are negatively impacted by family involvement in the patient's care. Clinician variances may be due to a staff member's failure to consult expert resources; lack of timely response to a consult, or omission of a key intervention by an individual or the health care team. System issues include: when a department's schedule is overbooked, surgery is canceled due to an emergency case, unavailability of a bed in an extended care facility, or inability to find essential home care services.

Variance analysis occurs at two levels: concurrent or the individual patient care level, and retrospective or the aggregate case type level. At the concurrent level, variance from the CareMap® provides a cue that it is essential to re-evaluate the multidisciplinary plan of care for the individual patient. The variance, its cause and action taken are recorded on the variance-tracking sheet. The action plan must also be recorded on the CareMap® tool if the variance sheet is not a permanent part of the medical record. As a result of this concurrent process, it may be possible to reverse or avoid negative variance.

Retrospective data is collated by case type. The data are aggregated, analyzed and addressed where demonstrated to be significant. To control the volume of data and better measure and understand the impact of variance data, many program Steering Committees now select to focus on outcomes, length of stay, and key quality indicators (interventions) demonstrating significant impact on resource consumption (Henry, in press). In addition, variance analysis is an essential component of a CQI initiative. Because this system provides data which is extracted directly from patient care, it provides an opportunity to develop strategies for improvements in the overall delivery of patient care. Actions taken as a result of the information generated through variance analysis enhance quality clinical outcomes and minimize costs. Therefore, variance analysis is integrated into the hospital system CQI structure.

Variance management is organized in a variety of ways, often with a project manager, nurse manager or case manager accountable for the data. In many institutions, this quickly becomes unmanageable when data are hand-tallied, due to the volume of data generated. In other institutions variance is computerized with data entry support through nursing, medical records, utilization review or quality management departments using personnel computers. The software currently used includes commercial spreadsheet and data base programs, medical record abstracting programs or programs internally constructed by computer programmers. Computerization of data leads to greater efficiency and better information on which to base decisions, when entered into stand-alone PCs, however, it remains difficult to link this data to other internal data management systems. When CareMaps® are computerized on health information networks, and variances are captured in real time and stored in permanent data bases with linkage to financial, acuity, and quality data, the ability to micro- and macro-manage patient care will be greatly enhanced.

Case Management

CareMap® and Case Management systems are designed to focus on the achievement of patient outcomes within effective and appropriate timeframes, while making efficient use of resources. The primary emphasis of the CareMap® tool is continuity of plan. In case management, the primary emphasis is both continuity of plan and provider (Center for Case Management, 1992a). In addition, case management continuity extends to include multiple geographic settings including acute, ambulatory, home and extended care settings. Case management is often implemented as a strategy to coordinate disciplines and services across the episode or continuum, monitor quality outcomes, manage the cost of care, strengthen clinical programs, and expand external market contracts (Bower, 1992). Programs may target highly complex, high-cost and high-risk popula-

tions. The specific activities with which the case manager is involved include:
• case finding and screening clients
• coordinating care, services and payment sources
• performing a comprehensive assessment
• developing a plan of care using the nursing process
• creating a professional network across the continuum of care
• monitoring and evaluating the plan of care using variance systems, cost accounting, acuity, utilization review and quality management data.

To be effective and efficient, case managers are demanding new levels of integration from information systems. The merging of clinical and financial data is required. There must be interfaces with existing ADT, order entry, financial costing and reimbursement systems. Case management and CareMap® systems have demonstrated effectiveness in reducing costs and improving client outcomes and satisfaction in spite of the primitive paper and computer systems in place.

Making the Transition from Paper-Based Case Management Tools to Computer-Based Systems

The Center for Case Management estimates that as many as 90 percent of American hospitals have developed some form of critical paths or CareMaps® to guide and monitor patient care outcomes (K. Zander, personal communication, November 22, 1993), and a recent survey of 581 hospitals revealed that 57% of respondents not using pathways currently are actively exploring their use for the future (Lumsdon and Hagland, 1993). The majority of these institutions, however, do not integrate case management tools with existing information systems. The two major barriers to such integration are: (1) the hospital has no existing patient care information system with which to integrate, or (2) the current patient care information system cannot yet support the use of pathways. A third, more subtle barrier occurs when system designers, policy makers, and vendors fail to see any value in such integration of care. This portion of the chapter describes the successful use of information technology to support CareMap® tools and case management systems in three facilities. In addition, several potential computer-based linkages of pathways with acuity, cost accounting, and order entry are explored. Finally, potential barriers to future information systems' product development for case management support are discussed.

The Pathway-Information System Linkage: Success Stories

As discussed in an earlier section, the inter-relatedness of pathways and patient care documentation systems cannot be underestimated. Virtually every agency which implements pathways will have to address their impact on the existing documentation system fairly quickly. The issues which typically arise include:
• How and where do we document variances?
• How do we reconcile today's medical and nursing orders with those predicted by the pathway?
• What is the pathway's relationship to the Medication Administration Record?
• How can we avoid redundant charting (i.e., documenting the same data in two or more places)?
• How can we reduce the overall documentation demands, especially for nurses?

Vanderbilt University Medical Center began in 1989 to explore these and many other issues related to efficiency and effectiveness of patient care delivery. Through the use of a pilot program on one unit, a team of providers, administrators, information systems analysts, and consultants began to reconfigure how work is done to care for patients. A complete description of the entire project is beyond the scope of this chapter; however, a major development of the experiment was a new, computer-based documentation system for bedside care providers which directly links the Collaborative Pathway (the name of Vanderbilt's tool) with a charting-by-exception system.

The system was initially developed to run on a local area network on the patient care unit, using IBM personal computer workstations. The lack of a medical center network infrastructure at that time, however, resulted in a PC stand-alone system. A four-month timeframe for development necessitated the use of prototyping tools. Clarion Professional Developer (Clarion Corporation) and LPM (Logix Corporation) were used (Ashworth and Aubrey, 1993). According to the developers, the Clarion product speeds up and simplifies the use of data base applications. They reported that LPM used in conjunction with Clarion allowed more control over source code generation, development of large systems in a modular approach, and smaller, faster programs. Ashworth, the user analyst on loan from the Information Management Department who did the development work, is also a registered nurse. Communication among team members working on the documentation project with Information Management was greatly enhanced by Ashworth's background in clinical care.

Collaborative Pathways are stored in the computer's hard drive. When a patient is admitted to the unit, the medical receptionist must key in certain data elements related to patient demographics and diagnosis because there is currently no linkage to the hospital's mainframe system. (Planning is underway to accomplish that linkage.) The screens are simple to use and the cursor moves automatically to the next field. Demand fields are used for certain data which must be entered. The user cannot pass the field without completing it. The average time to admit a new patient to the system is five minutes, according to Irene Hatcher, BSN, RNC, Documentation Specialist, at VUMC.

After the patient is entered into the system, the nurse must assign a Collaborative Path. There is a menu selection screen for assistance. Once the assignment is made, the predicted tasks, activities and outcomes for DAY 1 are reviewed in conjunction with the admission medical orders and the nursing admission assessment data. The nurse then reconciles these data with the pathway, adding or deleting tasks and activities in order to customize the day's patient-related work. Patient outcomes, predicted by the Collaborative Pathway, cannot be altered.

After customization, a copy of the revised pathway is printed for use by nursing, medical ancillary, and clerical staff. In addition, a 24-hour flowsheet is generated. The flowsheet is used by the patient care staff to document graphic data (T,P,R, B/P, weight, I&O), chartable tasks and activities (e.g., activities of daily living, treatments, diet, teaching, consults, lab work), physical assessment findings, and any incidental one-time orders. All of the data, except for graphics, are recorded as completed (or "normal") by a check mark in the appropriate box on the form. If the task was not completed or, if the physical assessment finding was abnormal, an "*" is placed in the box. No narrative charting is required *unless* there is an exception to what was predicted by the Collaborative Pathway (tasks and activities) OR to the physical assessment standards specific to the unit.

At the end of each 24-hour period, the nurse must evaluate patient progress toward specified outcomes on the Pathway, and document any variance (or exceptions). This is accomplished by selecting "Generate Flowsheet" from the menu. The program prompts the user to document whether or not the outcome was met. If the answer is "no," the program prompts the nurse for the reason. The program uses a four-category classification system for variance: patient/family, provider, system, or community. When the nurse first selects a category, a list of subcategories appears on the screen for further selection.

For example, if the predicted outcome was that the patient would be "OOB in chair for 15 minutes BID," and the patient was unable to do so because of post-operative hemorrhage, the nurse would make the following selections:

COMPUTER PROMPT: OOB in chair for 15 min. bid? Y or N?

USER RESPONSE: keystroke "N"

COMPUTER PROMPT: Select category:

Patient/Family
Provider
System
Community

USER RESPONSE: Highlight "Patient/family" using arrow keys; hit "enter"

COMPUTER PROMPT: Patient/Family reasons, select one:

pain
non-compliant
teaching incomplete
family refuses
physiologically unstable
psychosocial
other

USER RESPONSE: Highlight "physiologically unstable" using arrow keys; hit "enter"

The program automatically saves the information in a file as each outcome is addressed. The nurse cannot advance the patient to the next day on the Collaborative Pathway and customize it, nor can the nurse generate the next 24-hour Flowsheet until all outcomes are addressed and variance data have been recorded. This assures automatic, essentially effortless, variance capture on all patients in the system. These variance records are downloaded periodically and used internally for quality monitoring and improvement. No variance data appear in the chart as such. The nurse does make a narrative entry on the patient's record for each exception which occurs, describing the event and the action plan for correction.

In contrast to the PC stand-alone system described above, in California the Hemet Valley Hospital District (1991) reported development of a mainframe system to support the use of pathways and their integration with both order entry and documentation. Known as "Coordinated Patient Outcome System," it required six months to develop and another six months to "fine tune." The system uses an IBM AS400, Model B-60; RPG-3 language; GTE software; and interfaces with ADT and pre-admission, all clinical departments, utilization review, medical records and coding, and order entry (Spellman, 1992).

The primary tool is called a MAP, or Multidisciplinary Action Plan, which predicts tasks and activities for specific diagnoses. Due to the interface with Order Entry functionality, potential variances from expected tasks and activities are detected by the computer. According to Spellman, if the MAP predicted that a complete blood count should be obtained on DAY 6 for a certain patient, yet the Order Entry function recorded that no test was ordered that day, the MAP automatically highlights the task on the screen, notifying the nurse of this omission. The nurse has the ability to accept the variance alert and allow the computer to record the variance permanently, or to override the system if, in his/her judgement, this is not a variance situation. As was the case with the Vanderbilt PC system, variance capture is again assured. Such automatic capture of variances is a distinct advantage over manual CareMap® systems because no variance is lost. When integrity of the data is maintained, the contribution of variance and variance analysis to CQI of patient care is invaluable.

Montclair-Baptist Medical Center has developed a mainframe program which assists the Cardiovascular Case Managers in capturing, analyzing, and addressing variances. Written by programmers within the medical center system, the program runs in conjunction with the existing SMS patient information system. Called "CareMap® Program," it supports the paper CareMap® tool described earlier (see Figure 1).

When the patient fails to meet the benchmark goals prescribed by the pathway, the Case Manager enters this exception into the program. Within the program there are lists of goals, by day of stay, from which the Case Manager may select. After selection of the specific goal which the patient did not meet, the program then lists interventions and conditions which are often associated with failure to attain this particular goal. These predetermined barriers were derived from the cardiac team's more than two years of case management experience using paper and pencil variance capture systems and hand tabulations to record variance patterns and trends. The Case Manager can select the apparent reasons why this patient has not been able to attain the goal as prescribed. If none of the interventions or conditions listed apply to this particular patient, the Case Manager can use free text entry to describe the reason for the variance. Variances are categorized as one of four types: patient/family, provider, system, and placement. The information system generates reports on the frequency of variances by type and by day of stay, associated with the apparent reasons for the variances. These patterns and trends are reviewed by the multidisciplinary cardiac care team to determine where improvements in care can be made (P. Midyette, personal communication, November 29, 1993). This use of information technology clearly demonstrates the valuable integration of pathways and case management tools with CQI efforts.

The Pathway-Information System Linkage: Future Directions

Continued linkage of pathways with information systems is critical if their real potential to enhance quality in a resource-constrained environment is to be achieved. The previous examples of technology supporting the daily use of pathways in clinical practice represent a fraction of the integration which is not only possible, but compelling, as the health care industry moves into a national, managed care system. The health care network of the future will be successful only to the extent that costs of care are understood, monitored, and managed; and to the degree that patient care information, including monitoring of desired patient care outcomes, is shared by all providers within the network of care. Care pathways are tools which can readily enhance such cost and quality management.

Linkage of pathways to patient acuity measurement systems through information technology is a logical step in monitoring cost and quality. When such linkage occurs, daily customization of the CareMap® by reconciling medical orders and nursing assessments to the predicted task and activities should automatically capture workload. Currently, workload is captured by nurses manually checking off a list of tasks and activities on each patient every 8 or 24 hours. This list is then either manually tabulated into a score or is read by a scanner into a PC where it is scored. The score is translated into workload in most institutions. Workload data are used in various ways, but in all cases they can be translated into nursing costs. What if the workload were captured by the task, activities, and outcomes generated on the pathway, in a patient care information system? There are a number of advantages to such an idea. First, nurses would not have to classify patients manually. The computer could do the work for them, by reading the current task, activities, and outcomes from the CareMap® file on each patient at predetermined intervals (e.g., every 8 or 24 hours). Second, the information system could compute workload for each patient and for groups of patients by referencing the tasks, activities, and outcomes

Figure 3.
Pathway Linkage with Acuity Measurement

Computer Screen

Day 3
Activity
Up in chair bid
Treatments
Chest tube care
Central line care
Cardiac monitor
VS q2h
Foley catheter
I & O q shift
Diet
Full liq.c̄ assist

Database File
Vital sign routines
q 15 min .... 45 u wkld
q 30 min .... 30 u wkld
q 1 h .... 15 u wkld

Database File
Chest tubes .... 75 u wkld
Central lines .... 50 u wkld
Peripheral line .... 20 u wkld
Cardiac monitor .... 15 u wkld
I & O routines
q 30 min .... 25 u wkld
q 1 h .... 18 u wkld
q 2 h .... 12 u wkld

to a data base file which contains weighted workload values for each entry, mimicking the process used by commercial patient classification systems currently (see Figure 3). Such a system eliminates a repetitive, time-consuming task for bedside care providers. Further, by using the pathway to drive the acuity measurement system, redundancy in documentation is reduced since the task and activity list of most patient classification systems is very similar to those found on CareMaps®. Nurses would only have to handle and document the data one time to complete multiple tasks.

Another possible and intriguing linkage is the use of the pathways to drive the cost accounting system. Hospitals have difficulty in determining their costs per case, in part because financial information systems traditionally have focused on charges and reimbursement ratios per insurer. In a capitated environment, charges have no value. Rather, the emphasis is on understanding and controlling costs. What if the tasks, activities, and outcomes on the pathway were referenced to a data base file which contained dollar values for each? In such a system, the actual cost per case could be computed daily. Patients who are cost outliers could be concurrently monitored. Case managers, attending physicians, and patient accounting staff could receive daily updates on financial high risk cases, automatically, through the information system. In institutions where such monitors exist now, they are labor intensive, involving hours of utilization reviewers' time. Properly integrated, the data contained on the care pathway can substantially reduce that effort, while enhancing accuracy. Earlier identification of cost outliers, who tend to be the most complex patients, should lead to better control of patient care costs and quality of care.

Integration of pathways with order entry is another linkage not yet adequately explored. As described in the Hemet Valley example, such interface allows monitoring of compliance between the pathway and the actual orders. There are other advantages, however. Pathways could drive order sets. For example, if the patient is on DAY 2 of an acute myocardial infarction pathway, and the predicted medication orders include "D_5W 500cc to keep open" and "MS 2-4 mg. q4h prn pain," when the physician begins to enter his/ her orders into the computer, these orders would appear under the medication section for verification. The physician can elect to accept the orders "as is," with one keystroke, or can change the orders as desired. For each medical order on the pathway, the same process is followed. In this scenario, the pathway is suggesting the order set for physicians, who may then accept or alter them. This facilitates order entry for physicians and updates the pathway automatically as well. This is time-saving for physicians, nurses, and clerical personnel, and more importantly, should result in more accuracy in customizing pathways. It should also support more consistency in treatment plans for patients and a more focused approach to outcome-based practice. Finally, such a system has potential to greatly reduce dosage and transcription errors.

Issues in the Integration of Information Systems with Managed Care

The value of information systems in health care is not a subject of great debate. Points of contention, however, do arise when implementation strategies are developed. One of the toughest issues in the 1990s involves language. Nursing as a discipline has worked diligently for more than a decade to develop a distinct set of diagnoses and interventions which belong solely to the discipline. How should that identity be protected yet simultaneously merged into an increasingly collaborative, multidisciplinary document such as a CareMap®? The efficacy of patient maps and pathways is best served when one document is shared by all caregivers. It provides the basis for agreement, not only on each day's activities, but perhaps more importantly, on the desired outcomes for patients. All musicians in an orchestra know when to enter and exit the symphony, making their unique contributions to the music seamlessly. The problem for health care systems, which the orchestra does not share, is that nursing has its own language while other disciplines may have their own as well. Whose language will be used on the pathway—yours, mine, or ours? Some institutions have ignored the problem by viewing pathways and case management as nursing models of care delivery only. Others have taken a somewhat bold stand and declared that no discipline-specific language should dominate; indeed standard English is the language of choice. This indecision and conflict has kept information system vendors from investing heavily in case management support systems. They make money by selling products, and profits are maximized when one product is sold to many customers. Until the health care industry comes to more agreement on language standards, and on the need to move maps and pathways out of the nursing department and into the mainstream of health care, vendors will not be willing to risk development capital. Market demand is currently too fragmented, and therefore, product development is slow.

A second issue which begs resolution before information systems can support CareMaps® fully has to do with outcomes of care. To date, there has been no agreement that all maps and pathways must address outcomes or goals. Some institutions continue to monitor tasks and activities but do not address patient outcomes on a daily or ongoing basis. Further, goal or outcome statements are not universally stated in measurable terms (as they should be), nor is there agreement on how they should be stated. For example, should goals always be patient goals? Is there ever a time when it is appropriate for the actor in the goal/outcome statement to be the caregiver? Until these issues are resolved, vendors will again be wary of bringing a product to market.

Summary

The integration of information technology with case management will produce a number of benefits: time savings for nurses and other health care personnel; a decrease in errors; enhancement of collaborative team efforts to achieve patient outcomes; and the ability to closely monitor cost and quality outliers. Health care administrators, case managers and staff are dependent on development of sophisticated information systems which have the capability of computerizing demographic data, test results, CareMap® tools, fiscal reports generated concurrently, resource management reports and profitability of contracts on a daily and quarterly basis, and generating variance data in real time across multiple settings with simultaneous access by multiple providers. When these information needs are addressed, there will be decreased fragmentation of care, an increased access to services, and assistance in capturing outcome and cost management data, as well as the foundation for applied clinical research. The lack of highly effective information system products to support pathways and case management, however, results from the combined effects of (1) a rapidly changing health care industry which is experimenting with new ways of organizing care, and (2) a general lack of agreement on the language and syntax for expressing care needs and results. As the need for computer support continues to grow with the expansion of pathways and case management across all health care settings, greater consensus will be reached among professionals about how the information is best expressed and communicated. As uncertainty is diminished, the development of new and better products should proliferate.

References

Ashworth, G. B., and Aubrey, C. (1993). Collaborative care documentation by exception system. In M. E. Frisse (Ed.), *Proceedings of the Sixteenth Annual Symposium on Computer Applications in Medical Care* (pp. 109-113). Manchester, MO: McGraw-Hill Book Co.

Bower, K. A. (1992). *Case Management by Nurses.* Washington, DC: American Nurses Publishing.

Center for Case Management, Inc. (1992a). *Case Management.* South Natick, MA: Author.

Center for Case Management, Inc. (1992b). *Definitions.* South Natick, MA: Author.

Center for Case Management, Inc. (1992c). *Variance Management.* South Natick, MA: Author.

Hemet Valley Hospital District. (1991). *Managed Care Through Coordinated Care: Coordinated Patient Outcome System.* Palm Springs, CA: Author.

Henry, S. A. (in press). In P. L. Spat (Ed.), *Critical Path Implementation and Applications in Health Care: A Case Study.* Chicago: American Hospital Publishing, Inc.

Lumsdon, K., and Hagland, M. (1993, October 20). Mapping care. *Hospitals and Health Networks, 67*(20), 34-40.

Spellman, D. (1992, January). Presentation at the Expert Users' Forum, The Center for Case Management, Charleston, SC.

Spitzer, P. G. (1993). A comprehensive framework for I/S strategic planning. *Computers in Healthcare, 13*(May), 28-33.

Zander, K. (1992). Critical Pathways. In M. M. Melum, and M. K. Sinioris (Eds.), *Total Quality Management: The HealthCare Pioneers.* Chicago: American Hospital Publishing, Inc.

Zander, K. (1993). Dear vendor. *Computers in Healthcare, 13*(June), 34.

Maximizing Technology for Cost-Effective Staff Education and Training

Susan K. Newbold, MS, RN
Doctoral Student, Nursing Informatics
School of Nursing
University of Maryland at Baltimore

Introduction

The use of technology for education purposes in clinical settings outside the traditional educational arenas is a new challenge for health care administrators. The nurse executive, for example, is faced with perplexing choices of whether and how to integrate instruction technology into the health care organization. This chapter explores how the nurse executive can best use technology for cost-effective staff education and training.

Essentially one hundred percent of nursing schools across the nation use computer technology for instructional purposes (McAfooes and Bolwell, 1994). Generally, health care settings, including hospitals, health maintenance organizations, clinics, home health care, and physicians' offices have been slower to take advantage of the capabilities of the computer for staff education and training. Reasons for the slow dissemination of computer-based education include: cost, benefits that are difficult to quantify, fear, resistance to change, and lack of knowledge of how to integrate technology into staff education and training.

Business corporations have documented savings using computers to train in areas such as policies and procedures, business practices, and specific job knowledge. Nursing executives, too must determine how technology may be appropriate for their setting in this age of cost savings and attention to quality.

Availability of Software, or What Would I Do With A Computer If I Had One?

Selecting a computer system for an organization should begin with a definition of the purpose for the system. One organization might want to integrate automation into a nurse refresher course; another might seek to off-load mandatory annual classes, such as cardiopulmonary resuscitation, universal precautions, and fire safety to free the instructors for other work. Still another might elect to test the competencies of newly hired nurses during orientation.

The problems that nurse executives face in choosing a computer system can be defined in terms of budget cuts in educational staff, students coming out of schools without certain skills, the need to test new employees, the need for remedial work in medication administration, yearly required in-services, and the repetition of information needed to be taught in each orientation. Instructors may face a backlog of work and burnout from teaching the same repetitive information.

Styles of computer-assisted instruction (CAI) that health care organizations could use include: simulations, drill and practice, authoring tools, games, tutorials, and tests. The programs can be used to fill educational gaps, practice repetitive tasks, supplement orientation, and refresh and enhance skills.

After the computer needs are defined, software can be selected to satisfy the need. It is suggested that health care organizations first attempt to seek out software that is currently available and can be purchased. Developing one's own software may be appropriate in some cases, but should probably not be one's first venture into educational software.

A compendium of computer-assisted learning packages can be found in Bolwell's 1994 *Directory of Educational Software For Nursing* (4th ed.). Although many of the programs listed are targeted for nursing students, many titles are appropriate for use in hospitals and other health care settings. They include programs for teaching and testing clinical practice subjects such as pharmacology, anatomy and physiology, universal precautions, and wellness concepts. The most recent version contains over 700 titles with peer reviews of the programs. Other sources for information about software packages can be found in each issue of *Computers in Nursing,* published by the J. B. Lippincott Company.

One exciting project using instructional technology for nurses in medically underserved communities is now being conducted by the American Journal of Nursing Company under the direction of Dr. Mary Anne Rizzolo and Karen DuBois, RN, MS and funded by the United States Public Health Service Division of Nursing. This program features continuing education programs available through the Internet electronic network or through a dial-up service. The program directors envision that users will download programs onto their own computers, paying a small fee to use the program a limited number of times. This state-of-the-art program is especially useful for rural nurses and small hospitals without adequate educational support on staff.

Currently educational programs are available over the Internet. Information stored on a computer at the University of Washington can be transmitted over telephone lines for use by nurses with Internet access.

The University of Maryland School of Nursing offers independent study on Internet, Healthpro, Novalink and Delphi. Similar to independent study offered in journals, each network independent study module is approved for two contact hours of continuing education. The participant downloads the content material, reads it, completes the forms and quiz and submits them with a fee to the University for grading. A broad range of topics are available.

CAI programs can be purchased or developed for both DOS-based and Macintosh personal computers. The average CAI program will run on a 286 personal computer with EGA or VGA graphics, 640K memory and a hard drive. Newer programs require the use of a mouse. Interactive videodisc (IVD) programs require specialized equipment and cost more than the average personal computer.

Computer hardware should be selected following the purchasing standards of the organization. Ask for assistance from the information systems department in organizations large enough to have one. Vendors of packages will indicate what type of hardware including memory is needed to run the products. Buy hardware from a reputable dealer who will be available for technical support. Specialized equipment may be needed to run IVDs. Also the organization may elect to purchase computer attachments to project the computer screen onto a large over-head screen. This enables multiple viewers to see what is on the instructor's computer screen.

What is This Alphabet Soup?

As with all disciplines, there are acronyms associated with instructional technology. Computer-assisted Instruction (CAI) is instruction delivered via computer. Other common acronyms are: computer-assisted learning (CAL), computer-based instruction (CBI), computer-managed instruction (CMI), and computer-based learning (CBL).

For use of computers in testing, common acronyms are: CAT (computerized adaptive testing), CBT (computer-based training) and CST (computerized simulation test). Formats for computers include CD-ROM (compact disc-read only memory), CD-I (compact disc-interactive), Photo CD (photo compact disc), and IVD (interactive videodisc).

How Do I Know I am Purchasing Quality Software?

The quality of instructional technology is improving in terms of attention to adult learning principles, instructional design perspective, user interface, cognitive styles and use of graphics and sound. Early versions of CAI appear to be primitive when compared to programs now available. The buyer should be aware that there is no accrediting body for the production of instructional technology and no standards published so quality may vary greatly.

Programs are evaluated by peers in Bolwell's 1994 book mentioned previously. The *Interactive Instruction in Nursing and Other Health Sciences: Review of Evaluation Instruments* (Sparks and Kuenz, 1993), a monograph, is a digest of evaluation instruments for the appraisal of instructional technology. Included are instruments for the evaluation of CAI and interactive video as well as those media that do not fit into any category. *Computers in Nursing* includes a column in each issue entitled, "Software Reviews."

Other sources for expert advise on programs to consider include council members from both the National League for Nursing (Council for Nursing Informatics) and the American Nurses Association Council on Nursing Systems and Administration. The American Medical Informatics Association has a Nursing Informatics Working Group which can be solicited for advise. Talk to peers, attend staff development and nursing informatics conferences, and consult with local groups such as the Washington, D.C. Capital Area Roundtable on Informatics in Nursing for information on purchasing software for staff education and training.

E.T. Net is a bulletin board system run by and for nursing. It includes a conference at which participants can investigate software reviews.

In all cases the purchaser should expect to be able to preview software before purchasing. Each vendor will differ as to how copies of the software can be previewed. Some send the full working copy of the software, charge the customer and then expect payment or the returned software within 30 days. Other vendors send a preview copy which may not be a full working copy which self destructs after a limited number of uses.

What Are The Pitfalls of Which I Should Be Aware?

When reviewing a contract for purchase of instructional technology, examine the fine print, particularly the wording in license agreements. Make certain that the license fits your organization's needs. If the license is for one site, the software cannot legally be used for a multiple-site facility. Some licenses allow for unlimited copies of the software to be used, but only at one facility. The onus falls on the buyer to know the restrictions of the contract.

Ascertain the equipment needed to run the software. Some may require upgraded color monitors to obtain the full effects of the graphics. Some may require the use of a hard disk drive. Many programs run on a 286-based hardware, but others require 386 speed. Some programs only run in an IBM-compatible environment, others work only with Macintosh, but many are designed for both computers. Compatible hardware and software must be ordered. Also, the correct size disks (5 $1/4$ inch or 3 $1/2$ inch) must be ordered.

What Else Can I do With Computers Related to Education?

Computers can be used for the documentation of educational courses. Programs can be purchased to maintain attendance information or a simple application can be designed using a data base management system such as Paradox by Borland or Dbase IV by Ashton Tate. Word processing can be used to create handouts, develop outlines, learning objectives, etc. Spread sheets may be used to model projected costs and corresponding benefits.

Presentation methods can be enhanced by using instructional technology. Creative, attention-getting overheads and slides can be devised using Harvard Graphics by Software Publishing Corporation, Freelance Graphics for Windows by Lotus, Powerpoint by Microsoft, or Persuasion by Aldus. Consider using them to accompany lectures on hospital policies or during introductions to new equipment. This collection of desktop presentation software can be used create slides with the services of a commercial slide developer. Visual aids can be used to communicate messages more effectively if designed correctly.

Electronic mail within and outside of hospital can be an adjunct to learning. Organizations associated with universities can have free access to the Internet. Access to Internet can also be a purchased service through Prodigy, American On-Line, CompuServe, or Delphi. Some educational classes are available for downloading from the Internet. On the Internet, users can subscribe to a conference that discusses nurse managed centers or subscribe to a daily White House electronic bulletin on activities and speeches related to healthcare in the United States. A copy of the Health Security Act of 1993 can be obtained free of charge via the Internet.

Through electronic access, usually through the hospital library, or any computer with a modem, the appropriate software and a password, one can search MEDLINE an index to biomedical journal articles via the National Library of Medicine in Bethesda, MD or CINAHL (Cumulative Index of Nursing and Allied Health Literature). Electronic mail was used to submit some papers from the United States to an international nursing informatics conference in Australia.

Using Computers to Train for the HIS

Most hospitals have computer systems to assist in administrative, financial, and clinical patient care. In the clinical area terminals are on the nursing units or at the point of care and are connected to a central computer generally for the purposes of entering orders, retrieving patient results, care planning, assessments, and scheduling. Nurses are a prime user of hospital information systems (HIS). Training on how to use the computer systems and accompanying changes to policies, procedures, and work flow are needed when first implemented and during the orientation of new employees. Several HIS vendors, such as HBO and Company and TDS, offer products that assist with the training of staff to use the HIS.

In some cases where the vendor does not offer a product, hospitals, such as The Johns Hopkins in Baltimore, Maryland have purchased a training program authoring tool and develop their own CBT. The cost of the additional software and hardware needed to develop the CBT was approximately $6,000. Now the education department has turned over training for the Patient Identification System to the Medical Records department (Rae Skidmore, personal communication, February, 1994). Development of the application took one and one half months. Training that one took eight hours with an instructor now can take place in a four hour period. The software that copies sample screens from the mainframe application is appropriate only for computer-based classes and not other orientation or continuing education subjects. The hospital has used the software to develop programs for training staff or laboratory and radiology results, discharge summaries and notes, and nutrition. Further options are to use CBT for all training modules or only offer it to those who cannot attend the scheduled class or those who have difficulty with the traditional classroom situation. Although a specific cost-benefit study has not been done, Ms. Skidmore believes she spends less time in the classroom, but more students are being trained and more classes are being held ("Computer-based training," 1993).

Evaluating Cost Effectiveness

Using technology for staff education and training will, no doubt, have to be cost justified to evaluate the potential return on investment. The cost "related to health care computing, ... is the total expense associated with the acquisition of a computer system or with the use of computer resources, plus all other project-related non-computer costs" (Covey, Craven, and McAlister, 1985). Cost-effectiveness according to Covey et al. (1985) refers to the salutary health care or societal effects of establishing a new process. While a cost-benefit analysis is expressed in quantifiable terms; cost-effectiveness is usually qualitative, subjective, or subject to disagreement.

To justify the cost of using technology for staff education and training, the nursing executive with the assistance of staff education personnel must determine the perceived benefits of using computers. Then costs and savings can be determined as accurately and completely as possible.

Sample benefits for automated training for computer system users include consistent instruction, less time required of instructors for training, and less instructor burnout. Drawbacks include development time and cost for the initial set up. When using an authoring tool to create CAI, programs may require 200 hours of development effort for each hour of instruction.

Sample costs include hardware, software, hardware maintenance, software maintenance, staff, supplies, environment costs, miscellaneous costs, and inflation. Sample savings include the possibility of decreasing staff, increasing staff efficiency, reducing staff turnover, saving supplies, and decreasing the use of more expensive methods. Some vendors offer discounts for hospitals and educational institutions.

Start by investigating the number of instructor hours spent for each individual class. Determine how these hours can be reduced by the addition of computer based instruction.

Integrating Educational Computer Technology into the Organization

Once selected, guidelines must be created for the successful integration of computer technology into staff development or continuing education curricula. Sometimes computers and software have been purchased and then not used. A nurse education consultant (*Nurse Educators Microworld*, 1993) advises that the objectives, content, and other course assignments be reviewed. Select software that is consistent with the defined learner outcomes. Then define leaner outcomes for the software assignments and design guides for students when using the program. Select an evaluation method that will indicate content mastery.

Adult learning theory, user interface, and cognitive learning styles must be considered when integrating computers into education. Change theory can be used as a framework to address potential fears and negative attitude towards computers. Some hospitals use strategies to reduce fear and negative attitudes by holding open houses to announce the use of instructional technology and incentives or prizes for those who complete the first program.

Support for the Use of Instructional Technology

Several organizations have supported nursing in the use of computer technology. The Helene Fuld Health trust has awarded more than $80 million in grants for nursing education, including computer education. As of April, 1994, The National Council of State Boards of Nursing now administers nursing examinations on the computer. In the recent past, International Business Machines Corporation organized a consortium of universities to develop IVD technology programs for the nursing environment which is known as the Healthcare Interactive Video Consortium.

The Sigma Theta Tau Virginia Henderson International Nursing Library is a computerized collection of databases and knowledge resources that can be accessed electronically. One objective of this electronic library is to enhance access to nursing information. The data bases include an information resources data base which may be valuable in the clinical environment.

The National Institutes of Health Learning Center for Interactive Technology at the Lister Hill National Center for Biomedical Communications, located in Bethesda, Maryland, has the sole purpose of developing and supporting innovative methods for training health care professionals. This Center has published a series of monographs, such as *Interactive Technology, Computer-Based Education in Nursing*, and *Videodisc Repurposing*. A hands-on laboratory is available to visiting health sciences educators and researchers. In the early 1990's Drs. Susan Sparks, Educational Research Specialist at Lister Hill and Dr. Mary Anne Rizzolo, Director, Interactive Technologies, the American Journal of Nursing Company, conducted a series of invitational workshops to encourage the dissemination of computer technology for nursing education.

Summary

Instructional technology has the potential to revolutionize staff education and training in healthcare organizations. The state of the art in the use of technology for education purposes in clinical settings has been presented along with suggestions for the nurse executive to maximize technology and, at the same time, provide cost effective staff education and training.

References

Bolwell, C. (1994). *Directory of Educational Software for Nursing* (4th ed.). New York: National League for Nursing.

Computer-based training gains convert. (1993). *Healthcare Informatics, 10*(11), 30.

Covey, H. D., Craven, N. H., and McAlister, N. H. (1985). *Concepts and Issues in Health Care Computing.* St. Louis: C. V. Mosby Co.

McAfooes, J., and Bolwell, C. (1994). *Nurse Educators Microworld, 8*(1).

Sparks, S. M., and Kuenz, M. A. (1993). *Interactive Instruction in Nursing and Other Health Sciences: Review of Evaluation Instruments.* Bethesda, MD: U.S. Department of Health and Human Services, Public Health Service, National Institutes of Health.

The Value of Bedside Computer Systems in Restructuring Nursing Care

Karen E. Dennis, PhD, RN
Associate Professor
School of Nursing
University of Maryland at Baltimore
Associate Director for Education and Evaluation
Geriatric Research Education and Clinical Center
Baltimore Department of Veterans Affairs Medical Center

Introduction

Continuous evolution in the health care environment has brought tighter fiscal constraints and changes in reimbursement, as well as complex advancements in technology, increased patient acuity, shorter length of stay, and a heightened demand for registered nurses (RNs). Working synergistically to spur fundamental changes in the way hospitals do business, these factors contribute to the nursing profession's current emphasis on restructuring organizational patterns and refocusing resources to engender the most effective use of nurses' time and expertise. The list of systemic, organizational problems that hamper the efficient and effective delivery of patient care is seemingly endless. Many of these problems, however, reflect inadequate resources that diminish professional time in direct patient care and use professional staff dollars to complete non-professional tasks.

Restructuring within hospital nursing departments has taken many forms, including decentralization, professional practice models, shared governance, matrix schemes, and clinical centers plans. Within these organizational formats, the quest for the optimal model of nursing care delivery has moved from functional to team nursing, then to primary nursing, and now to case management. Patient-centered care as a restructured organizational format has sweeping implications for all hospital departments, including nursing. Another important component of restructuring is the configuration of nursing staff mix and the redefined roles of RNs, licensed practical/vocational nurses, and assistive personnel in a manner that recognizes the competencies of each (D. L. Gardner, 1991). Clearly, the restructured future of nursing departments has resounding implications for the professional practice of nursing.

As nursing departments move toward restructure, advances in computer technology move toward supporting the work of nursing departments. Exponential increases in the speed, memory, and storage capacity of desktop computers and the capabilities of software programs have increased the efficiency of completing nursing administrative tasks such as scheduling, establishing and monitoring budgets, and tracking professional license renewal. Stand-alone capabilities are enhanced even further when there is network connectivity to hospital information systems for sharing administrative data with other departments. Less widespread is the adoption of information systems that support the work of clinicians at the point where care is delivered. Marginal increases in the adoption rate of bedside computer systems reported by hospitals, from 3% to 5% over five years, will increase significantly in the future if the institutions claiming plans for significant investments in computers for patient care follow through (Hard, 1992; Packer, 1987).

✓ Benefits of Bedside Computers

The cost-benefit ratio is a considerable factor in the adoption of bedside computer systems, with inherent costs much more clearly defined and defended than benefits. In terms of costs, bedside computer systems may reach $5,000 per bed on a medical/surgical unit and $30,000 per bed in an intensive-care unit (Welsch and Nicholson, 1991). In terms of benefits, time savings is the most common parameter that has been studied and therefore claimed.

Because work sampling studies in nursing may include only RNs or all nursing personnel, and may use different definitions for direct versus indirect care, incomparability of results makes them difficult to interpret. A study of 24 RNs in three hospitals across entire eight-hour shifts, however, found that approximately one third of nursing time was spent in direct patient care, one half in indirect care and unit management, and about 14% in personal time (Prescott, Phillips, Ryan, and Thompson, 1991). With the implementation of bedside computers, estimates of time savings related to the nursing staff's performance of clerical work range from 30 to 90 minutes of time per person, per shift (E. Gardner, 1990; Herring and Rochman, 1990; Korpman, 1991). Additional studies evaluating different types of computer systems corroborate the time savings of clinical information systems, particularly when these systems: (1) emphasize communication rather than simply on-line charting (Hendrickson and Kovner, 1990); (2) are located at the bedside rather than clustered in pods or placed at the nurses' station (Halford, Burkes, and Pryor, 1989); and (3) account for variations in workload volume (Lower and Nauert, 1992). The growing capabilities of bedside computers and their integration with hospital information systems spark have stimulated innumerable projections of benefits to professional practice which must be evaluated through future research. Until there is convincing and replicated empirical evidence for the posited benefits, it is likely that educated conjecture rather than data-driven decisions will guide the immediate future of the use of bedside computers in nursing and health care.

Capabilities of Bedside Computers

Bedside systems that are integrated with hospital information systems can be programmed to send key information to other departments automatically as it is recorded. Elevated temperatures and notations of wound drainage can trigger a message to the electronic mail cue of the infection control nurse, and documentation of a patient's fall can transmit to the desktop terminal of the quality improvement/risk manager. Computers can enable laboratory and radiographic tests to be ordered from and returned to the bedside as well as alert physicians and nurses that incompatible medications have been ordered. Bedside computers can prompt nurses that assessments and care plans need to be updated or that certain aspects of care need to be performed, and staff members can prompt one another by highlighting important occurrences so that other care providers are notified immediately of this information at sign-on.

System software typically links different screens so that information entered on one screen appears in other forms, eliminating the need to record data more than once. For example, a patient's temperature entered in familiar numeric form can be displayed in graphic version to reveal a trend across several days, and some systems even eliminate nurse entry of certain data by recording values directly from blood pressure cuffs, cardiac monitors, and infusion pumps. Computer-generated summary reports, such as lists of patients on IV therapy that also include solution and flow rate, as well as the date of the last insertion site and tubing changes—along with lists of all patients with elevated temperatures—help the staff track the status of patients in groups as well as individually. Systems that generate a task list for each patient for each shift and produce a shift report for each patient further streamline the flow of information and ultimately, the workload. The value of bedside computers becomes more pronounced when users go beyond the mere transformation of paper forms into computerized versions and use these systems to restructure and support professional practice.

Data-Based Evaluation

The scarcity of studies that provide empirical evidence to support or refute the anecdotal claims (Cassassa, 1990; Randall, 1991) and verify the perceived benefits for nurses in hospital settings (Staggers, 1988) is not surprising. The low adoption rate of bedside systems impedes the much-needed evaluation research, and the emphasis on cost savings for nursing personnel, support department functions, and paper forms shifts the focus away from professional practice and the conservation of one of hospitals' most valuable resources: registered nurses.

One recent study, however, systematically evaluated the impact of a bedside computer system on nursing staff in two major areas: the efficiency and effectiveness of their work, and their satisfaction with this technology (Dennis, Sweeney, Macdonald, and Morse, 1993). MedTake (developed by Micro Health Systems and marketed by Baxter Healthcare Corporation) was tested for 3 months on a 30-bed medical unit in a Department of Veterans Affairs Medical Center. One terminal designed to serve no more than two patients was installed in each patient room and another terminal was located at the nurses' station; all were hard-wired to a central information server and printer. At the bedside, categorical function keys facilitated the entry and retrieval of information by activating screens for each of 12 modules: care plan, vital signs, intake, output, hygiene, activity, assessment, significant other, safety, diet, respiratory care, and wound care. Each screen was replete with a broad array of terms which staff members selected by entering the numeric digit provided for each term or highlighting the terms with the cursor. The computer system subsequently strung together the selected terms and phrases in a grammatically correct and linguistically sophisticated format to record the information.

Chart monitoring, a self-report questionnaire, and individual interviews comprised the major forms of data collection in this study. Pre- and post-implementation, a random sample of patients' charts was monitored to assess compliance with standards issued by the Joint Commission on Accreditation of Healthcare Organizations (JCAHO) (Joint Commission on Accreditation of Healthcare Organizations, 1991), to determine charting frequency, and to evaluate the technical aspects of charting such as legibility and format. The 23-item Bedside Computer Impact (BCI) questionnaire was collected from all nursing staff assigned to the unit. Developed and tested by the investigators for use in this study, the BCI (Cronbach's Alpha 0.80, Content Validity Index .90) tapped the dimensions of work efficiency, effectiveness and satisfaction. Semi-structured, tape-recorded interviews elicited staff members' in-depth perceptions regarding the system's implementation and outcomes.

Quality and quantity

The bedside computer system brought significant improvements in compliance to 11 (34%) of the JCAHO standards for nursing documentation that were monitored. Although two of these criteria addressed formatting techniques, such as giving titles to notes, the majority reflected substantive aspects of patient care, such as nursing assessments and patients' responses. The number of narrative entries that nursing staff made in patients records increased significantly ($p<.001$) from an average of seven entries per patient using the manual system to an average of 92 entries per patient with bedside computers. Licensed Practical Nurses and Nursing Assistants made a significant 21% increase in the frequency of their documentation, versus a non-significant 5% increase for RNs who already did the majority of the manual charting. Charts were striking for their legibility, which resulted in a marked ease in the ability to read narrative comments, distinguish numbers, find specific information, and identify care givers. Similarly, with the computerized format, completions and omissions in documentation were obvious. Because gaps in flowsheets were glaring, nurses could discern whether vital signs had been taken in a timely manner and whether other aspects of care had been completed and recorded.

Analysis of the BCI questionnaire revealed that the nursing staff was significantly more satisfied and viewed the total impact of the system significantly more favorably than they had anticipated prior to implementation. Many of the themes related to work efficiency and effectiveness that emerged from interview data have implications for restructuring nursing care: availability, timeliness, comprehensiveness/accuracy, and communication.

Availability

Availability meant that nurses no longer spent precious yet unproductive time in perpetual searches for patients' charts, nor did they have to find a place to write or wait to make their notations until patients returned from another department. Literally and figuratively, documentation and information were always at their fingertips, and nurses noted that they could redirect this "found" time into other, more important aspects of patient care. Moreover, other members of the health care team needing information about the patient had immediate access to the written documentation. Nurses perceived availability as the pre-eminent benefit to their work efficiency, for the bedside computers reduced frustration as remarkably as they eased work flow.

Timeliness

Timeliness was enabled by immediate documentation of the assessment of patients' conditions, development of plans, completion of tasks, and evaluation of care. No longer did nurses resort to notes scribbled on pieces of paper pushed into pockets or inked onto backs of hands, with data to be recorded at the end of the shift, or after the end of the shift, if indeed one could decipher what had been written hours earlier. Turning to the terminal after giving care meant that anyone who needed the most recent information about the patient would be able to find it.

Comprehensiveness

Comprehensiveness and accuracy markedly increased with the use of bedside computers. Nursing staff made significant improvements in documenting such areas as patients' responses to care, the early identification of continuing care needs, and the capabilities of the patient and/or significant other to manage those continuing care needs after discharge. Explanatory comments added to flow sheet notations gave a more complete picture of the patient's status. The computer-driven menus that filled the screen with a striking array of terms and phrases and provided a wide range of cues from which to select documentation terminology were particularly helpful to ancillary nursing staff who did not have to create written descriptions of their observations and tasks. They merely had to select what appeared on the screen before them. Accuracy was a concomitant feature of comprehensiveness, since staff members could look at the patient while charting and remember to document assessments or interventions that they otherwise might have forgotten. Accuracy also was enhanced by timeliness and elimination of redundant documentation, since the risk of transcription error increases every time information is transferred from scrap paper to flow sheet to narrative note.

Communication

The bedside computer system also facilitated the entire process of communication exchange. On-line review of patient information enabled the staff to retrieve information that might have been missed; nurses frequently used the review feature to locate, clarify, or confirm information they had missed earlier in the change-of-shift report. Likewise, physicians consistently used the review function to obtain the most current information about patients to include in treatment decisions. With point-of-care technology, staff members always knew that the information they needed about a patient had been entered, and they always knew exactly where to find it—unlike the manual charts with multiple pages, sometimes out of order or reversed back-to-front after perusal by multiple health care providers.

Restructuring: Computers, Nurse Extenders, and the Nursing Process

The capability to acquire, interpret, and analyze information at the bedside is a major support to redefining roles and restructuring nursing practice. With workers fewer in number (and more expensive), workload greater, patient throughput faster, intensity higher, and demands relentless in the 1990s (Fralic, 1992), attention is shifting to the greater use of "nurse extenders" or "assistive personnel" as an element in restructuring hospital nursing departments. The appropriate use of assistive personnel within nursing departments and the appropriateness of their use at all is the focus of much discourse (D. L. Gardner, 1991; Neidlinger, Bostrom, Stricker, Hild, and Zhang, 1993; Prescott et al., 1991). However, a crucial factor is the employment of these individuals in a manner that enables and enhances the professional practice of nursing, versus one that brings parceled-out, disjointed care and moves nurses further away from patients. Nurses' accountability for direct nursing care and management of care through interdisciplinary collaboration and coordination are not ameliorated by the introduction of nurse extenders. A redefinition of nurses' roles needs to be concurrent with the adoption of assistive personnel.

The results of a study on the incorporation of nurse extenders into a professional practice model suggest that nurses need greater knowledge and sharper skills both in delegating tasks and in supervising unlicensed personnel in various job descriptions (Neidlinger et al., 1993). To the degree that nurse extenders support an enriched role redefinition for RNs, so that nurses use their time and resources to meet the identified needs of patients rather than make difficult decisions regarding what care is completed and what is left undone (Prescott, Dennis, Creasia, and Bowen, 1985), the current trend toward assistive personnel may have positive outcomes. Rather than seen as substitutes for RNs, nurse extenders who have highly focused training rather than extensive formal education can enable the realignment of nursing versus non-nursing tasks, as well as assist or relieve nurses in a number of direct patient care activities. In this manner, they support rather than undermine the nursing process.

Assessment

The assessment phase of the nursing process is comprised of multiple components related to information, including collection, assembly into a meaningful form, analysis, synthesis, and interpretation. The collection of some, although certainly not all, information about patients can be done by trained nurse extenders who are further cued to observation and documentation comprehensiveness through terminology displayed on bedside terminals. When given the verbiage for documentation and not hampered by deficits in written language skills, nurse extenders can assume responsibility for recording the aspects of care for which they have been delegated responsibility and do it well (Dennis et al., 1993), thus relieving RNs of this additional time and workload demand. With the ease of information retrieval enabled by bedside computers, nurses can use the timely, written documentation of nurse extenders along with more traditional verbal interchange to enhance, not supplant, their own information acquisition. This process is not dissimilar to that used by physicians who rely heavily on the observation and patient monitoring by nurses for their medical treatment decisions (Dennis and Prescott, 1985).

Planning

Automation makes care plans or critical pathways used in case management easy to develop and revise at the bedside. Computers not only facilitate recording and format techniques, they also foster the integration of diverse and complex information required to meet patients' needs. Having up-to-date care plans readily available at the bedside enables nurse extenders to consistently review patients' care needs and goals and verify that all of their delegated responsibilities for care have been completed. Documentation of observations and tasks according to the problem list and care plan further underscores the potential of nurse extenders to facilitate the RN's ongoing responsibility for developing and refining the plan of care. Having critical paths constantly accessible at the bedside enables all members of the interdisciplinary health care team to insure that plans are current and consistent with the patient's progress and the established goals.

Implementation

Implementation is the nursing process component that is most appropriate for extensive delegation to assistive personnel. Helping patients with hygiene, ambulation, and other activities of daily living does not necessarily have to be done by a RN, nor do certain circumscribed tasks such as inserting intravenous lines, drawing blood, and placing urinary catheters. Rather than abrogation of responsibility for implementation and direct patient care, however, selected delegation to others by nurses in redefined roles means that an even greater onus is placed on the RN for insuring the conduct, correctness, and documentation of these patient-care activities. By providing uninterrupted availability of the patient's chart, fostering timely and comprehensive documentation, and enabling completions and omissions of care to be noted immediately upon rapid review of patients' information, bedside computers permit nurses to easily determine the status of care at any point in time throughout their tour of duty. While computers do not rule out verbal follow-up, they do eliminate the time nurses spend in trying to locate assistive personnel for status reports, just as they eliminate nurses' perpetual search for patients' charts to complete their own documentation.

Evaluation

Information central to patients' status and welfare that is integrated and displayed by bedside computers markedly contributes to the evaluation of care and patients' responses to it. Once again, observations made by nurse extenders that are comprehensively documented with the aid of menu-driven computer screens can contribute markedly to this evaluation process. Reviewing the plan of care at the bedside while concurrently evaluating the patient can enable the nurse to more accurately and comprehensively align needs, progress, and goals. Variance from designated timeframes within critical paths can be readily identified and corrective steps immediately incorporated into a new plan of action. When bedside terminals are connected to hospital information systems and used by all members of the health care team, evaluation and modification of interdisciplinary care is supported by treatments initiated or terminated, tests ordered, and discharge decisions contemplated in an expeditious manner (Welsch and Nicholson, 1991), without nurses' spending inordinate amounts of time attempting to make telephone contact with other providers.

Actual and Projected Outcomes

Whether bedside computers, redefined roles, and restructured organizational formats actually refocus nurses' time to improve patient care remains to be demonstrated, since saved time for nurses may not necessarily translate into greater benefits for patients. However, data collected during the implementation and integration of a bedside computer system and a professional practice model begins to capture the dynamics (Miller and Sheridan, 1992). Because a professional practice model and bedside computers were implemented almost simultaneously in this study, it is not possible to discern how much of the effects can be attributed to each factor. Nevertheless, the integration of a professional practice model and bedside computers, versus an unrestructured model with manual documentation system, provides insight into the value of bedside computers in restructuring nursing care. Nurses on the restructured units with bedside computers experienced an increase in the time they spent in direct patient care, and a change in the types of their activities. Indirect care rituals were replaced by professional activities such as conferring with and supervising nursing staff, as well as direct care concerns including treatment, communication, and patient education. Given this prologue, additional studies are needed that systematically evaluate the impact of bedside computers on nurses' time, the ways in which nurses spend their time, and their efficiency and effectiveness in restructured roles.

Summary

While the adoption of bedside computers can eliminate redundant paperwork, increase productivity, and make drastic cuts in nurses' performance of non-nursing tasks, the major benefits accrue not from the technology per se but from the revised procedures and restructured practice that these systems can engender. Strictly transferring paper products to electronic mechanisms without re-engineering professional practice will not markedly enhance professional autonomy and accountability or patient outcomes. Moreover, distinctions between hospital information systems and clinical information systems will need to blend into patient care information systems. Bedside computer systems for nursing documentation will need to become systems for interdisciplinary collaboration and documentation to realize their fullest potential in health care settings. In summary, the greatest value of bedside computers is likely to emanate from supporting professionals in acquiring and analyzing information, making collaborative treatment decisions, and coalescing integrative roles around patient-centered care.

References

Casassa, E. (1990, May). Bedside computing positively impacts patient care. *Computers in Healthcare*, 26-31.

Dennis, K. E., and Prescott, P. A. (1985). Florence Nightingale: Yesterday, today, and tomorrow. *Advances in Nursing Science, 7*, 66-81.

Dennis, K. E., Sweeney, P. M., Macdonald, I., and Morse, N. A. (1993). Point of care technology: Impact on people and paperwork. *Nursing Economic$, 11*(4), 229-237.

Fralic, M. F. (1992). Into the future: Nurse executives and the world of information technology. *Journal of Nursing Administration, 22*(4), 11-12.

Gardner, D. L. (1991). Issues related to nurse extenders. *Journal of Nursing Administration, 21*(10), 40-45.

Gardner, E. (1990). Hospitals not in a hurry to plug in computers by the bedside. *Modern Healthcare, 20*(28), 31, 34, 39-40.

Halford, G., Burkes, M., and Pryor, T. A. (1989). Measuring the impact of bedside terminals. *Nursing Management, 20*(7), 41-42, 44-45.

Hard, R. (1992). More hospitals move toward bedside systems. *Hospitals, 56*(19), 72, 74.

Hendrickson, G., and Kovner, C. T. (1990). Effects of computers on nursing resource use. *Computers in Nursing, 8*(1), 16-22.

Herring, D., and Rochman, R. (1990). A closer look at bedside terminals. *Nursing Management, 21*(7), 54-61.

Joint Commission on the Accreditation of Healthcare Organizations (1991). *1992 Joint Commission Accreditation Manual for Hospitals (Vol. 1, Standards)*. Oakbrook Terrace, IL: Department of Standards, JCAHO.

Korpman, R. A. (1991). Patient care automation: The future is now. Part 6: Does reality live up to the promise? *Nursing Economic$, 9*(3), 175-178.

Lower, M. S., and Nauert, L.B. (1992). Charting: The impact of bedside computers. *Nursing Management, 23*(7), 40-42, 44.

Miller, E. R., and Sheridan, E. A. (1992). Integrating a bedside nursing information system into a professional nursing practice model. In J. M. Arnold, and G. A. Pearson (Eds.), *Computer Applications in Nursing Education and Practice* (pp. 62-70). New York: National League for Nursing (Pub. No. 14-2406).

Neidlinger, S. H., Bostrom, J., Stricker, A., Hild, J., and Zhang, J. Q. (1993). Incorporating nursing assistive personnel into a nursing professional practice model. *Journal of Nursing Administration, 23*(3), 29-37.

Packer, C. L. (1987). Point-of-care terminals: Interest abounds. *Hospitals, 61*(18), 79.

Prescott, P. A., Dennis, K. E., Creasia, J., and Bowen, S. (1985). Nursing shortage in transition. *Image: Journal of Nursing Scholarship, 17*(4), 127-133.

Prescott, P. A., Phillips, C. Y., Ryan, J. W., and Thompson, K. O. (1991). Changing how nurses spend their time. *Image: Journal of Nursing Scholarship, 23*(1), 23-28.

Randall, A. (1991). Bedside systems offer positive incentives. *Healthcare Informatics, 8*(8), 26-28.

Staggers, N. (1988). Using computers in nursing. *Computers in Nursing, 6*(4), 164-170.

Welsch, E., and Nicholson, S. (1991). Bedside terminals: Panacea or gadget? *Nursing Economics, 9*(6), 437-440.

Communication Technologies for Nurse Executives

LTC(P) Nancy T. Staggers, PhD, RN (Army Nurse Corps)
Deputy Director for Clinical Policy Support
Health Affairs
Health Services Operations
Office of the Assistant Secretary of Defense

Introduction

Facsimile (fax) machines, voice mail, and electronic pagers are crucial to effective information management among nurse executives today. These single-mode communication technologies have been adopted quickly into the work flow of nursing organizations, meshing easily with existing business methods. Much more promising but more slowly being adopted are interactive technologies such as electronic mail (e-mail). E-mail and related enabling technologies empower users at all levels in organizations but can mandate new communication and work design methods. If e-mail represents a step into the evolution of nurses' work design, then even newer technologies such as work flow and integrated media, will represent a new stage in this evolution. The overview of communication technologies presented in this chapter concentrates on messaging forums, builds on an e-mail foundation, introduces applications beyond e-mail, moves on to integrated technologies, and ends with a discussion outlining the implications of using advanced messaging for managing information.

Basic Interactive Messaging Technologies

E-mail: The Foundation

Nurse executives and other nurses can use e-mail to send electronic messages to other individuals or groups located in different geographical areas. Using a modem or networked computer, system users can electronically send, receive, forward, print, and/or store personal documents and messages by accessing mail options on their computers. Messages are communicated nearly instantaneously to recipients and replies are attached to the original message, forming an automatic audit trail for issues addressed.

E-mail is especially useful for routine communications in large organizations or in any organization with geographically separated personnel. Meeting minutes, agendas, policies, announcements, position papers, and general inquiries can be sent electronically to system users. Along with its administrative uses, health care e-mail applications can include routine consults, on-line educational offerings for CEUs, and can even provide non-urgent laboratory results retrieval. As organizations emphasize ambulatory areas and have fewer workers inside their walls, e-mail will be an invaluable tool for maintaining communications among personnel. In fact, Reinhardt (1993) believes it is only a matter of time until e-mail is as pervasive and as easy to use as the telephone.

E-mail is not limited to private, intra-organizational communications. Executives may choose public e-mail services such as AT&T, MCI, CompuServe, or Internet to communicate with others. Using public networks has the added advantage of linking users to anyone else with access to the service, opening a world of connections. For instance, nurse executives may use Internet, an international network of universities and government agencies, to consult with academic counterparts located in another part of the country or the world. Other applications on three networks of interest to nurses, Internet, FidoNet, and BITNET, are described in a 1993 article by Sparks and in her chapter in this book. For more information about e-mail basics, readers are referred elsewhere (Perry, 1992; Reinhardt, 1993; Staggers, 1989, 1990).

The Impact of E-mail

Computer messaging creates a domain freed of time, distance, and political boundaries (Perry, 1992). Nurses may communicate asynchronously, completing messages as time allows during a day. Recipients may then respond as time permits during their busy schedules. Spanning time zones is no longer a barrier to completing business. Nurses in other time zones read and respond to mail, eliminating the need to connect by mutually convenient telephone hours. As Ball, Hannah, Jelger, and Peterson (1988) noted, their book was created by international authors using e-mail and networks to send electronic manuscripts. Dealing with other executives in distant areas and time zones is facilitated with e-mail. For instance, Army nurse executives and consultants have used e-mail for several years to communicate with colleagues in Hawaii and Germany simultaneously, making collaboration across several oceans possible.

E-mail affects both individual and organizational productivity and accountability. This convenient method of communicating allows executives to effectively eliminate telephone tag, many routine meetings, and the need to communicate using "live" exchanges for all matters. Personal contact may be preserved for more urgent or sensitive issues. Besides the convenience and speed of e-mail, this technology gives executives flexibility and organization in their schedules by allowing them to read mail at any time from nearly any location. Executives can touch the pulse of their organizations by accessing e-mail even while they are away at conferences. Or they may choose to read e-mail on a Sunday evening to prepare for the Monday morning rush of activities. For employees like community health nurses, using a modem allows them access into organizations without returning to the parent building. The reliability of e-mail prevents memos from getting lost in the system, provides an automatic record of discussions and has the potential to decrease the number of interruptions in an executive's day. Access to experts is easy and uncovering hidden expertise is more likely. Not atypically, executives using Internet could poll 10,000 people for help with a dilemma using a question beginning with, "Does anybody know . . . ?" E-mail dissolves rank and hierarchical boundaries because messages from everyone appear without the usual titles or rank, creating a more democratic viewing of information (Brown, 1993). Open access permits connections to experts that were never possible in the past and allows more diverse ideas to emerge. This same access ends the isolation of some nurses, such as rural health care workers, giving them a connection to other opinions and expertise. More important, a study done by Hewlett-Packard found that the average cost of an e-mail message, $0.22, was less than a letter, $0.51, or a fax, $1.66 (Perry, 1992).

No new technology is without negative implications, however. After surmounting the equipment barrier, probably the most evident disadvantages of e-mail relate to the volume of information, the readability of e-mail text, and privacy issues. For more mature users of e-mail systems, disadvantages occur when using multiple systems and managing volumes of information. Executives and workers at one hospital received an average of 20 to 50 messages per day (Gardner, 1993) while the president of a company received as many as 100 to 200 messages and spent 30% of the day processing mail (Baker, 1993). My own work involves reading e-mail in five different systems; a colleague uses as many as nine! More critical than accurately recalling nine unique access codes to sign on to systems is managing the volumes of information generated. Executives returning after a vacation may be confronted with several hundred messages to read. Some federal e-mail users complain about the volume of what they perceive to be "junk mail" on one system. E-mail includes a new level of productivity for executives, but the corresponding open access means interacting with more users and issues than ever before. The disadvantages can be partially solved, however, by generating organizational policies about sending clear, concise and relevant messages (Baker, 1993) and choosing e-mail systems with a message screening tool for triaging mail.

The readability of e-mail text is a more difficult issue to resolve. Many current e-mail systems are text-based, although this is changing. Without different fonts and graphics, e-mail can be uninteresting to read (Magia, 1993), and some users miss critical points or misread issues while skimming through mail. Of course, e-mail text masks the usual cues of interpersonal communication so message meaning can be misinterpreted by users who then react inappropriately or negatively (Anderson and Shapiro, cited in Perry, 1992). Partially in response to this problem, e-mail users have developed "emoticons" (Amirrezvani, 1993) or rudimentary codes to convey feelings. Meant to be read at a 90-degree angle, a sample of codes follows (Perry, 1992):

    :-)   a smile or a joking comment
    ;-)   a sarcastic or flirtatious comment
    :-(a frown or being upset or depressed
    %-)   confused
    :-D   a laugh

A third issue, privacy, is the most sensitive issue for e-mail users. Individuals may assume e-mail is as private as traditional mail. It is not. For instance, message recipients typically have the ability to forward mail to others. Forwarding messages can occur without the original writer's permission or knowledge, broadcasting to an audience other than the one the original writer intended. Even if there is the option to block forwarding on some messages, recipients still can print out or download messages and distribute them. Because e-mail resides on computers and networks, its very existence in electronic form makes it available to an audience.

E-mail privacy issues have caught the attention of lawmakers. In fact, employers have a legal right to periodically monitor e-mail use in their organizations (Jensen, 1993). The Electronics Communications Privacy Act of 1986 allows employers to monitor messages on a company network. As more users come on-line, privacy and security remain critical and as-yet unresolved issues for all information systems, including e-mail.

E-mail Use

Outside health care, e-mail use is flourishing. With an estimated 25.9 million users today (Baker, 1993), revenues of $1.6 billion are projected for public e-mail services in 1996 (Gardner, 1993). No specific statistics about e-mail use in health care organizations are readily available other than one study reporting e-mail usage over a week's time (Sands, Safran, Slack, and Bleich, 1993). If the health care literature is any indication, e-mail is at a very early stage of adoption, for only a few articles have addressed e-mail applications in health care (Gardner, 1993; Sands et al., 1993; Sparks, 1993; Staggers, 1989, 1990). Yet, interest in using electronic communications is strong. Sparks (1993) calls for nurse participation in electronic networking. The Department of Veterans Administration and federal workers, including nurses, have used e-mail as an organizational tool for several years.

Despite some disadvantages, e-mail provides a communications infrastructure unlike any previously available. In fact, the federal sector sees so much potential in e-mail, it is planning a global mail network infrastructure, to be called the Defense Message System, a system designed for over two million users (Masud, 1993). For nurse executives, using e-mail may not be a question of whether to begin, but rather when to use the technology. Resources available about programs may help ease organizations into electronic communications. For instance, Marshall (1993) evaluated seven e-mail programs, rating Lotus' cc:Mail first for its basic message handling capabilities, interface appearance, ease of use, and available tools. Once e-mail use is established in the organization, more advanced interactive technologies build upon the foundation these basic e-mail programs create.

Advanced Interactive Messaging Technologies

Workgroup Software

As its name suggests, workgroup software supports collaborative efforts among groups of individuals with personal computers or workstations. Several years ago this type of software was called groupware or group productivity software. Although the first versions were somewhat slow to be adopted, newer versions are being more quickly accepted because of their impact on workers' productivity. Typically, workgroup software such as WordPerfect Office or Microsoft Windows for Workgroups offers a suite of applications, including e-mail, time management for group scheduling, integrated calendars and a task manager for project management. Users may keep public calendars that show available meeting times with blocked information about unavailable times. Group members can then have the computer poll several group members for the first mutually available time for a meeting. Workgroup software options vary from vendor to vendor but include basic functions such as shared documents, shared messaging and document handling features, and data bases for information such as telephone directories. Also, group members can share files, comment on and even mark up documents during on-line meetings. Lastly, workgroup software can allow access and importing of non-text files such as spreadsheets.

Workgroup software with its e-mail foundation allows geographically distant group members to share information and collaborate on projects, large or small. One way to think of this type of software is that it allows islands of individuals with information on their separate computers to evolve to groups of people collaborating on shared information. For instance, Digital Equipment Company (DEC) used a team of 53 engineers in Massachusetts, Colorado, Arizona, Singapore, and Germany to design a new disk drive. Using e-mail, DEC estimated it was able to finish the project in a year's less time with 40% fewer people than with traditional methods (Perry, 1992). One way the group saved time was by shifting work across time zones. Engineers in one location would work on a problem until late in the day. Then, they would summarize their progress, along with any continuing difficulties for their colleagues in another time zone. Those workers would continue work on the problem while the original group of engineers slept. The next day, the original group of engineers would begin work where the others left off. Group productivity was maximized by 30% using this technique, group members estimated.

Using workgroup software makes work teams in different locations, even countries, commonplace (Perry, 1992). Applying this to nursing, nurse executives could assemble teams of individuals despite their location, time zone or affiliation. Workgroup software could be especially useful for large or less structured groups, crossing organizational boundaries and maximizing use of part-time group members.

Workflow Software

Workflow software can be considered a subset of workgroup software in that it provides intelligent routing of documents within a specified group of employees. It is a tool that can digitally replicate existing business processes, or it may be used to reinvent new processes and create new structures. Workflow software guides users through tasks, tracks tasks, issues reminders, and routes information. Using the more advanced type of workflow software, a business or organization begins using the software by first understanding and diagramming the flow of information within a specific process, e.g., requesting prn or agency nurses through the organization's contracting department. Doing this analytic work allows organizations to carefully examine processes and streamline them as appropriate. After that, the processes are automated by adding intelligence to information/documents at each step of a process. In the case of requesting prn nurses, nurse managers would fill out electronic forms that are automatically directed to their supervisors for approval. Next, the forms are electronically routed to contracting for execution. Ideally, the contracting office would be networked to the agency providing prn nurses. The request would be received automatically in their computers, scheduling could occur, and the proper monies would be billed back to the contracting department's computer. These processes all occur without human intervention in routing. Preprogrammed rules allow the forms to flow as prescribed (Reinhardt, 1993).

Reinhardt (1993) described three different architectures for workflow software: (a) user-based, (b) object-based, and (c) action-based. User-based systems have tools for individuals to complete interactions with other people and applications, for example, e-mail. The interactions are defined by a rules mechanism or engine that allows filtering and sorting of mail. Users define how they would like to manage a process by accessing mail and then adding various functions to the messages. For instance, users may want messages designated as urgent to be routed to an "urgent" folder for immediate processing. User-based systems represent an informal, decentralized method of automation.

Object-based and action-based systems are more centralized in their approach to workflow methods. Object-based software integrates intelligence into documents to allow users to correctly process forms. With these programs, active fields within a document can even be designated to automatically access an appropriate data base for current values. Rules for processing are based on both time and events. As well, information about each form is transmitted to a data base for tracking. The routing mechanism is programmed using both graphics tools and text (scripts). Then the programmed objects can flow through an organization in the prescribed manner. This type of workflow program can be integrated with other applications so that users may access data bases or spreadsheets while working with a particular document.

The most conceptually advanced programs are action-based software systems built around understanding the flow of work in an organization and providing an underlying framework for completing tasks. The core of the application is a data base representing a center of actions or tasks. These automatically connect to a set of tools for managing transaction processing. Together they create a workflow management center. The status of each document is stored in the data base. Other tools allow users to manage work flow and monitor performance. An example of this kind of technology is Action Technologies' Workflow Management Systems that includes a graphical workflow designer and an applications builder to connect workflows into external applications (Reinhardt, 1993).

Workflow software is especially useful for applications such as processing purchase-order documents, travel and vacation requests. Obviously, these routine applications are a large part of administrative business in nursing organizations as well. The more advanced types of workflow software allow organizations to re-engineer business processes. A good workflow tool should help both analyze and automate information-based activities. The user-based workflow applications provide a small advance over basic e-mail, but the object- and action-based applications provide a global approach to supporting work.

The Impact of Workgroup Software

While basic e-mail is messaging between people, workgroup software is messaging between people and processes (Reinhardt, 1993). These advanced applications have generated much excitement because of their potential impact on the way work is done. The usual positive impacts of automating processes are evident. Communication speed, reliability, and accuracy improve. In addition, productivity and resource management are particularly affected by workgroup software. Second, workgroup software allows worker knowledge to be concentrated more on decisions than rules about information flow. Productivity is enhanced by the automatic routing of documents, the streamlining of superfluous activities, and tracking forms. The e-mail and document sharing portion of workflow software can increase productivity by improving the stock of ideas, providing leads for solving issues, unusual references, and other information. Individuals can offer on-line ideas and notions for others to digest and get nearly instant feedback (Perry, 1992). Groups have the potential to solve some issues in a compressed amount of time, as with the example of the DEC engineer. The group scheduling and calendar features allow optimizing scarce resources such as audio-visual equipment or consultants. Most importantly, the advanced features of action-based workflow software allow organizations or groups to re-invent the business operations, as well as analyze and streamline processes.

By design, this software reduces the amount of low-level tasks nurses would need to cognitively process. Then, nursing information is transformed from paper-based "rules" of processing information into concentrating on the decision about information instead. The low-level knowledge of who and where to send a document and tracking its progress can then be replaced by higher-level information needs.

The most obvious negative impact is the setup and analysis time required to implement workflow software. Before optimizing the use of the more centralized workflow software such as object and action-based software, nurses will need to critically examine workflow patterns, design processes, and define them within the software. Of course, analyzing and computerizing workflow in an incremental method is one way to manage the seemingly overwhelming setup time.

Another negative impact concerns on-line decision-making. Complex issues can be difficult to resolve on-line if no one person acts as a facilitator or group leader. More access to documents may mean more discussion and longer process times to come to closure. Lastly, workgroup software blurs central decision-making and may create difficulties for managers and organizations more accustomed to centralized structures (Yager, 1993).

Despite the analytic and setup times, workflow software offers the potential to redefine business operations in nursing organizations. Redesigning workflow could alleviate superfluous tasks and increase efficiency, complementing other quality management efforts in organizations. Then, what will remain in health care organizations is the industry of managing work and managing the value of information.

Integrated Technologies

One of the most frustrating activities for technology-oriented executives is buying and learning to use these various interactive and single-mode tools. In the computer realm alone, executives may have to buy, learn, and retain information about word processing, spreadsheets, data base, presentation software, communication, and e-mail packages. The executive's environment can contain a myriad of equipment: a cellular telephone, standard telephone, computer terminal(s), modem, fax machine, copy machine, and perhaps teleconferencing equipment. These diverse and time-consuming technologies are becoming more integrated, especially in the new age of wireless communications.

Integrated Desktop Computing Devices

This technology integrates voice, video, and communications technologies into a desktop computer. Using systems such as MINX (Datapoint Corporation of San Antonio), Apple AV Technologies or PictureTel LIVE, users may sit at their desktop computers to dial-up videoconferencing for conducting business. After dialing another user, individuals may view each other through small windows on the computer screen. Sitting in front of their computers, users speak into built-in microphones. Stored computer files may be accessed from shared work space and displayed on the main area of the screen. One individual may send a document to another by merely dragging it into a folder icon. If hardcopy material needs to be displayed, a user may hold it up to the camera for others to see.

Other technologies are being integrated into computers. Apple advertises two new Macintosh products that integrate video, TV, messaging, voice recognition, text to speech, and voice/fax telephone communications with computing. Users may now point and click on phone messages or tell the computer to read the phone message, e-mail, spreadsheet values or documents. Individuals may give voice commands to open an application, fax a document, play a CD, or begin recording a video program. A built-in microphone allows users to place telephone calls while sitting in front of the computer.

Personal Communications Devices

Personal communications devices bridge the gap between cellular phones, pagers, and more traditional computer files (Ziegler, 1993). Unlike the desktop versions of integrated technologies, these personal communication devices are portable. Two examples are the Eo and Newton technologies. Eo was built around a pen and paper metaphor with nine applications bundled into one technology (Smotroff, 1992), including fax, phone, e-mail, note-taking, calculator, scheduling, and an address book. With Eo, individuals can make phone calls, send faxes, and do typical computing tasks by tapping an electronic pen on icons (Skrzycki and Burgess, 1993).

The Newton, released in Summer 1993, is similar in that it reads and transforms handwritten notes, sends and receives faxes, and allows access to e-mail via a wireless connection but it also transforms rough sketches into more formal structures. This device has received mixed initial reviews on its handwriting recognition abilities in particular, but certainly these devices are unique in that they allow for mobility, immediacy of information access, and relative economy (Ziegler, 1993). Telecommunications experts give the personal communications devices cautious reviews, calling them "mediocre and pricey" (Skrzycki and Burgess, 1993). To the contrary, these are the first in a line of enabling technologies that will likely follow into nurse executives' lives.

Implications of Using Interactive and Integrated Technologies

As nurse executives take advantage of basic, advanced, and integrated messaging technologies, several issues are likely to emerge.

Access

Messaging technologies allow unparalleled access to people and organizations across time zones and distances. With integrated portable technologies, systems will provide communications capabilities to nurse executives, no matter their location. This increased access makes two fundamental assumptions: (a) nurses want more access, and (b) they want more information. With more access and information, the lines between home and work have the potential to blur, for these technologies can easily facilitate increased hours of work. The change to more access and more information will be insidious. Exactly *how much* access and information nurse executives will tolerate may be an issue. Unlike in the past, off-site conferences or vacations may not be retreats from interruptions. With personal communications devices and cellular phones, individuals traveling between locations is no longer a barrier to access. Executives may feel there is little escape and little uninterrupted time. In fact, one executive expressed regret for missing time to think (Rossheim, 1993). In the future, nurse executives may have to plan for uninterrupted periods of time and sanctuaries away from messaging technologies.

New Organizational Work Design

Messaging technologies have the potential to create virtual offices and virtual users. With mobile technology, there is less need to be based in one location to do nursing's business. Nurse executives armed with personal communications devices can be as accessible while touring off-site patient units as when they were stationed by a telephone in an office.

Nursing may find these technologies create more loosely structured organizations, using workgroup software to create and manage many tasks. Messaging technologies may allow easier use of consultants and part-time experts in solving particular issues. Hierarchical boundaries will be softened. Dialogue can occur between the CEO and a new staff nurse without adhering to the usual staffing channels. Powerbases will be redefined by information and knowledge expertise rather than position in the organization. Interactive messaging technologies easily support the shift to more flattened organizations. In fact, e-mail supports very loosely organized and fluid organizations, based on team approaches that shift and change. E-mail could be a facilitating tool for case managers. The flexibility of messaging allows time and location independence in communicating, so that a new culture and work design is possible. Organizations could become more idea-oriented and less tradition-bound (Rash, 1993). There is the potential to be based on knowledge-processing rather than data/information processing in nursing.

Workers' roles may be redefined. Executives who use integrated technologies will have less use for secretaries with traditional skills. Executives will do their own word processing or dictate to a computer that translates speech into text. A secretary may be replaced by an information managing assistant. This worker would keep information organized for the executive and complete more advanced tasks than in the past. Certainly, basic technology skills will be requisite for this person, as well as for the executive, and a communications equipment infrastructure will be mandatory for organizations.

The Pace of Change

The number of new messaging products is startling. For even techno-prone executives, maintaining status as an informed consumer is a challenge. The rate of change in technology may be quicker than organizational budgets and nurse executives can implement, for many executives have only recently adjusted to voice mail. However, the rate of adoption of messaging technologies in nursing organizations is keyed to the support of nurse executives. After completing an assessment of organizational communications needs and making a decision about appropriate technology, installing the tool is only the beginning. Executives set the example and tone by using the tool as well. If executives assign their secretaries to read and write e-mail, subordinates will not take the technology seriously either. On the positive side, the vast numbers of new individuals on e-mail will force vendors to make more usable products. Information-stressed executives will demand products that are intuitive to learn and use.

Summary

Messaging technologies impact the productivity and accountability of workers in nursing organizations and have the potential to transform the way nurses work. The change to advanced messaging technologies and beyond may be incremental, but the age of evolution of nurse executives' information management begins with the advent of these tools.

References

Amirrezvani, A. (1993, November). Tips for taming e-mail. *PC World*, pp. 284-287, 290, 295.

Baker, M. S. (1993). E-mail sidesteps time-wasting meetings. *Budget Sound Business Journal, 14*(10), 32-37.

Ball, M. J., Hannah, K. J., Jelger, U. G., and Peterson, H. (1988). *Nursing Informatics: Where Caring and Technology Meet.* New York: Springer-Verlag New York.

Brown, B. P. (1993, April 5). Data super highway will open up information. *Capital District Business Review*, p. 14.

Gardner, E. (1993, February 1). Hospitals giving e-mail a stamp of approval. *Modern Healthcare*, pp. 45-46.

Jensen, D. (1993, March 6). For government and business, e-mail isn't as private as you might think. *The Business Journal-Milwaukee*, p. 4.

Magid, L. J. (1993, October 18). Software combines power of graphics with the ease of e-mail. *The Washington Post* (WashTech section), p. 16.

Marshall, P. (1993). Making the most of messaging. *Info World*, pp. 76-77, 80, 82, 84, 86, 88, 90, 92, 94, 96, 98, 100.

Masud, S. A. (1993, October 11). DOD thinks big in its plan for global e-mail. *The Government Computer News*, pp. 1, 76.

Perry, T. S. (1992). E-mail: Pervasive and persuasive. *IEEE Spectrum, 29,* 22-33.

Rash, W. (1993). Remote computing in the enterprise environment: How far can it go? *OS2 Professional, 1*(7), 41-42, 44, 46-48.

Reinhardt, A. (1993, March). Smarter e-mail is coming. *Byte, 18*(3), pp. 90, 92, 94, 96-98, 100, 102, 105-106, 108.

Rossheim, J. (1993, June 28). Cellular phones: Some like 'em and some don't. *PC Week*, p. 211.

Sands, D. Z., Safran, C., Slack, W. V., and Bleich, H. L. (1993). Use of electronic mail in a teaching hospital. In C. Safran (Ed.), *Symposium on Computer Applications in Medical Care* (pp. 306-310). New York: McGraw-Hill Book Co.

Skrzycki, C., and Burgess, J. (1993, July 1). New generation of personal communicators goes on sale. *The Washington Post*, pp. 1, 11.

Smotroff, M. (1992, November 4). Eo unveils world's first personal communicators. *Business Wire*, p. 11.

Sparks, S. M. (1993). Electronic networking for nurses. *Image: Journal of Nursing Scholarship, 25*(3), 245-248.

Staggers, N. (1989). E-mail basics. *Journal of Nursing Administration, 19*(10), 31-35.

Staggers, N. (1990). Communicating in the 1990s: A technology update. *Nursing Economics, 8*(6), 408-412.

Yager, T. (1993, March). Better than being there: Desktop video teleconferencing could change how you do business. *Byte*, 129-130, 132-133.

Ziegler, D. (1993, June 6). System bridges cellular's gaps. *The Denver Post*, p. 1.

Nurse-Designed Voice-Activated Computer Systems for Nursing Documentation

Joan Trofino, EdD, RN, FAAN
Vice President, Patient Care Services
Riverview Medical Center
Red Bank, New Jersey

Do not follow where the path may lead. Go instead
where there is no path and leave a trail.
—Anonymous, Motivational Quotes

Introduction

Voice-reporting technology represents one of the last computer frontiers in an information-dominated society. Since human speech is an immediate and natural method of communication, the use of voice technology will become common in the future as an easy method to enter and convey computerized information (Bertolucci, 1990; Kurzweil, 1989; Lange, 1991; Smarte, 1989).

New voice-activated systems capable of recognizing words through sound and then reacting to them with voice output are enhancing communication possibilities. Since these new systems eliminate the need to use the hands to type or write, they permit immediate single-word input to generate sentences and phrases, and do not require computer literacy to operate (Lange, 1991), it is not surprising that they are rapidly coming into use by business, industry and health care.

The usefulness of automated medical records to improve patient care and to serve as an assessment tool for medical personnel has only recently been discovered. Voice report technology may assist in reducing malpractice litigation and the need for physicians to practice defensive medicine, which often results in increased and costly diagnostic testing (Belton and Dick, 1991).

The U.S. health care industry is probably the most data-intensive in the world. Our patient records contain more descriptive and tracking information than most records developed by other industries (Belton and Dick, 1991).

Surprisingly, on the brink of the 21st century, the data-rich health care industry remains one of the least automated and least computerized. Computer systems entered the field of health care finance more than a decade ago; however, the bulk of health care practices relating to patient care documentation are still managed primarily by obsolete methods, i.e., handwritten notes.

Belton and Dick (1991) identified the following reasons for this:
• the belated recognition of the importance of the medical record, principally its relationships to quality and consistency of medical care and malpractice exposure and rates;
• the non-profit stance of health care providers, which makes it difficult to widen investment in computer-based systems for the creation and storage of medical records; and
• the inability of equipment suppliers to provide easy-to-use systems that could be accepted by a clear majority of medical staff members. (p. 27)
In today's fast-paced health care environment, the medical record, which is primarily a narrative chronicle, requires a paradigm shift from handwritten or taped transcription to

accurate, accessible, cost-effective, computer-based patient records. Widespread computerized documentation and analysis of current health care procedures and practices may answer questions about the efficacy of treatments and protocols. Such accountability from health care providers serves to strengthen practices and reduce malpractice litigation and/or claims of nursing negligence, while providing government and other third-party payers with value-laden, high-quality, cost-efficient care for patients.

The Voice Process: Historical Overview

In the late 1980s, advances in automated speech-recognition (ASR) made it possible for physicians in specialties like radiology, pathology and emergency medicine to create, edit, store and print medical records by speaking directly into a computer (Belton and Dick, 1991). Government reports have indicated that voice-controlled patient reporting can "minimize changes in the way physicians practice medicine, while also providing a cost-effective, timely, and efficient way for hospitals to record patient data." (General Accounting Office, 1991, p. 19).

Bakst (1987) predicted that the cost of these systems will drop to approximately $1,500 to $2,000 for systems that offer a 250-word vocabulary. By the end of the 1990s, voice-activated text processing systems compatible with word processors, personal computers, and electronic typewriters will be commercially available (Bakst, 1987).

Nurses Also Need Automated Speech-Recognition

Nurses, like physicians, have found themselves increasingly overwhelmed by ever-growing documentation demands. In this era of limited resources and exploding technology, now is the time to take a new look at the methods nurses have used to document patient care. (Trofino, 1993a).

Documentation Issues in the 1990s

Current nursing knowledge requires the development of a comprehensive patient care plan based upon a nursing diagnosis. Technology demands have resulted in an ongoing process of data gathering, sorting and recording of information, tasks often completed by nurses. Growing regulatory expectations by the State Health Department and Joint Commission on Accreditation of Healthcare Organizations include random visits to the health care agency and retrospective chart reviews. Conclusions about quality, appropriateness of treatment and the responsiveness of health care providers to standards of patient care is obtained to a great extent from the documentation entered into the medical record by physicians and nurses.

A New Documentation Methodology

In this new era of technology, nurses, like physicians, require a computer-based documentation methodology. The new system should enable anyone, including computer novices, to produce flawless documents that would pass all regulatory surveys, as well as help increase job satisfaction and productivity among nursing personnel.

In direct response to the nursing shortages experienced in the 1980s, the New Jersey Department of Health established the Nursing Incentive Reimbursement Award (NIRA) Program. This award was aimed towards improvement of the work environment for nurses practicing in New Jersey Hospitals. In 1990 and 1991, the Riverview Medical Center Nursing Division applied for and received $1,000,000 in NIRA grants. The following study indicates how ASR served as the technological change agent in creating complete and virtually flawless nursing documentation by voice (Trofino, 1993a; 1993b).

Vendor Selection

Transformational leadership over two decades has promoted an involved and committed nursing culture at Riverview Medical Center. Staff nurses make decisions that affect their governance and practice. Thus, it was considered only natural for staff nurses to fully participate as members of the Computer Nursing Advisory Committee. This committee focused initially on a review of the literature and then the establishment of technology objectives for nursing documentation.

The committee objectives included a user-friendly system that:
- contained a large vocabulary
- permitted end-user customization
- was cost effective
- could interact with the planned hospital-wide computer system (Trofino, 1993a; 1993b).

A speech recognition system for emergency medicine had been introduced into the department earlier, with good acceptance by physicians. Thus, it seemed logical to begin to build voice recognition for nursing documentation into the Emergency Department (ED). The physicians' medical vocabulary could be used as a data base, and this new nursing concept would be developed in a clinical area where voice-recognition technology had already been well received by the physicians.

The initial focus was to follow an orthopedic emergency admission through triage, emergency assessment and into the operating suite. Elective admissions for orthopedic surgery were also included later in our study.

Creating a Cadre of Nursing Experts

With the financial support from our grant, we were able to purchase three voice-activated computer development systems. "Domain experts" from the Operating Room (OR) and ED attended a comprehensive four-day training program offered by the vendor.

Initially, these expert nurses were to develop the nurses' notes documentation program. Through a process known as "knowledge engineering," selected domains of nursing were identified for the computer. A software program that includes words, phrases, report forms and the necessary logical thought processes required to develop nursing documentation was created by the domain expert nurses.

Nursing personnel were educated by nurses knowledgeable in the use of the system, in a computer-learning laboratory. Estimates indicate that the training of nurses in the use of the voice-recognition computer requires between one and three hours to obtain proficiency.

Developmental Phase

The automated speech-recognition technology underlying the nurses' notes program permits command and control of personal computer functions by voice with little use of the keyboard required. Users speak into a telephone handset and their words appear instantly on the computer screen. This system facilitates computer use, especially for people with little or no keyboard skills (Trofino, 1993a; 1993b).

An important component of this knowledge-engineered software program is the "trigger phrase." When such a phrase is spoken into the system, it "triggers" a much longer passage of text. Thus, in documenting an intra-operative nursing care plan for a patient who has been assessed as "anxious," the nurse only speaks the single word, "anxiety" and the following completed care plan appears on the computer screen:

Intra-operative Nursing Care Plan

Diagnosis and prescription: Anxiety and fear related to impending surgical intervention and lack of knowledge.

Design and plan: Patient will be able to verbalize concerns and ways of coping with them and therefore have the ability to cope with anxiety.

Production and management: Assess the patient's perception of the surgery and answer questions.

Explain pre-operative, intra-operative, and post-operative routines and activities. Listen to patient's concerns and reassure patient as necessary. (Trofino, 1993a, pp. 42-43)

This single-word trigger phase, "anxiety," triggers the system to produce a 75-word report. Additionally, the outcomes of this documentation method are far superior than traditional handwritten notes, because the printout is virtually flawless and ready to stand the survey test for clarity and completeness of documentation.

The trigger phrase system reflects the high degree of standardization in clinical reporting. Clearly, as health care providers continue to standardize care delivery through the use of critical paths, guidelines or protocols, software programs designed by the user to reflect standard care patterns will be most beneficial and time saving to the documentation process. Voice-recognition technology can permit the user to customize the report text to describe a particular patient.

The knowledge-engineering process that we employed in our study combined a trigger phrase with fill-ins and multiple-choice passages. For example, to generate a nursing assessment of the patient who presents with a laceration, the nurse says, "nursing assessment," then "laceration," and the following text appears on the screen (parenthesis indicates fill-in text):

Laceration: This patient presents a (#) (inch, centimeter, linear, superficial . . .) laceration on the (location). There is (no, controlled, uncontrolled . . .) bleeding at this time. This injury was caused by a (N) (animal bite, auto accident, fall, glass, knife . . .) (#) (minutes, hours, days) ago. (up to date, not current).

In order to fill in the blanks in the text and thereby customize the standardized text to a particular patient, the nurse says the following words:

two; centimeter; superficial, left third knuckle; no; fall; 30 minutes; not current.

This produces the following report, which accurately describes the nursing assessment for this particular patient.

LACERATION: This patient presents with a two-centimeter superficial laceration on the left third knuckle. There is no bleeding at this time. This injury was caused by a fall 30 minutes ago. The patient has not had a tetanus booster within the last five years.

Just 12 words were used to create a 44-word text that is accurate and in accordance with standard guidelines for nursing assessment of an individual patient.

A singular advantage to the use of a voice-recognition system is its malleability. The user may edit a document to reflect specific departmental guidelines for documentation. Additionally, the introduction of a nursing theory to describe care provided or planned can be easily assimilated into this system. Considering the vast array of changing documentation requirements, the ability to easily shape or change the software must be considered a strong asset of the system.

Should the need to create a document for a highly complex patient condition occur, the trigger-phrase system can be suspended temporarily, allowing the user to dictate text word by word, using the system's free-text mode. In this mode, the system has the flexibility of a tape dictation system, with the added advantage of immediate availability of the corrected and completed report (Trofino, 1993b).

Developmental Barriers

Cost may be considered a barrier when evaluating the usefulness of a voice recognition system for nursing documentation. The cost of the system, however, is roughly reflective of the annual cost of salary and benefits for a transcriptionist. Further, the system is available 24 hours a day, seven days a week. The cost may not be considered excessive when compared to other high-tech systems. Additionally, a general purpose system that is used by both physicians and nurses would also assist in producing increased cost-effectiveness.

Placement of computer equipment in the OR environment presented an initial barrier in this study. However, the computer, which is standard size, was successfully placed in the operating suite, permitting the circulating nurse to document care during the operative procedure or immediately upon its completion (Trofino, 1993a; 1993b).

Outcomes

Documentation time of operating room nurses using voice-activated computers has decreased over the past two years by 66%. Operative reports that originally took 15 to 18 minutes to complete manually have been reduced to a mere five minutes and are virtually flawless. Still unexplored is how this time savings can be translated into the increased use of the ORs, accommodating more patients on an average day without incurring nursing overtime costs.

Furthermore, during this study, a nursing knowledge base-development program was completed, three voice-reporting systems were installed, and domain experts were educated along with others in the operating and emergency departments.

Voice-report nursing documentation systems have been completed for orthopedic procedures performed in the emergency and operating departments. The staff at emergency triage has completed initial patient assessment data by the nurse, using voice-recognition software. Nursing domain experts in other areas like the Surgical Day Stay and Outpatient departments are also developing the documentation screens needed for their particular clinical units. The use of the original Voice Emergency Medicine System, along with the completed ED and OR nursing screens, greatly assist the new applications by providing an established nursing language/vocabulary. The domain experts from other specialties need only reorganize the vocabulary to respond to their own documentation requirements.

Future Visions

Voice-activated nursing documentation has been introduced in areas where high volume, standard reporting is required. As a managed health care system drives us towards increased standards of care, however, standard reporting will increase, reflecting critical paths, protocols or practice guidelines. Consequently, this system may prove as useful on general medical/surgical units and in critical care units.

Smaller, more compact equipment will emerge in the future. The use of a telephone line and a screen linked to a central mainframe will help to streamline present equipment clutter. The benefits identified over the past three years while using voice-activated nursing documentation include:

• Comprehensive nursing documentation with little nursing effort
• Decreased charting errors and omissions
• Increased compliance with regulatory standards, which are included in the software
• Consistent documentation practices
• Clear, concise legible documentation
• Increased interdisciplinary communication
• Considerable time savings for nurses
• A nurse-driven, malleable software program

•A first step towards the computer-based patient record of the future. (Trofino, 1993a, p. 42)

The introduction of a nursing documentation computer system is one of the most important decisions a nurse executive will make. Staff nurse involvement from the early stages of selection through full implementation can help ensure a smooth introduction and more complete acceptance of computer technology by nurses.

The usefulness of computer technology is becoming increasingly evident to staff nurses. However, their ability to play a key role in complete design and implementation of computer software is still a relatively new concept. This demonstration project is ample evidence of the outstanding achievements possible when empowered staff nurses are motivated towards greater goals, some still undeveloped.

By engaging the entire nursing staff, executives in health care organizations can release the energies of a giant cadre of new leaders who are knowledgeable of clinical practice demands and equally prepared to solve some of the most difficult problems.

In such an empowered environment, the nurse executive serves as facilitator, coach, guide, supporter, never as director or task master. By clearing the road of obstacles, " . . . those frightful things you see when you take your eyes off your goals" (*Motivational Quotes*, p. 16), nurse executives set the stage for staff nurses to rise to new levels of productivity, goal achievement, and professional and personal satisfaction.

Summary

The urgent need for methods and procedures that save time, are cost effective and have excellent outcomes will only increase in the future. Early evaluation of the usefulness of voice-activated nursing documentation seems to indicate a positive response in all three areas. Continued use and development by clinical nurses will finally demonstrate if we have created a simple useful method to conserve nurses' time, improve job satisfaction, produce close to perfect documents and ultimately enhance patient care. It seems likely that voice-recognition systems which provide the most natural means of communication between professional and machine will become the new technology frontier as we approach the 21st century.

References

Bakst, S. (1987). Voice recognition system: Are they ready to listen? *Office Systems, 4*(4), 70-71.

Belton, K., and Dick, R. (1991). Voice recognition technology: Key to the computer-based patient record. *Journal of Automated Medical Record Association, 62*(7), 27-32.

Bertolucci, J. (1990). Mike will replace mouse, Apple executive says. *Byte, 15*(4), 28.

General Accounting Office. (1991, January). *Medical ADP Systems: Automated Medical Records Hold Promise for Patient Care.* (GAO/IMTEC-91-5). Washington, DC: Author.

Kurzweil, R. (1989). Beyond pattern recognition. *Byte, 14*(13), 277-288.

Lange, H. R. (1991). The voice as computer interface: A look at tomorrow's technologies. *The Electronic Library, 9*(1), 7-11.

Motivational Quotes. (1984). Lombard, IL: Great Quotations, Inc.

Smarte, G. (1989). Sounds. *Byte, 14*(13), 246.

Trofino, J. (1993a). Voice-activated nursing documentation: On the cutting edge. *Nursing Management, 24*(7), 40-42.

Trofino, J. (1993b). Voice-recognition technology applied to nursing documentation. *The Journal of the Health Care Information and Management Systems Society, 7*(4), 41-45.

Automated Systems for Staffing, Scheduling and Resource Management

P. J. Maddox, EdD, RN, CNAA
Associate Professor
College of Nursing and Health Sciences
George Mason University
Fairfax, Virginia

Introduction

In the 1990s, both the health care industry and the roles and responsibilities of its managers and executives have changed significantly. By any measure, though, few professions have seen as dramatic a change in their role in recent years as have nurse managers. (Finkler and Kovner, 1993). While nurse managers have long been responsible for effectively managing clinical activities and objectives, today's nurse manager must effectively manage clinical care with fewer resources. Indeed, an increasing part of the professional role is to efficiently manage a variety of scarce resources. This expectation requires that both nurse managers and executives have well-developed managerial skills and organizational tools that support decisions concerning the use of organizational resources to control or reduce costs, along with expertise in their chosen profession. According to Finkler and Kovner (1993),

> . . . the financial aspects of the job of every nurse manager are growing and becoming more sophisticated each year. Nurses are expected to develop and justify budgets, to use appropriate computer technology and to minimize the cost of staff and supplies. (p. 3)

Within the last decade, the use of computers and the information they can generate to support managers and essential management functions has increased dramatically. Today's nurse manager must be familiar with and facile in the use of computerized data and information that supports management decision making and important functions, such as human resource management. Nurse managers and executives require unique data sets and a system of integrated information to facilitate their management work (Fralic, 1992). The quality of the decisions that they make is directly linked to the quality of the information available to them.

Computers may assist managers to prepare budgets, identify and analyze variances, create reports, forecast program conditions and manage productivity. In the area of effective and efficient human resource management, the use of computerized support for staffing, scheduling and productivity analysis is considered essential by many nurse executives and managers (Porter-O'Grady, 1987). In response to these issues, this chapter provides basic information about the acquisition, development and use of computerized nurse staffing and scheduling systems.

Computerized Systems

All components of staffing (obtaining, distributing and scheduling human resources) can be computerized. Any computerized staffing and scheduling system will include similar essential components. Because there is variance in the availability of computer technology to managers throughout health care organizations, an overview of the essential components of computerized staffing and scheduling systems follows.

Equipment and Software Components

Computerized information systems that support staffing and scheduling consist of computer equipment (hardware) and instructions (software). Software is specifically programmed to manipulate data in accordance with the institution's own practices and preferences.

Four types of hardware components are necessary for a computerized staffing and scheduling system. The first component, the computer itself, may be either a freestanding minicomputer (personal computer) or a mainframe computer. One of two general types of personal computers are most frequently used for this purpose: IBM or MacIntosh. The second type of system components are devices that allow users to enter data into the computer (keyboard, mouse, light pen, bar code-scanner). The third type of components are storage devices (discs and magnetic tapes). The fourth component consists of devices that allow users to retrieve information from the computer (display monitor and printer).

The software components of computerized staffing and scheduling systems consist of text processing instructions (word processing program); data base management instructions (data base program) and "number-crunching" instructions (spreadsheet and statistics programs).

Word processing programs support text management for document, form and report preparation. WordPerfect, Microsoft Word and WordStar are three widely used word processing programs.

Designed to replace manual accounting ledgers, spreadsheet programs are used to record and manipulate numerical data. They organize numbers in ledger format and perform calculations in accordance with mathematical instructions (formulae). Spreadsheets consist of cells that are made by intersecting rows and columns. Cells may contain text or numbers and may be programmed with mathematical instructions for automatically treating numerical data (e.g., summing the cells in one column). Excel, Quattro-Pro and Lotus 1-2-3 are widely used spreadsheet programs.

Statistical programs contain instructions for calculating recurrently used statistics such as frequencies, means, standard deviations, correlations, regression analyses and more. Statistical Package for the Social Sciences, SAS, and GB-Stat are widely used statistics programs. SmartForecastsII is a specialized program designed to support statistical analyses used in forecasting.

Data base programs support the organization and retrieval of large amounts of informational data. These programs consist of one or more files composed of records from data fields. Data bases support the manipulation and arrangement of all or selected data in an established sequence. Figure 1 illustrates a data base field. Paradox and dBase are two widely used data base programs.

The computer equipment described above is commonly used in business and health care organizations to support a wide variety of financial and management functions. While a contemporary health care facility is likely to possess basic computer equipment, additional equipment must usually be purchased and used exclusively to support the staffing and scheduling system. It is necessary to dedicate equipment solely for this use in order to manage time-intensive computer access for data inputting, to ensure data base security and to manage computer capacity effectively. (A detailed discussion of the technical and organizational specifications of computer components are contained later in this chapter). Staffing and scheduling systems may be custom developed using the software application programs described above or may be purchased from a vendor as a

Figure 1.
Database field example

Number	Field Name	Entry
1	NAME	
2	STR_ADDR	
3	CITY	
4	STATE	
5	ZIP_CODE	
6	PHONE	
7	SEX	
8	EMP_TYPE	
9	LICENSED	
10	LICENSE_NO	
11	LIC_REN_NO	
12	LIC_DATE	
13	EXP_DATE	
14	LIA_INS	
15	INS_AMOUNT	
16	PRIM_AREA	
17	UNIT_ASSG	
18	PRIM_SHIFT	

predesigned system. A detailed discussion of many issues and requirements that support a facility's decision to develop or purchase a staffing and scheduling system is also found later in this chapter.

Staffing Functions and Processes

Certain basic functions and processes are managed by individuals (or in the case of automation, by computers) when any staffing and scheduling are done. Staffing consists of three functional components: Personnel planning, shift scheduling and staff reallocating (Bergmann and Johnson, 1988; Budd and Proptnik, 1989). Figure 2 illustrates these functions.

The first component, personnel planning, requires the use of detailed personnel data. Information in the personnel data base includes staff position, professional qualifications, special experience, training, unit assigned and scheduling preferences of each staff person. This information is expanded to include planned absences (e.g., vacation and sick leave), planned training and current staff schedule requests at the time that schedule planning is underway. In addition to personnel-related data, data concerning planned and current unit manpower needs are also used.

The second component, shift scheduling, requires matching information about unit shift workload and staffing requirements with information about staff available on a week-to-week, day-to-day basis. Taking into consideration unit manpower needs and individual preferences and capabilities in accordance with institutional scheduling policies, a preliminary schedule can be derived. This is a complex function, given the importance of ensuring that the needs of both are met and that the right staff are assigned at the right time to provide anticipated patient care. Spreadsheet and statistical programs are used to generate the preliminary staffing plans and unit schedules that are explained above.

The third component involves changing unit staff allocations to respond to current unit staffing needs. This may involve allocating more or less staff or changing staff sched-

Figure 2.
Staffing and scheduling functions

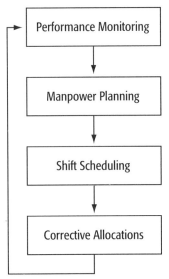

ules because of staff skill mix changes, or to respond to unplanned changes in staff availability (e.g., sick leave).

Whether a manual method or a computerized system is used, the functional components of decision making for effective staffing and scheduling remain the same. Considerable complexity is involved in managing the interaction and sequential decisions made by each functional component. When computerized, the first two components involve programming to support preplanning or projecting staff, based on assumptions or predictions about unit manpower requirements. Planned projections are generated in accordance with the institution's personnel policies and professional standards governing staff assignments and scheduling. The third functional component must use real-time information about unit needs and staff availability. It calls for changing or ratifying the projected schedule to match available staff with current unit staffing requirements.

Hospital personnel policies and nursing standards contribute to the complexity of system decisions. Thus, the degree of flexibility in managing staff preferences, planning timetables, supervisor prerogatives in schedule changes and cost/quality decisions are all affected and must be appropriately managed to meet organizational expectations and achieve acceptance (Behner et al., 1990). It is imperative that institutions have established written policies that govern personnel assignments for productive and nonproductive purposes, scheduling prerogatives and goals, and staffing standards (including the skill mix of personnel). If these do not exist prior to implementing a computerized system, such policies will need to be developed to support the programming of decision parameters that support the staffing function. These parameters are institutionally driven and unique.

Data Access and Reports
Following the entering of required/necessary data and the development of planning schedules, the schedule must be reviewed and accepted on a preliminary basis. This may be done via a computer display monitor or via printed paper copy made available to the individual responsible for unit scheduling. Given the institution's preference, the first re-

view may be delegated to an administrative support person before being approved by nursing supervisory staff. In any case, an institution must determine who receives this document (and all documents), and when. Later in the scheduling cycle, schedules will be modified and approved for final unit posting. If managers are expected to work from printed copies of schedules and other computer outputs (as opposed to the display monitor), the institution must assign responsibility for and manage the distribution of such documents. Document and report printing and distribution can be both time consuming and costly. Most institutions will elect to work from a printed paper system, given that the alternative requires ready access to the system's computer terminal(s) and display monitor(s). Access to the staffing and scheduling computer may also be achieved via local area network access (a basic system configuration issue).

The report capabilities of staffing and scheduling systems are limited only by the data available. The organizing of data into meaningful reports is a particularly important decision. Data must be presented and manipulated in such a way as to be useful and understandable. Proprietary systems will usually offer a series of standardized reports and documents as part of the basic package. Customized reports may also be programmed. If the staffing and scheduling system is custom developed, special and recurring documents and reports must be a part of the system's programming. Keep in mind that data (no matter how good) is only useful to the institution and its managers if it is accessible. Also, keep in mind that these systems will have more data and report capabilities than any institution can readily use and store. In addition to unit schedules, the following types of documents are often selected for regular management reports:

• productivity reports
• summary of hours worked and paid (broken down by type of productive and nonproductive hours)
• overtime hours (by unit, position)
• personnel budget variance analysis
• licensure and certification expirations
• workload and utilization tracking (historical).

A myriad of special request reports may be programmed and made available on an as-needed basis. Who has access to request and receive reports is an important institutional decision issue. Another related issue is the institution's decisions concerning access to the data base and reports as it affects system security and confidentiality.

Custom-Developed and Proprietary Systems

The decision to acquire a computerized staffing and scheduling system brings with it an important organizational decision: whether to develop a custom system or to purchase an established staffing and scheduling system. An established system is most likely to be proprietary and available by purchase agreement through a vendor. Typically, the purchase agreement is a license to use software for a specific period of time. The software is not owned by the hospital. The decision of whether to purchase a proprietary system or develop one's own should be based on extensive, disciplined organizational research and an analysis of organizational need, resources and expected costs and benefits. If a nursing organization has access to adequate technical expertise and computer hardware and software, a system to support staffing and/or scheduling can be developed. Essential software requirements include an electronic data base application and a spreadsheet application (discussed earlier in this chapter), as well as dedicated hardware. At a minimum, such an effort requires expertise in application programming and large data base management. This usually requires the expertise of computer programmers and system analysts, as well as one or more staffing management expert(s). Following system development and implementation, there will be ongoing support needs for system troubleshooting, updating and maintenance which will also require skilled system support staff.

The alternative to developing an in-house system is to purchase a proprietary system to support staffing and scheduling. A number of proprietary systems are available today. ANSOS and RESQUE are two commercially available systems in wide use. All systems use a set of preprogrammed functions, along with the hospital's own standards and processes, to perform essential staffing and scheduling operations. Vendors of such systems usually offer consultative services to assist in implementing their systems (from installation, to user training, to trouble shooting, and maintenance). While using a proprietary system reduces the hospital's need for a skilled programming staff, it does not lessen the hospital's obligation to provide policies and standards that govern staffing and scheduling. Nor does it obviate the need for staff to support the day-to-day operations and management of the system.

Trade-offs exist, of course, between developing a customized system and acquiring a proprietary one. Advantages of custom-designed systems include the ability to design a system to meet all organizational requirements and specifications. Additionally, the custom-developed system may be readily updated to accommodate organizational changes. The advantages of acquiring a proprietary system may include better user acceptance and faster turnaround time for implementation.

The remaining part of this chapter provides an overview of the complexities and issues associated with successfully acquiring, installing and using computerized staffing and scheduling systems.

Organizational Need

When it has been determined that the effectiveness and efficiency of the nursing service might be facilitated by a computerized staffing and scheduling system, the organization should engage in a disciplined needs-analysis process. A needs-analysis typically serves three purposes: First, it identifies the nursing organization's goals and management expectations for use of the system; second, it may serve as the basis upon which the institution evaluates the need and thus allocates financial support; and third, specifications may assist the organization in selecting hardware and software and/or consultant vendor services.

The needs-analysis begins with the establishment of clear and realistic organizational expectations for a computerized staffing and scheduling system. The information derived from this process will be useful to the organization for several purposes. It begins the system specification process that will lead to the development of the request for proposal (RFP) from vendors or will identify the expectations of a custom-designed system. Essential content of the needs-analysis will include all technical and performance requirements and organizational specifications, including system application, scope and purpose, installation and use requirements, training and user support requirements and evaluation criteria. (Content that is required for the RFP is discussed later in this chapter.)

An important fact to remember is that computer systems do not perform management functions; they are a management performance tool. Therefore, it is essential to involve working nurse managers in the needs-analysis. Included in the analysis should be existing and projected information, and report requirements of nursing service managers and executives. Other important information that assists in determining the requirements of the system is the identification of processes and procedures used in current nurse staffing and scheduling activities (e.g., description of personnel, personnel data base content and record management, staffing procedures and unit/department scheduling policies). Organizational characteristics determine system capacity requirements and programming complexity. At a minimum, the following organizational information should be identified: The number and type of work units; number, type and description of personnel; and, unit scheduling parameters. Special requirements such as data security, backup systems and data archiving requirements should also be identified.

The needs-analysis also includes the expected costs and benefits to the organization for acquiring, installing, maintaining and using the system. For instance, any anticipated savings or costs associated with personnel should be projected. Worth noting is the fact that many institutions have undertaken computerization anticipating personnel reduction savings that are not realized. Computerization does not usually eliminate the need for staff (clerical or managerial). Depending upon how the institution handles staffing and scheduling manually, as well as the computer system's characteristics and operational support requirements, additional staff (such as clerical staff with data-entry skills) are often required. In terms of managerial impact, many organizations are quick to assume that computerization of staffing and scheduling functions will save managers considerable time. While time planning and constructing schedules may be reduced, new demands on the working manager's time usually surface. For instance, a refocusing or shifting of managerial work often occurs from schedule drafting to schedule approval and schedule change management. Because staff data, schedule requests and unit staffing requirements are continually changing, nurse managers will find themselves spending time managing data (e.g., updating personnel data and unit scheduling parameters). One potential benefit is in the area of productivity management.

Computerized systems usually offer real-time analysis of data for managers to use in making day-to-day staffing decisions. Such information may be very useful in improving the efficiency of personnel staffing decisions on a shift-by-shift basis, thereby reducing personnel costs. Additionally, working managers and executives also report that regular and special reports facilitate budget variance analysis and budget planning. Managers and executives often report improvement in record keeping for meeting accreditation requirements and special data retrieval projects. Such benefits usually accrue from increased timeliness, accuracy, completeness, accessibility and standardization of staffing and scheduling data and reports.

Regardless of the expected benefits, there will be costs associated with system development, acquisition and management. Potential projected costs include the cost of system acquisition and installation, as well as new system support costs. It is particularly important to evaluate projected costs against the organizational value of projected benefits.

System Specifications and the Request for Proposal

If an organization decides to acquire a proprietary computerized staffing and scheduling system, the organizational needs-analysis is used not only to justify the purchase of the system, but to generate the system specifications and organizational expectations of a system. This is useful information and essential content for the RFP that will be developed. The RFP serves to organize the institution's system requirements for purposes of conveying this information to prospective vendors. It is also useful to the organization in making preliminary and final vendor selections. The technical, functional, and financial specifications recommended for inclusion in the RFP are as follows:

•A comprehensive description of the system application requirements. This includes: the number and types of users, system functions and organization; data, file and report requirements; and system security requirements. Product upgrade acquisition expectations

and new product availability should also be specified.
- System reliability and backup requirements. This includes electronic medium for data archiving, battery backup for power failures and the need for a redundant capability to support functions in case of failure.
- Service requirements (during and after warranty). Beyond repairs and maintenance, this also includes implementation consultation, training and support.
- Hardware and software features and requirements, such as disk capacity, number and capabilities of printers, and number of working data entry terminals. Number and types of documentation documents. Requirements for site preparation to support installation (e.g., cable installation and temperature or humidity controls should also be specified).
- Evaluation criteria
- Vendor site visit and system demonstration requirements
- Implementation schedule
- General price constraints
- Instructions for preparing and submitting proposals (including format, submission deadlines and contact person(s)
- Information about the vendor. This includes staff capabilities, company size, similar completed projects, financial statements, and a list of clients and references (Hicks, 1984).

System Selection

The final selection should be based upon an organization's assessment of the vendors' product, abilities and performance track record. Will they be able to meet the organization's technical requirements? Are they likely to provide service after implementation that is timely and in accordance with the organization's specifications? Keep in mind that most computer systems have a life span of between five and ten years. Business relationships with the vendors are likely to be at least this long. Sales promises and marketing materials and claims are not an adequate basis for vendor evaluation. Neither should price alone determine your selection. A thorough review of the vendor's personnel, capabilities and the track record of their product(s) and performance with similar installations are important evaluation considerations. Information from visits to existing vendor installations (site visits) and thorough reference checks are also important considerations.

Successful System Implementation

Successful implementation of a computerized staffing and scheduling system requires extensive organizational commitment and comprehensive planning. Figure 3 illustrates the process from planning through evaluation. Preparation and involvement of staff at all levels and in all phases of the project will be critical to system acceptance and use (Drazen, 1983). The following organizational recommendations are made:
- Ensure that organizational expectations of the system are up-front and realistic for staff nurses, support staff and managers. Keep in mind that computers do not compensate for organizational limitations such as poor management practices or inadequate administrative support staff.
- Do not implement a computerized system with expectations to reduce manpower. Usually, the same number of staff will be required, with a change in their skills and responsibilities. In some cases, additional support staff may be required to support system operations.
- Executive management must be enthusiastic and committed to the computerized system

Figure 3.
System justification, design and implementation process

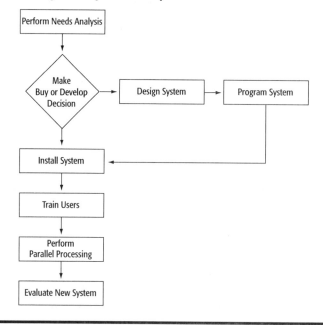

and visibly supportive of staff efforts at all levels throughout this organizational change. This means support in the form of space, time and financial resources for training, as well as support for responsibility and performance changes.
•Actively involve nurse managers and support staff from the beginning of the project through evaluation. This includes participation in the needs-analysis, work and functions analysis, identification of learning needs, system design, implementation planning and evaluation.
•Select for regular, recurring distribution only those reports that are relevant to personnel receiving them. Do not print and distribute every report available from the system. Make other reports available on an as-requested-basis.

Training

While there are many recommendations to ensure the successful implementation of a computerized staffing and scheduling system, none is more important than education and training. Two types of training are recommended: system overview training and detailed user training.

System overview training is necessary to prepare nursing staff throughout the organization for what is expected in supporting the system and to explain how it will be used. It is important to include an explanation of any changes in data management, scheduling flexibility and procedures (including deadlines for requests and timetables for publishing draft and final schedules). This type of training is primarily informational and can be conducted in large groups.

Detailed user training, on the other hand, should be conducted in small groups composed of similar staff, to teach skills by application function (e.g., managers and administrative and support staff). It is essential that skill training employ a "hands-on" practice approach with the specific applications that individuals will be using. Training content should be customized for each user group, as well. Basically, it should include system terminology and overview, hardware operation, explanation of user responsibilities, demonstration of user-specific functions, explanation of policies, procedures and documentation for using the system and for executing staffing and scheduling functions, explanation and use of the backup system, explanation of printouts and reports available and instructions for system troubleshooting and/or problem reporting. Adequate time for detailed user training (8 to 24 hours) needs to be allowed. Also, sessions should be spread out to prevent overload (e.g., four 2-hour sessions over a one-week period).

All training should be completed prior to system implementation. Arrangements must also be made for training new staff after implementation. Typically, vendors will provide initial system training as a part of the installation of the proprietary system. Thereafter, or in cases where systems are developed on-site, organizations must decide whether to handle system orientation and skill development using "in-house" resources or by other mechanisms such as consultants or outside training programs.

System Testing and Evaluation

Following the system's initial installation, the next step is to make the system operational. If the computerized system is replacing a manual system, it is recommended that a period of parallel operations be conducted. This requires a one-to-three-month use of the computer system in tandem with the manual system. Use of parallel systems is costly and frustrating for staff, given that workloads increase and productivity is temporarily decreased due to duplication of work efforts. The effort is worthwhile, however, in that it ensures the new system's reliability and builds personnel skill and confidence in using the new system. Especially, this includes confidence in problem-solving in using the system and user difficulties without adversely affecting essential operations. Once the period of testing is successfully completed, use of the manual system can be terminated.

Following full implementation of the system and after a reasonable period of use, the new system should be evaluated. The development or acquisition and implementation of the system will have required a detailed planning process. At this point, it is important to ascertain whether the new system is meeting the original goals and objectives identified in the needs analysis. Is the system performing according to specifications? Additionally, user impact and use should be evaluated. Are staff using the system to its full, intended capacity? Are there any work flow problems? Are procedures working well? Are there any significant user issues (acceptance, skill performance)? Are all features being used? Are reports meaningful to those receiving them? Significant adverse findings should be changed or problem-solved at this time to optimize user cooperation and system performance in the long run.

Summary

The purpose of this chapter was to provide an overview of the requirements for developing and working with computerized staffing and scheduling systems. Recommendations for optimizing implementation and successful use were presented. Implementation of a computerized staffing and scheduling system involves considerable organizational effort and expense. Extensive planning for system design and implementation is required to achieve an organization's expectations. Such a system will have a significant effect on the work and expectations of clerical, managerial and clinical staff alike. Highly visible top management support, staff involvement, extensive training and open communication will be important to achieving successful implementation. The benefits of computerized systems are realized only when systems are used to their full intended purpose. The ability to collect and retrieve accurate and uniform data is particularly advantageous for accreditation requirements. And lastly, computerization is not a substitute for managerial competence or decision making. What an organization does with the data it collects ultimately determines the benefit of the system to that institution.

References

Behner, K. G., Fogg, L. F., Fournier, L. C., Frankenbach, J. T., Robertson, S. B., et al. (1990). Nursing resource management: Analyzing the relationship between costs and quality in staffing decisions. Health Care Management Review, 15(4), 63-71.

Bergmann, C., and Johnson, J. (1988). Managing staffing with a personal computer, Part I. Nursing Management, 19(4), 28-32.

Budd, M. C., and Proptnik, T. (1989). A computerized system for staffing, billing and productivity measurement. Journal of Nursing Administration, 19(7), 17-22.

Drazen, E. L. (1983). Planning for purchase and implementation of an automated hospital information system: A nursing perspective. Journal of Nursing Administration, 13(9), 9-12.

Finkler, S. A., and Kovner, K. T. (1993). Financial Management for Nurse Managers and Executives. Philadelphia: W. B. Saunders Co.

Fralic, M. A. (1992). Into the future: Nurse executives and the world of information technology. Journal of Nursing Administration, 22(4), 11-12.

Hicks, J. O. (1984). Management Information Systems: A User Perspective. New York: West Publishing Co.

Porter-O'Grady, T. (1987). New age information: Beginning with a Data Base. In Nursing Finance: Budgeting Strategies for a New Age (pp. 17-36). Rockville, MD: Aspen Systems Corp.

Professional Perspectives on Information Issues

Ethical Issues in the Management of Patient Data: Maintaining
Confidentiality in a Reformed Health Care System 257
Confidentiality: Computer Security and Data Protection 264
The Role of the Professional Association in Policy Development
Related to Information Standards 272
Standards of Practice and Preparation for Certification 280
Nursing Informatics: Education for a New Specialty and
Career 288
Research Focus Areas in Informatics 295
A Global Perspective on the Future of Informatics 303

Ethical Issues in the Management of Patient Data: Maintaining Confidentiality in a Reformed Health Care System

Sara T. Fry, PhD, RN, FAAN
Henry R. Luce Professor of Nursing Ethics
Boston College
Boston, Massachusetts

Gail Ann DeLuca Havens, MS, RN, CNA
Doctoral Candidate, Nursing Ethics
School of Nursing
University of Maryland at Baltimore

Introduction

The professional obligation to protect the privacy of health care patients has a long tradition (Veatch, 1981). Most professional codes of ethics refer to a duty to protect patient privacy by keeping patient information confidential. These codes limit exceptions to this obligation to the requirements of law and the protection of innocent third parties (Beauchamp and Childress, 1989). Privacy, defined as a state or condition of inaccessibility to others, is highly valued by our society (Allen, 1988). Individuals expect that their person, his or her property, and information about them will be inaccessible to others unless they authorize access to specific others and for particular reasons. This is especially true in such special relationships as the health care provider/patient relationship.

Unfortunately, today, the traditional professional obligation to maintain patient confidentiality is in danger of erosion by increasingly sophisticated methods of health care data collection, vast networks of electronic data exchange, and new proposals to further computerize patients' health care records (Flaherty, 1989; Westin, 1976). Indeed, when one considers the number of people who can gain legitimate access to computerized health care records as they currently exist, one sees that the potential loss of personal privacy through use of information exchange systems assumed in health care reform proposals is a tremendous threat to all citizens. With the potential for the loss of patient privacy, there is also a potential for loss of the ethical integrity of the health care provider-patient relationship. Proposed health care reforms, however, make it difficult, if not impossible, for health care providers to keep patient information confidential. Confidentiality, defined as the ethical obligation to keep someone's personal and private information secret from the knowledge of others is the cornerstone of the trust relationship between health care provider and patient. As others point out, effectively responding to potential privacy losses in new health care information exchange systems throughout the world may well be one of the most difficult ethical challenges to be faced in the 21st century (Alpert, 1993).

Given these concerns, this chapter responds to the following questions and issues:
- Why is loss of patient privacy a serious moral issue in health care?
- How do new proposals for exchange of health care data threaten the ethical integrity of the health care provider-patient relationship?
- What are the specific ethical challenges to the maintenance of professional confiden-

tiality posed by health care reform proposals?

• What should be the nursing profession's ethical agenda when potential loss of patient privacy through health care reform measures an issue?

The Importance of Personal Privacy and its Protection

The privacy of the individual can be defined in many ways (Schoeman, 1984). Most scholars, however, agree that the concept of privacy is highly valued by society and should be protected by law as a property right or a personal right. In other words, all citizens should be able to expect their mental processes, psyche, possessions and property, physical body, and personhood to be legally protected from unwanted surveillance by others. To state that a person has or enjoys privacy is to state that a person's body, mind, personality and property are inaccessible to others. We value privacy because it is the state and/or condition within which relationships of trust, friendship, love, and mutual respect occur (Fried, 1968). Since any threat to privacy has the potential to threaten a person's ability to maintain the integrity of significant relationships that help define that person's individuality, society has devised means to protect personal privacy.

In the United States, the value of privacy and the need for its protection have centered on developments in constitutional, statutory, and case law. The need for privacy protection has centered on legal judgments concerning abortion (*Roe v. Wade,* 1973), contraceptive use by married couples (*Griswold v. State of Connecticut,* 1965), removal of life-sustaining technologies (*In re* Quinlan, 1976), and the sterilization of incompetent persons (*In re* Grady, 1981). Viewpoints about the use of medical records in health research, screening for genetic disease, and the use of computerized personal information for epidemiological research, all assume that protecting privacy is of utmost importance in society (Gordis and Gold, 1980; Riskin and Reilly, 1977; Watson, 1981).

Given the important role that privacy plays in our society, it is no surprise that protecting privacy in health care relationships is of concern to both health care providers and patients. Privacy is necessary to the development of trust and mutual respect between a patient and his/her health care provider. Because privacy is important, health care providers have a moral obligation to hold in confidence what they know about a patient and what the patient has revealed to them. For example, the American Nurses Association's *Code for Nurses* states, "The nurse safeguards the client's right to privacy by judiciously protecting information of a confidential nature" (American Nurses Association [ANA], 1985, p. 4). In the *Code for Nurses,* the patient's right to privacy is considered an inalienable right, and the nurse is obliged to safeguard confidential information about a patient learned from any source. Likewise, the American Medical Association's *Principles of Medical Ethics* state, "A physician . . . shall safeguard patient confidences within the constraints of the law" (American Medical Association, 1992, p. 10). Thus, physicians are obliged to maintain confidentiality of patient information in the same manner as nurses.

The reasons for these expectations of confidentiality from nurses and physicians vary. First, maintaining confidentiality enables individuals to seek help without fear of public knowledge. If patients can expect that all information known about them will be held in confidence by the health care provider, then they will be more willing to fully disclose their health problems. Fuller disclosure enhances treatment resulting in more effective and efficient health care. In this sense, confidentiality has utilitarian value—it advances the overall goal of health care and benefits the well-being of patients. By helping to maintain trust between patients and health care providers, confidentiality performs an important social function.

Second, maintaining confidentiality enhances a patient's right to make health care choices free from the influence of others. When information about patients is held in confidence, patients retain the moral authority to determine what will and will not be known about them by others. Patients determine *who* will know information about them, and *what* information will be known and under which circumstances. Maintaining confidentiality thus supports the notion that privacy is essential to an individual's sense of identity and well-being in the same way that self-determination is essential to personal identity and individual well-being (Benn, 1971).

Is it reasonable for patients to expect that *all* information about them will be held in confidence by health care providers? Not always. There may be instances when confidentiality should be broken to protect other interests of the patient or even the welfare of other parties (Beauchamp and Childress, 1989). In addition, there may also be instances where confidentiality should be broken to meet the requirements of law. Overriding obligations of confidentiality for these reasons may understandably create a considerable ethical conflict for the health care provider.

This is an additional reason why privacy loss is a serious moral issue in health care. Health care providers need to be clear about their ethical obligations to ensure that they do not promise society, as well as individual patients, more than they can deliver when protecting the confidentiality of patient information. Patient expectations about confidentiality and professional obligations to maintain confidentiality need to be carefully reevaluated as health care reform proposals are assessed. This is necessary to determine precisely what patient information health care providers will be required to release and what privacy protection patients can reasonably expect from the health care system.

Health Care Information Management and the Ethical Integrity of the Health Care Provider/Patient Relationship

Individuals come to the health care system because they need immediate health care; to obtain that care, they give information to the health care provider. The ability of the health care provider to provide individualized care to the patient is always dependent, to a large extent, on the accuracy and amount of information that the patient volunteers to the provider. This information is gathered through a health history, physical examinations, and laboratory tests and procedures. If the patient is reluctant to provide information, or withholds permission to gather essential information through tests and procedures, the health care provider's ability to treat or provide care adequately is seriously hampered. Without full knowledge of the patient's condition, the health care provider cannot do his/her job effectively and efficiently. Health care providers cannot provide the "best of care," the patient's health may deteriorate or not improve, and treatment and/or care that is not designed for the right reasons might cost more in the long run.

Obtaining full information about the patient through history, tests, and procedures is the key to providing the most expert and cost-effective health care possible. But here is the ethical dilemma: Patients are reluctant to provide information *unless* they can be assured that this information will be held in confidence. Health care providers, on the other hand, usually cannot guarantee that patient information can be held in confidence because currently there exists little legal protection of health care record information. Patients have expectations that information about them will be held in confidence, and health care providers are assumed to have obligations to keep patient information confidential (by professional codes of ethics), but few mechanisms are in place to meet these expectations or support presumed professional obligations where confidentiality of health record information is concerned (Alpert, 1993).

In the United States, only a few states have adopted laws to protect health care records, so this ethical issue looms very large. While some states have laws to protect highly sensitive information (AIDS test results and/or mental health records), only a few states (California, Washington, and Montana) have actually enacted laws that define access to health records, in general (Alpert, 1993). Most state regulations regarding health care records concern health care insurance transactions or promote information exchange for insurance purposes rather than protecting patient privacy. Federal law protects confidentiality of health care record information only in relation to substance abuse and for those records under custody of the federal government (Alpert, 1993). While the unauthorized sharing of health care record information is considered unethical throughout our society, in the majority of states, it is not illegal. Furthermore, there is no widely accepted standard across all states for disclosure of health record information.

With the growing potential to store health care information in multiplying electronic media, this lack of disclosure standards takes on alarming dimensions. In the past, loss of patient privacy through breaches of confidentiality could be relatively confined because the majority of information was paper bound and stored in such a manner that access to the information was controlled. Now, however, electronic data interchange and networks of health record information systems provide easier, quicker access to personal information and make it harder to detect when unauthorized access has been gained. True, most information storage systems employ security measures to protect individual privacy and to hamper unauthorized access to the information. These measures, however, are not uniformly applied, and, in fact, there is little agreement on who should have legitimate access to health care information and for what specific reasons.

The lack of controls and standards, and the lack of consistent protection by law, are serious threats to the integrity of the health care provider/patient relationship. Surely, the failure to maintain the integrity of the relationship today may influence the cost effectiveness of health care delivery in the future. These concerns are doubly important when one considers proposals for health care reform that rely on computer technology and highly advanced information processing systems to speed health care information exchange and billing for services ("New Medicare claims," 1994).

Ethical Challenges of Health Care Reform

The two most difficult ethical challenges in health care reform are: (1) the protection of patient privacy, and (2) the protection of confidentiality in the patient/health provider relationship. These challenges are created by several assumptions about the use of computer-based patient records (CPR) in health care reform implementations and the feasibility of new technologies for electronic storage of health data. For example, most health care reform proposals call for the use of electronic cards—a card similar to an Automated Teller Machine card or a "smart card" that functions as a microcomputer ("Smart card technology," 1988). The cards will be carried by the individual patient and will allow provider access to information about the patient, his health care insurance, and (in the case of the "smart card") health record information stored on up to as many as several hundred pages. The danger of this technology is that a great deal of private, non-medical-use information about the patient and his family is also available in the health care record and can be accessed by unauthorized persons through use of the electronic cards (Alpert, 1993). The information gained can be used to make decisions about an individual and family members that go far beyond their health needs. Further, the fact that this information has been accessed by unauthorized persons may not be known by these patients for many years afterwards. The ethical implications of using electronic cards to store personal health care information are quite clear.

The control of third-party access to health care records is an additional concern in the coming health care reform. To improve efficiency of health insurance operations, as well as to know more about employees' health status, employers undoubtedly will be tempted to computerize health care records and to ask employees to authorize release of this information, without specifying the uses and limitations of the information gained. In turn, employees may find it difficult to challenge employers' efforts to computerize their employee health records for fear of losing employment. Since studies confirm that many companies use health record data to make employment-related decisions, there is good reason to be concerned about the ethical intentions of employers who request release authorization for the use of the stored data (Linowes, 1989).

Patients' health records can also be accessed through electronic information storage without their knowledge for entirely non-medical uses. Prescription information in the patient's health care record may be accessed by data collectors and then sold to pharmaceutical companies, a practice with little state and no federal regulations. For instance, when a person applies for life insurance, the Medical Information Bureau, a New England non-profit association formed for the purpose of preventing insurance fraud, stores information about this person that will eventually be shared with all member insurance organizations (Alpert, 1993). It frequently stores and shares information about one's health record, lifestyle, and driving record, although most of this has been gathered without the individual's knowledge and has never been verified by any legitimate source.

An Ethical Agenda for the Nursing Profession

The members of the nursing profession have a responsibility to work with elected representatives and with all other health care providers to: (1) understand the value structures of health care reform proposals, (2) reach consensus on a standard of care that can be supported by procedures to store health record data, and (3) promote protection of stored data by strict federal regulations.

Values of Health Care Reform

Different values inform the various health care reform proposals currently being discussed. Some proposals favor traditional values such as individual choice and assert that health care is basically a private enterprise. Other proposals favor the value of equity and emphasize the social dimensions of providing health care and the need for equal access to health care. The different values supported by these proposals are all good values in that they promote morally worthy goals. As a society we value the collective good, public support for health care, and equal access for all, while at the same time we value individual choice, and the protection of decisional privacy and information about our health.

Will it be possible to preserve these values to the same degree or provide an efficient and cost-effective health care reform system without foregoing the importance of other values? Probably not. The real challenge is to design a reformed health care medical record system that will protect and even enhance our most important health values while *not* ignoring other values important to human dignity and the right to privacy. In this computer era, members of the nursing profession need to support values consistent with our obligations to protect patient privacy and to put forward every effort to maintain confidentiality of patient information.

Consensus on a Standard of Care

To maintain and protect important values, all health care providers need to reach consensus on a *standard of care*. Unfortunately, current discussions about the implementation of various health care reform proposals threaten to eclipse this very important patient need.

Before any proposals are implemented, their likely outcomes and the implications for both patients and health care providers need to be known. Furthermore, the standard of care these proposals will be measured against needs to be made explicit. Before we can agree on a standard of care, the various care standards already being maintained by current health care plans need to be discussed and subjected to ethical analysis. In short, before additional proposals are placed before us, we need *more* information about the present status of health care in this country and the various health care delivery systems through which care is provided. To look at even one more proposal without this information is unwise. To discuss how to implement any proposal or insurance billing mechanism without a standard of care to serve as an ethical Rosetta Stone is foolhardy. We are on the threshold of making important changes in this country's health care system, but are in danger of doing so without necessary consensus on the values to be protected and agreement on a standard of care that can reasonably protect these values.

Nursing's Agenda for Health Care Reform (ANA, 1992) outlines a standard of care supporting many of the values important to the health consumer. This document provides a value structure supported by the *Code for Nurses* (ANA, 1985), and *Nursing: A Social Policy Statement* (ANA, 1980), and follows respected traditions of nursing care. Further, it provides the values base for designing measures that will be used to assess the outcomes and cost effectiveness of health care. Most importantly, this document provides the standard of care that must be central to storage and sharing of patient record information. This agenda needs to be seriously considered by those designing health care reform proposals and implementation of the CPR. Nurses and other health care providers will bear personal responsibility for the moral quality of the reformed health care delivery system once it is available to the public. The nursing profession's standard of care needs to be constantly brought before the legislators working on health care reform proposals.

Federal Regulations for Health Record Storage and Use

Protecting patient privacy while providing essential health care is absolutely necessary. New federal regulations are needed for the collection, use, storage, access to, and disclosure authorizations of the CPR and electronic data storage innovations of health care reform. The nursing profession should encourage legislation that protects patient privacy and delineates expectations of health worker confidentiality. Patients need to be informed of their rights to their health record information and their right to be notified of its use. Likewise, regulations should carefully define what constitutes legitimate access to this information by whom and for what purposes. Most importantly, it is also necessary to define what constitutes improper access and illegitimate use of data, and how the use of the CPR and electronic data storage of health information will be monitored.

Finally, the enforcement of regulations to protect the values standards of health care needs to be embedded with specific civil and criminal penalties. In addition, the legitimate means for patients to collect damages when unauthorized use of their health information occurs needs to be established. With its expertise and political clout, the nursing profession can work to ensure that measures to protect patient privacy and confidentiality of the health care provider-patient relationship will be implemented in health care reform. Through its support of these ethical measures, the nursing profession will have fulfilled an important professional responsibility to the public.

Summary

Loss of patient privacy is a serious moral issue in health care. New proposals for exchange of health data threaten the ethical integrity of the provider-patient relationship. Health care reform proposals also present ethical challenges to the traditional bond of confidentiality between patient and provider. The nursing profession can have a significant role in helping to establish consensus on the values that should be protected in health care and on a standard of care that can reasonably protect these values.

References

Allen, A. L. (1988). *Uneasy Access: Privacy for Women in a Free Society.* Totowa, NJ: Rowman & Littlefield.

Alpert, S. (1993). Smart cards, smarter policy: Medical records, privacy, and health care reform. *Hastings Center Report, 23*(6), 13-24.

American Medical Association (1992). *Current Opinions of the Judicial Council of the American Medical Association, Including the Principles of Medical Ethics and Rules of the Judicial Council.* Chicago: Author.

American Nurses Association (1980). *Nursing: A Social Policy Statement.* Kansas City, MO: Author.

American Nurses Association (1985). *Code for Nurses with Interpretive Statements.* Kansas City, MO: Author.

American Nurses Association (1992). *Nursing's Agenda for Health Care Reform.* Kansas City, MO: Author.

Beauchamp, T. L., and Childress, J. F. (1989). *Principles of Biomedical Ethics.* New York: Oxford University Press.

Benn, S. I. (1971). Privacy, freedom and respect for persons. In J. R. Pennock, and J. W. Chapman (Eds.), *Nomos XIII: Privacy* (pp. 56-70). New York: Atherton Press.

Flaherty, D. H. (1989). *Protecting Privacy in Surveillance Societies.* Chapel Hill, NC: University of North Carolina Press.

Fried, C. (1968). Privacy. *Yale Law Journal, 77,* 475-493.

Gordis, L., and Gold, E. (1980). Privacy, confidentiality, and the use of medical records in research. *Science, 207,* 153-156

In re Grady, 426 A.2d 467 (N.J. Sup. Ct. 1981).

Griswald v. State of Connecticut, 381 U.S. 479 (1965).

Linowes, D. F. (1989). *Privacy in America.* Urbana, IL: University of Illinois Press.

New Medicare claims system to speed billing, slash red tape. (1994, January 20). *The Baltimore Sun,* p. 7A.

In re Quinlan, 355 A.2d 647 (N.J. Sup. Ct. 1976).

Riskin, L. L., and Reilly, P. P. (1977). Remedies for improper disclosure of genetic data. *Rutgers-Camden Law Journal, 8,* 480-506.

Roe v. Wade, 410 U.S. 113 (1973).

Schoeman, F. (1984). *Philosophical Dimensions of Privacy: An Anthology.* New York: Cambridge University Press.

Smart Card Technology: New Methods for Computer Access Control. (1988, September). Washington, D.C.: National Institutes of Standards and Technology.

Veatch, R. M. (1981). *A Theory of Medical Ethics.* New York: Basic Books.

Watson, B. L. (1981). Disclosure of computerized health care information: Provider privacy rights under supply-side competition. *American Journal of Law and Medicine, 7,* 265-300.

Westin, A. F. (1976). *Computers, Health Records, and Citizen's Rights.* Washington, DC: United States Department of Commerce.

Confidentiality: Computer Security and Data Protection

Patricia C. McMullen, MS, JD, RNC
Uniform University Services
Washington, D.C.

Nayna C. Philipsen, PhD, JD, RN
Compliance Analyst
Board of Physicians, Quality Assurance
Baltimore, Maryland

Introduction

The fundamental essence of privacy is the right of individuals to control unauthorized access to information about themselves (Curran and Curran, 1991). Unauthorized access embraces the right to confidentiality. Confidentiality is the duty of health care providers to protect the secrecy of information about patient condition, regardless of its source. This chapter discusses potential pitfalls in confidentiality that may occur when health care providers have access to patient medical records, especially in the use of computerized records in health care settings. In addition, this chapter offers practical suggestions to protect patients' privacy rights.

Since the fourth century B.C., the Hippocratic Oath has encouraged physicians to protect patient confidentiality (Weir, 1992). Until recently, however, patients had little legal recourse when the privacy of their medical records was breached. Today, state and federal laws provide patients with legal avenues to compensate them for violations, and simultaneously present providers with legal, as well as ethical, duties to protect patient privacy. The policy behind such laws is to protect the caregiver-patient relationship by encouraging patients to feel free to seek health care, to reveal sensitive information, and to request screening for contagious diseases without fear of the breach of confidentiality.

In a computerized age, the ability to control dissemination of confidential patient information is increasingly difficult. Prior to the use of computerized medical record keeping, the potential for abuse of information was limited to those who had access to a limited number of "hard" copies of the patient's record. With the advent of computers, access to patient records has broadened to anyone with access to the system. Because of computerization of patient records, the uses of these readily available patient records have also expanded. No longer do records consist of the one copy at the nurse's station or the doctor's office used exclusively for treatment. Today, patients' records are not only reviewed by multiple health care team members, but they are also used for a wide variety of purposes in addition to medical treatment; e.g., institutional quality assurance, licensing quality assurance, biomedical research, third-party insurance reimbursement, credentialing, litigation, court-ordered release, and regional and national data banks.

Over time, both health care providers and patients have come to regard the computerization of medical records as a double-edged sword. True, computerization facilitates rapid access to data for treatment, for research, and for credentialing, as well as other legitimate and desired goals. Questions arise, however, concerning who should have access to medical records, how affected patients can correct misinformation generated into computer data banks, and what remedies should be available to patients who are harmed by incorrect computerized records, or by abuse of their confidential information. Anyone who has tried to correct misinformation in a computerized credit record can identify with the frustration and harm that such misinformation can create. The broad generation of information from credit card companies to other sources has also raised public awareness of potential problems of abuse from any computerized data source of personal information.

Licensed professionals, including physicians and nurses, should also be wary about the inadvertent generation of confidential information into computer banks. In anticipation of possible confidentiality problems, the Health Care Quality Improvement Act of 1986 created the National Practitioner Data Bank (Philipsen and McMullen, 1993). Under this federal mandate, a computer information system related to professional competency of practitioners has been generated. Licensing bodies are required to report malpractice judgements, adverse state board actions, adverse privilege actions and adverse membership actions by professional organizations. Upon employing or credentialing professionals, hospitals and other health care employers are required to check this Data Bank, and to re-check every two years thereafter. Currently, physicians and dentists are the only health care providers listed in the National Practitioner Data Bank, but in the very near future, nurses and other health care professionals will be listed as well. Already physicians affected have expressed dismay about misinformation and use of information from the Data Bank. (Philipsen and McMullen, 1993). Examination of some recent legal cases concerning confidentiality and medical records demonstrates the reasons why confidentiality laws have developed.

Examples of Recent Problems with Medical Records and Confidentiality

Within the last few years, many legal cases have arisen concerning medical records and confidentiality. The following cases demonstrate valid concerns about medical record confidentiality.

Human Immunodeficiency Virus

Several recent cases have dealt with access to patient information on human immunodeficiency virus (HIV) diagnosis and treatment. For example, in *Doe v. Roe* (1993), a flight attendant requested that her attending physician not reveal her HIV status to her insurance carrier or to her employer, fearing such information might jeopardize her employment. According to the flight attendant, her physician orally agreed to protect information regarding her HIV status. Several months later, it was revealed that the physician had forwarded her entire medical chart, containing references to her HIV-positive status, to the attorney representing the flight attendant's employer in connection with her workers' compensation claim. The flight attendant sued the physician for breach of confidentiality and breach of his oral promise to keep the information confidential. The New York Supreme Court, Appellate Division, found that the release of the flight attendant's record violated both the duty of confidentiality and the expressed oral promise not to disclose the HIV information.

Likewise, in the case of *Doe v. District of Columbia* (1993), the U.S. District Court for the District of Columbia allowed prisoners with HIV to sue corrections officials who breached the medical confidentiality of their HIV status. And, in *Doe v. Shady Grove Adventist Hospital* (1991), the Maryland Court of Special Appeals held that an AIDS patient was entitled to anonymity in connection with a lawsuit concerning violation of the confidentiality of his medical records and for invasion of privacy.

Psychiatric Treatment

In *State v. Shiffra* (1993), Shaun A. Shiffra, on trial for sexual assault, claimed that his contact with the plaintiff, Pamela, was consensual; in preparing his defense, he sought all of Pamela's psychiatric records. He contended that her records were relevant on the issue of Pamela's consent to have sexual relations. The state opposed this request on the grounds that Pamela's psychiatric records were privileged information and that physical evidence corroborated Pamela's assertion that there had not been consent. The Wisconsin Court of Appeals found that Pamela's psychiatric records might be pertinent in terms of both her ability to tell the truth and whether she could accurately perceive the events that led to intercourse with Defendant Shiffra. Consequently, the Court ordered an in-chambers review of all of Pamela's psychiatric records. The court found that if the review disclosed that the records were too remote in time or were inconsistent with her current mental condition, they would not be given to the defense.

Another criminal case, *Commonwealth v. Moyer* (1991), also addressed the issue of confidentiality of psychiatric records. In that case, it was alleged that Clarence Moyer, Jr., had committed repeated sexual assaults on several minors. At trial, the administrator of a psychiatric hospital testified that Mr. Moyer had voluntarily committed himself following an alleged sexual assault. He read portions of Mr. Moyer's psychiatric record during the trial. One entry stated: "Patient was seen one-to-one and told writer he had just talked to his lawyer and was pleading guilty; that he didn't want to put the boy through a court hearing; that he couldn't sacrifice the boy. Patient seemed relieved." The jury convicted Moyer. However, the appellate court overturned Moyer's conviction on the grounds that his inpatient psychiatric records were confidential under Pennsylvania law and should not have been admitted into evidence at trial.

The case of *Siegfried v. City of Easton* (1992) concerned alleged police brutality. The couple who filed suit claimed that the City of Easton knew that one of the police officers named in the suit had a propensity for violence and, by taking no action, his superiors had acquiesced or condoned his actions. The plaintiffs sought the police officer's mental health records, contending these records were relevant to the issue of the City's knowledge of the officer's propensity for violence. The City of Easton claimed that mental health records were privileged under either the psychotherapist-patient relationship or by executive privilege. In determining whether the records should be protected, the court weighed the evidentiary value of the mental health records against the patient's privacy interests. The court found that the records were generated in conjunction with the officer's employment and therefore were not privileged.

Drug and Alcohol Treatment

In July of 1986, Valerie Ranft, a pedestrian, was struck by an auto driven by Thomas Lyons. A few hours after the accident, the defendant, Mr. Lyons, registered a blood alcohol level of 0.18 and was found guilty of operating a motor vehicle while intoxicated (*Ranft v. Lyons,* 1991). Ms. Ranft filed a civil suit against Mr. Lyons and sought his treatment records from Milwaukee Psychiatric Hospital, along with a court order compelling him to submit to a medical examination by a physician experienced in diagnosis and treatment of alcoholism. During his deposition, Mr. Lyons denied that he was impaired by alcohol. The court found that this denial constituted a waiver of his physician-patient privilege, and that Ms. Ranft could obtain his medical records. The court further found that Mr. Lyons should be subjected to a physical examination to determine the ability of his body to resist the effects of a high blood alcohol level.

A Charleston, South Carolina, physician also sought to withhold his alcohol and substance treatment records from the public record. In 1988, the physician was admitted to a private hospital for substance abuse treatment. Subsequently, he was sued by the survivors of a patient under his care who had died three months prior to the physician's hospital admission for substance treatment. The South Carolina State Board of Medical Examiners sought his substance abuse treatment records to determine if the physician had completed a 30-day treatment program at the facility and whether he was fit to practice medicine. The South Carolina Supreme Court found that the public's interest and need for disclosure outweighed the doctor's privilege, and ordered release of his substance treatment records to the State Board of Medical Examiners. However, the Court ordered the State Board to keep the information revealed in the records confidential (*State Board of Medical Examiners v. Fenwick Hall*, 1992).

Guidelines for Determining Control of Medical Records

In general, there is a strict level of confidentiality for patients receiving treatment. For example, in drug or alcohol abuse instances, providers are prohibited from disclosing whether someone is undergoing treatment in a federal facility. If a member of a health care team discloses that person is indeed a patient at the facility, such a disclosure constitutes a violation of a federal statute (42 CFR Part 2). According to the statute, not even family members, employers, or insurers are entitled to information concerning a patient's status (Philipsen and McMullen, 1993). Obviously, knowledge of the general rule, while providing a guideline for decisions, does not guarantee an outcome in any particular situation. Fortunately, there are also general guidelines for certain exceptions to the rule of patient control of information about care. For example, who has the authority to control access if a patient is incapacitated, incompetent, a minor, or deceased? The law has recognized these classifications of patients as deserving extraordinary consideration and therefore has created special designations to treat these patients as if they were competent adults.

The Incompetent Patient

If a patient is incapacitated or incompetent, the court appoints a guardian who is empowered to stand in the place of the patient. The health care team needs to be certain that this individual has been legally appointed, can produce a guardianship order, and is not just assuming guardianship on his or her own accord. (Philipsen and McMullen, 1993).

The Minor Patient

In the case of treatment of minors, parents generally control a child's medical communications. However, it is also a general rule that minors, under certain circumstances, are "emancipated," that is, treated like adults. Although emancipated minor laws vary from state to state, typically minors are treated as adults when they seek treatment for mental health services, venereal disease, abortion, family planning, pregnancy, and drug abuse, as well as treatment for their own minor children. Additionally, a court can declare a child to be an emancipated minor, in which case, that child is deemed to be an adult under the law. In emancipated minor cases, even if parents request access to the minor's medical records, they cannot be released without consent of the emancipated minor. Parents and health care providers often do not understand these laws, which exist to encourage minors to seek diagnosis and treatment for certain health problems.

The Deceased Patient

If a patient is deceased, the court appoints a personal representative to serve in his/her stead. This surrogate then controls the flow of confidential medical information about the deceased patient.

Exceptions to Control by the Competent Patient

Treatment of incompetent, minor, or deceased patients demonstrates that courts are willing to take extraordinary measures to keep medical records under the control of the patient. However, a number of the preceding case examples also demonstrate that there are instances where even the competent adult patient is unable to control access to his or her medical records. These exceptions to the general rule usually fall under one of a few legal tests applied by courts.

One test used to determine whether medical records can be released without direct consent of the patient is the Compelling Public Interest Test. For example, in the case of *Dr. K. v. State Board of Physician Quality Assurance* (1993), the Compelling Public Interest Test was used. The Maryland State Board of Physician Quality Assurance received several complaints that a certain Dr. K. , a psychiatrist, was engaged in sexual misconduct with a patient. The Board of Physician Quality Assurance sought to obtain the patient's records from Dr. K. However, both Dr. K and the patient contended that these records were confidential under psychiatrist-patient privilege. The Maryland Court of Special Appeals held that the patient's constitutional right to privacy had to be balanced against the Board of Physician Quality Assurance's duty to protect the welfare and safety of the public from misconduct by physicians. Consequently, the Court of Special Appeals ordered release of the patient's psychiatric records. The Charleston, South Carolina, case involving substance abuse by a physician, cited above, is a further example of the court's finding that the public interest can outweigh even the strictest confidentiality requirement.

Courts have also ruled that the *substantial interest of an individual* can outweigh the confidentiality rule. The case of *Diaz v. Lukash* (1993) concerned a registered nurse who was convicted and sentenced to death for the murder of 12 of his patients. It was contended that the nurse, Robert Diaz, had caused the death of these patients through administering massive doses of lidocaine. On appeal of his death sentence, Diaz sought to introduce evidence from autopsy records in New York. The prosecution, however, contended that the autopsy findings were confidential. The New York Court of Appeals found that Defendant Diaz demonstrated a substantial interest in the autopsy records, since these records were vital to his death sentence appeal. The Court of Appeals ordered the lower court to balance any privacy concerns against Diaz's interest in the autopsy records.

The case of the above Defendant, Thomas Lyons, is a good example of *patient waiver* of confidentiality. Although unwitting, Mr. Lyons effectively waived the confidentiality of his alcohol treatment records when he claimed under oath that he was not impaired at the time he struck pedestrian Valerie Ranft.

Statutes Protecting Medical Confidentiality

Medical Records Acts

Most states have a Medical Records Act which contains guidelines on the sharing of medical information. Typically, patients have absolute access to their medical records, provided they supply the treating facility with a written authorization to release requested information. Under these laws, health care providers are given a reasonable time to retrieve and reproduce patient records, and can charge a reasonable fee for this service. This means, of course, that a health care provider cannot block a patient's access to his or her medical records. Failure to provide requested records can result in provider civil liability, criminal penalties, and discipline by licensure boards. In one recent case, a Maryland hospital was found liable for $1 million in damages for failing to give the patient's representative her records (*Franklin Square Hospital v. Laubach*, 1991). In another case, an Oklahoma court allowed a civil suit by a patient against a dentist for failure to provide medical records as required by a state statute that also authorized criminal sanctions (*Bettis v. Brown*, 1991).

Licensing Statutes

All states have statutes governing the licensing of health care occupations, including a Nurse Practice Act and a Medical Practice Act. These acts typically require confidentiality, sometimes explicitly and sometimes by requiring that professionals act in an ethical manner, such as by incorporating the American Nurses' Association's Code of Ethics, or the Principles of Medical Ethics of the American Medical Association; both specifically assert the confidentiality of medical communications. Violations can result in revocation of a professional license or of limitations on it (Philipsen and McMullen, 1993).

Federal Computer Security Act

Computerized charting issues are a concern in all federal health care settings. The federal government has attempted to address some of these issues by enacting the Federal Computer Security Act (28 USC Sections 2671-2680). This detailed statute sets forth guidelines for limiting access to computerized information. Under the Act, The National Bureau of Standards has developed computer-processing standards. All federal agencies dealing with sensitive information must submit a computer security plan to the Bureau of Standards for approval. Each agency plan must also detail how sensitive data will be secured (See Martin, 1992; Soma and Bedient, 1989).

Other Statutes

Both federal and state governments continue to develop statutes which impose special duties of confidentiality for specific classes of patients, such as those undergoing treatment for alcohol and drug abuse, or patients diagnosed with AIDS. For instance, federal law requires a very high level of confidentiality for drug or alcohol abuse patients under Federal Statute 42 CRF Part 2. Providers need to be aware of statutes particular to their practice area.

The Americans with Disabilities Act

A recent concern in all future considerations of patient confidentiality centers around the Americans with Disabilities Act ("ADA," 42 USC Sec. 12131-12180). This Act prohibits discrimination of "qualified" individuals with disabilities. Although the ADA was not designed primarily as a medical confidentiality act, patients with qualified disabilities could use the ADA as a defense against arguments that their records should be released for the public welfare, because of a substantial individual interest, or under the doctrine of waiver. In one case already presented to a U.S. District Court, a physician-patient successfully used the ADA to block a state licensing board's inquiries into his substance abuse (*Medical Society of New Jersey v. Jacobs*, 1993).

Suggested Security Measures for Management of Computerized Patient Information

Although this is not an exhaustive list of security measures that providers can use to protect computerized medical records, the following tips should prove helpful in health care settings:

•Restrict access to patient information. All authorized users should have individual passwords and password lists should be available to only a few select people within the organization. (Collins, 1990). Passwords should be changed regularly.

•A key-operated power switch should be applied to all terminals to prevent unauthorized users from tampering with information (Collins, 1990).

•A "time out" device on each terminal that turns it off when it has not been used for a few minutes can protect data in the event of the unexpected distraction of an authorized user (Collins, 1990).

•Temporary employees or "floaters" should be assigned short-term passwords. (Collins, 1990)

•The system should be programmed to keep a record of who accessed what information, with the date and time of the activity. This allows the later tracking of possible breaches of confidentiality.

•Avoid use of the mainframe computer to store especially sensitive information; for example, information concerning AIDS testing (Wolfe, 1990).

•Be careful about where computer printouts are discarded. Confidential records need to be handled separately from regular paper disposal.

•When releasing data for research or to a national data bank, be sure to remove all identifiers of individual patients or of others whose identity should be protected; for example, a peer reviewer. (Prentnieks, 1992)

•Avoid the use of public domain software to minimize the potential for the introduction of a virus into your system. (Wolfe, 1990)

•When allowing researchers to access patient data, require written documentation of measures that they will use to protect the records from unauthorized disclosure, including their plan to destroy records upon completion of the study. (Prentnieks, 1992).

•Whenever you release an individual patient record, double check to assure that you have obtained a valid written release of medical information from the patient or a legally recognized representative of that patient. Remember that state and federal statutes will dictate the requirements of a valid release.

Summary

This chapter discusses potential obstacles that health care providers face when dealing with confidential patient information. Case examples are discussed to emphasize how the courts analyze confidentiality situations. Also, legal concepts used to determine whether confidential information is admissible under certain circumstances are reviewed. Finally, practical suggestions to protect the confidentiality of computerized medical information are offered.

References

Bettis v. Brown, No. 74.500 (Okla. Ct., App. October 22, 1991).

Collins, H. L. (1990) Legal risks of computer charting. *R.N. 53*(5), 81-86.

Commonwealth v. Moyer, No. 2314 (Pa. Super., July 26, 1991). Reported in *Health Law Digest,* 1991, *41.*

Curran, M., and Curran, K. (1991) The ethics of information. *Journal of Nursing Administration, 21,* 47-49.

Diaz V. Lukash, No. 241 (N.Y., November 16, 1993).

Doe v. District of Columbia, No. 92-635-LFO (U.S. District Ct. for D.C., April 13, 1993).

Doe v. Roe, No. 0369 (N.Y. App. Div., 4th Jud. Dept., May 28, 1993).

Doe v. Shady Grove Adventist Hospital, No. 1058 (Md. App., November 27, 1991).

Dr. K. v. State Board of Physician Quality Assurance, No. 138 (Md. App., November 2, 1993).

Franklin Square Hospital v. Laubach, 318 Md. 615, 569 A.2d 693 (1991).

Medical Society of New Jersey v. Jacobs, No. 93-3670 (WGB). (U.S. District Ct., N.J., October 5, 1993).

Martin, S. E. (1992). Analysis of the Computer Security Act of 1987 and its consequences for the Freedom of Information Act. *Communications and the Law, 14,* 73-90.

Philipsen, N., and McMullen, P. (1993). Medical records: Promoting patient confidentiality. *Nursing Connections, 6*(4), 48-50.

Prentnieks, M. E. (1992). Minnesota access to health records: Practical steps to complying with a confusing law. *Minnesota Medicine, 75*(9), 39-41.

Ranft v. Lyons, No. 90-2134 (Wisc., May 7, 1991).

Siegfried v. City of Easton, No. 91-2880 (U.S. District Ct., Pa., E.D., December 21, 1992).

Soma, J. T., and Bedient, E. J. (1989). Computer security and the protection of sensitive but not classified data: The Computer Security Act of 1987. *30 AIR FORCE L.R. 135-146.*

State Board of Medical Examiners v. Fenwick Hall, No. 23672 (S.C., June 8, 1992).

State v. Shiffra, No. 92-1986-CR (Wis., Dist. II March 31, 1993).

Weir, R. (1992) Patient confidentiality. *Iowa Medicine, 82*(2), 305.

Wolfe, K. (1990). Confidentiality and common sense. *AAOHN Journal, 38*(7), 338-340.

The Role of the Professional Association in Policy Development Related to Information Standards

D. Kathy Milholland, PhD, RN
Senior Policy Fellow, Research and Databases
Department of Practice, Economics and Policy
American Nurses Association

Introduction

Information systems and their applications to nursing in particular and to health care in general have been long-standing concerns of the American Nurses Association (ANA). The association's many activities in this arena, especially in the development of standards related to information systems, demonstrate its long and continued participation. The roles of professional associations in general are discussed briefly here in an effort to establish a framework for (1) ANA's interest in standards development, (2) ANA's view of the ANA mission, and (3) its functions, addressed in the context of standards. Following this, ANA's recent work with informatics, data bases, and other areas of standards development is discussed.

Professional Associations

Professional associations can be defined as voluntary, non-profit organizations comprised of individuals working in the same or related fields (Caruso, 1977). The main purposes of a professional association are to elevate professional standards, to educate members, and to strengthen their economic and general welfare (Caruso, 1977; Mack, 1991). In addition, a major purpose of an association is the enhancement of the professional climate wherein members carry out their disciplines. Enhancement includes representing and advocating the collective needs of association members with all those who have the power to influence areas affecting member needs. This kind of policy work must extend beyond the national and state government levels to the farthest reaches of public influence (Mack, 1991). The American Society of Association Executives states that professional associations are responsible both for information dissemination about the association and its members and for maintaining high professional standards (American Society of Association Executives [ASAE], 1988). Clearly, a professional association, like the ANA, has a significant role to play in the development, maintenance and enforcement of standards that affect its members, and association policies are often directed towards standards issues.

ANA was founded in September, 1896, by delegates from 10 alumnae associations. Its first bylaws were completed in 1897 when the association was called the Nurses Associated Alumnae of the United States and Canada. In 1911, the name was changed to American Nurses Association (American Nurses Association [ANA], 1991a).

The purposes of ANA are found in its articles of incorporation and bylaws. The purposes are: (1) to work for the improvement of health standards and the availability of health care services for all people; (2) to foster high standards of nursing; and (3) to stimulate and promote the professional development of nurses by advancing their economic and general welfare. The bylaws in themselves also identify many functions of the association. Those relating to policy work and standards are designed to establish standards of nursing practice, nursing education, and nursing services; to ensure a system of credentialing in nursing; to initiate and influence legislation, governmental programs, national health policy, and international health policy; and to represent and speak for the nursing profession with allied health groups, national and international organizations, governmental bodies, and the public (ANA, 1991a).

Standards

Established standards are necessary to protect the health and safety of consumers and to provide important information that might otherwise not be available. The development and enforcement of professional standards give consumers confidence in products and providers: standards facilitate comparisons among people and systems. Voluntary standards are an important method for standardization and are usually preferred to government regulation since voluntary standards are considered to be more flexible, adaptable, and affordable. A major responsibility of an association, then, is to contribute significantly to the development and certification of standards (ASAE, 1990). Following its own guidelines, ANA has been developing standards for the nursing profession since the late 1960s.

Within the ANA, standards are defined as "authoritative statements by which the nursing profession describes the responsibilities for which its practitioners are accountable" (ANA, 1991b, p.1). Standards of practice are divided into (1) standards of care, and (2) standards of professional performance. Standards of care address the competent delivery of nursing care as demonstrated by the nursing process: assessment, diagnosis, outcome identification, planning, implementation, and evaluation. A competent level of behavior in the professional role is addressed by the standards of professional performance. Activities in this arena include quality of care, performance appraisal, education, collegiality, ethics, collaboration, research, and resource utilization (ANA, 1991b).

The standards developed by ANA are generic standards applicable to nursing practice in all settings. They identify the responsibilities of all professional nurses. Further, these standards can serve as the basis for the development of quality management systems, data bases, regulatory systems, and many other systems, activities and structures within nursing and health care. These standards for clinical nursing practice serve as the foundation for ANA's policy activities related to standards for information systems.

In general, there are three types of information standards in health care: message standards, coding standards and content standards. Message standards address the communication of a specific unit of data (a "message") between two different computer systems. They define the fields, format and structure of the message containing the information (Workgroup on Computerization of Patient Records, 1992). Health Level Seven (HL7) is an example of a message standard. HL7 specifically addresses the exchange of data among health care computer applications. The goal of the message standards is to reduce or eliminate the need for custom interface programming and program maintenance. In this standard, the trigger events (e.g., patient admission, request for a particular piece of equipment, completion of a laboratory test) which stimulate the production of a message are defined, as are the formats for each message (Health Level Seven, Inc., 1991).

Coding standards focus on defining uniform terms and concepts (Workgroup on Computerization of Patient Records, 1992). In the clinical arena, this means defining diagnoses, interventions (procedures, treatments, actions, therapies), and outcomes. There can be single or multiple coding schemes, and some schemes address more than one aspect of the clinical practice process. The International Classification of Diseases (ICD) is a coding standard for diagnoses. In the United States' version of the ICD (the ninth version with clinical modifications or ICD-9-CM), for example, diseases of the circulatory system are assigned codes ranging from 390 to 459. Rheumatic fever without mention of heart involvement is coded as 390; rheumatic fever with heart involvement is code 391 (*St. Anthony's ICD-9-CM Book,* 1992).

The identification and definition of broad categories of information in the patient record are referred to as content standards. Work is under way, for example, to define the content and structure of an automated patient record and an automated longitudinal health record. Content standards should not be confused with data dictionaries which define the fields of information in a record. Content standards, as noted above, establish categories of information; they do not specify the internal structure of patient record systems (Workgroup on Computerization of Patient Records, 1992). In the work on the development of content standards for an automated longitudinal health record, now under way, various general content areas have been identified: demographics, administrative data (legal agreements, financial information, provider/practitioner information) and clinical data. A proposed minimum set of clinical data needed for a longitudinal health record is: problem list, immunizations, exposure to hazardous substances, patient and family health history, physical exam and assessments, orders and treatment plans, diagnostic tests, medication profile, scheduled appointments, and information about each encounter or episode of care. These are broad areas of information.

ANA Policy Activities

Since the 1970s, ANA has been actively addressing policy development related to information systems. Most of this work has been related to coding and content standards, although there has been a recent effort to establish message standards.

As early as 1976, the ANA supported efforts to develop a common language for identifying nursing problems. During this time period, ANA scheduled a series of regional conferences on nursing diagnoses. The focus of these conferences was to educate nurses about nursing diagnoses and to conduct actual development of diagnoses (ANA, 1977).

With the publication of the *Social Policy Statement* in 1980, ANA promoted a process-oriented model for nursing practice (i.e., the nursing process). The nursing process includes the following components: nursing assessment, nursing diagnosis, nursing interventions and nurse-sensitive patient outcomes. This framework was advocated by the association as the basis for developing a nursing practice classification system (ANA, 1980).

The 1986 House of Delegates adopted a resolution identifying the need for nurses to use information systems to collect essential data for clinical practice, management of nursing care and nursing resources, research, administration, education, and advocacy of public policy. This resolution also recommended that the Nursing Minimum Data Set (NMDS) be tested and implemented on a local, regional and national basis (ANA, 1986, pp. 171-172).

The following year, the 1987 House of Delegates developed further policy on the classifications of nursing practice (ANA, 1987, pp. 177-179); these 1987 policies are presented here. Through these policies, ANA promoted the classification of nursing practice by using the categories of assessment, diagnosis, interventions and outcomes (these are examples of a content standard). The Association is committed to the development of a single, comprehensive system for classifying nursing practice to be used in all nursing practice situations, and will seek collaboration with intradisciplinary groups as classification systems in nursing are developed. ANA will promote consistent use of classification systems in nursing education and delivery of nursing services. The Association will also promote the integration of nursing information with health care data systems. Development of an international classification system of nursing practice will be encouraged and actively supported. ANA will collaborate with interdisciplinary groups in the development of classification systems for health care.

Numerous activities within the nursing profession resulted from the adoption of these policies. The ANA Council on Computer Applications in Nursing developed the monograph *Computer Design Criteria for Systems That Support the Nursing Process,* published in 1988 (Zielstorff, McHugh, and Clinton, 1988). *A Computer Nurse Directory,* published by the Council on Computer Applications in Nursing, lists, by state and functional area, nurses involved in informatics (1988). Collaborative efforts by ANA continue with the North American Nursing Diagnosis Association (NANDA), and an agreement (with NANDA) has been reached on the process by which ANA councils may submit nursing diagnoses for review and adoption.

In January 1989, ANA published *Classification Systems for Describing Nursing Practice* (ANA, 1989). This collection of working papers is intended to assist the nursing profession in achieving the goal of a uniform nursing practice classification system. Nurses from all areas of practice, education, administration, and research will find the insights in this publication useful for understanding the necessity for and mechanisms needed to achieve this uniform system.

The Uniform Clinical Data Set (UCDS) has been developed by the Health Care Financing Administration (HCFA) for use by state Peer Review Organizations to review hospital care and to systematically acquire clinical data on patient characteristics and the process of care (Jencks and Wilensky, 1992). ANA has met with the leadership of HCFA to discuss the inclusion of nursing data elements in UCDS. In March 1989, ANA convened a meeting of nurse experts to make recommendations on specific data elements to include and how to use information on the effectiveness of nursing care in evaluating the quality and outcomes of care. This work with HCFA continues.

The 1990 House of Delegates established additional policy direction for the association regarding minimum data sets for describing nursing practice. The House of Delegates directed ANA to pursue collaborative efforts with national nursing organizations, major vendors of nursing information systems (NISs), and other health-related organizations to develop the essential minimum data elements for determining the costs and quality of nursing care (ANA, 1990b). The delegates also agreed that ANA will provide leadership for: development of uniform classification schemes for nursing; development, acceptance, and widespread use of a national nursing data set to support nursing practice; and encouragement for incorporation of nursing minimum data elements into clinical data sets and inclusion of a national NMDS in NISs (ANA, 1990a).

In November of 1989, the Steering Committee on Databases to Support Clinical Nursing Practice was convened. This committee, which reports to the ANA Congress of Nursing Practice, was charged with the following responsibilities: (1) to develop a uniform nursing language, (2) to incorporate nursing vocabularies into health-related data bases, and (3) promote the development of nursing vocabularies and taxonomies. With respect to information systems standards, the committee's primary focus has been on content and coding standards, although it provides oversight for ANA activities related to message standards.

The Steering Committee established two policies to serve as a framework and guide to its work: (1) classify nursing practice according to diagnoses, interventions, and nursing-sensitive patient outcomes; and (2) utilize the 16 data elements of the NMDS as the minimum elements for a NIS. The NMDS is defined as an essential set of information items with uniform definitions and categories concerned with nursing which meets the information needs of diverse multiple data users throughout the health care system (Werley and Lang, 1988).

In the arena of content standards, the Steering Committee has been working to develop a Unified Nursing Language System (UNLS). A UNLS identifies the semantic linkages among different nursing vocabularies (Milholland, 1992). It also extends these linkages to other health care-related vocabularies. This means that nurses in one setting, such as a hospital, may use one set of diagnostic terms to name a patient's health problems (e.g., NANDA diagnoses). In the home health care setting in that patient's community, nurses may use a different vocabulary of patient problems (e.g., Omaha System). The UNLS will automatically link the terms that refer to the same phenomenon. Thus, nurses can communicate about the patient's care without having to use the same naming system. In addition, the UNLS automatically will map the nursing diagnoses to other health care classification systems such as the ICD-9-CM.

As part of the development process for the UNLS, the Steering Committee has examined nursing nomenclatures with respect to their relevance and usefulness for inclusion in this system. Several nursing nomenclatures have been recognized by the Steering Committee as useful for inclusion in a UNLS:

•NANDA taxonomy of nursing diagnoses (North American Nursing Diagnosis Association, 1992);
•The Omaha System: a problem, intervention and outcome classification system for home health care (Martin and Scheet, 1992);
•Home Health Care Classification of nursing problems and interventions for home health care (Saba, 1990); and
•Nursing Interventions Classification system of nursing interventions (Bulechek and McCloskey, 1992).

These vocabularies provide the content basis for identifying the nursing terms that should be included in computer-based health care information systems. Using selected content from these vocabularies, an initial coding schema for problems has been developed and proposed to the World Health Organization, publisher of the International Classification of Diseases, for inclusion in the 10th edition of the ICD. These ANA-recognized vocabularies also are being included in the Metathesaurus of the Unified Medical Language System, a project under development by the National Library of Medicine (Humphries and Lindberg, 1989).

The Steering Committee has become the entity within the profession of nursing that denotes which nursing nomenclatures are to be integrated into external data bases and retrieval systems. ANA supports continuing development of nomenclatures and taxonomies for clinical nursing practice, and will provide letters of support to individual investigators with projects of merit. The vocabularies recognized to date, ANA points out, are viewed as a beginning, not an end.

Through the Steering Committee, ANA is actively involved in the development of message standards for communicating patient care information between computer systems. The HL7 Patient Care Special Interest Group is currently identifying an object-oriented model of the patient care process. This work will be used to evaluate the current HL7 standard, recommend changes to accommodate data needs related to patient care, and/or recommend new message standards. An ANA nurse staff member chairs the special interest group and provides regular reports to the Steering Committee.

ANA represents nursing at meetings of the Healthcare Information Systems Planning Panel, an organization formed to coordinate the multitudinous standards activities occurring in the health care information systems arena. This panel seeks agreement from various standards groups on the areas of standards developments for which each group will be responsible. Issues affecting all standards groups are discussed and recommendations are provided.

Nursing is represented by ANA members at meetings of the Computer-Based Patient Record Institute (CPRI) Workgroups on Codes & Structures and Systems Evaluation. An ANA member, Dr. Lucille Joel, represents the association on the CPRI board of directors. Activities of the ASTM (formerly the American Society for Testing and Materials) related to health care information systems standards are monitored and contributed to by ANA member liaisons. ANA was an active participant in the recent Workgroup on Computerization of Patient Records, sponsored by the American Hospital Association. This workgroup published a report of its recommendations for achieving a nationwide health information infrastructure, including necessary work on standards related to health care information systems and the patient record (Workgroup on Computerization of Patient Records, 1993).

Through its own publications, ANA provides perspectives and policy directions regarding the development and use of information systems as they relate to nursing practice. The ANA Council on Computer Applications in Nursing has published a series of monographs on computer applications: *Computers in Nursing Education* (Grobe, Ronald and Tymchyshyn, 1987), *Computer Design Criteria for Systems that Support the Nursing Process* (Zielstorff, McHugh, and Clinton, 1988), *Computers in Nursing Research: A Theoretical Perspective* (Abraham, Schroeder, and Schwirian, 1992), and *Computers in Nursing Administration* (Saba, Johnson, and Simpson, 1994). Through a joint effort with the National League for Nursing, the association has published *Next Generation Nursing Information Systems: Essential Characteristics for Professional Practice* (Zielstorff, Hudgings, and Grobe, 1993). This monograph, the outcome of a 1989 meeting of nurses and information systems vendors under the auspices of the National Commission on Nursing Implementation Project, provides useful and timely guidelines for nurses and information systems developers.

Also related to standards for information systems is the establishment in 1992 of nursing informatics as a distinct specialty area of nursing practice by the ANA Congress of Nursing Practice. Since that designation, a task force has been developing a scope of practice and standards of practice for this specialty. By 1995, the American Nurses Credentialing Center is expected to develop and offer a certification examination. Once this process is in place, certified informatics nurses will provide an excellent resource for nursing executives' purchasing and implementing information systems.

Summary

The American Nurses Association has a long-standing interest in the development and implementation of standards for nursing practice and for information systems that affect the practice of nursing. Policies and standards are identified through the activities of the ANA House of Delegates, task forces, liaison with national standards organizations, and the development of related publications. The association recognizes and takes seriously its responsibilities to represent the nursing profession in all of the numerous information systems arenas now and in the future. The Steering Committee and the Committee on Standards and Guidelines envision joint projects to promote the adoption of valid, comprehensive data sets to information systems vendors and users. The development of the UNLS is proceeding along several paths intended to accommodate current demands for nursing data sets, as well as the long-term need for a science-based language. The House of Delegates has clearly identified the computer-based patient record with its related systems and related activities as a priority for the association and for the profession. Thus, the role of the professional association in the development of policies for information systems standards has been, and will continue to be, significant and influential in the health care professions.

References

Abraham, I., Schroeder, M., and Schwirian, P. (1992). *Computers in Nursing Research: A Theoretical Perspective*. Kansas City, MO: American Nurses Association.

American Nurses Association. (1977). *Report of the Six Regional Conferences on Classification of Nursing Diagnosis.*. Kansas City, MO: ANA Board of Directors.

American Nurses Association. (1980). *Social Policy Statement*. Kansas City, MO: Author.

American Nurses Association. (1986). Development of computerized nursing information Systems (NISs) in nursing services. *Summary of Proceedings*. Kansas City, MO: Author.

American Nurses Association. (1987). Access to and utilization of nursing information resources. *Summary of Proceedings*. Kansas City, MO: Author.

American Nurses Association. (1989). *Classification Systems for Describing Nursing Practice*. Kansas City, MO: Author.

American Nurses Association. (1990a). Initiatives regarding the effectiveness of health care and national uniform nursing data sets. *Summary of Proceedings*. Kansas City, MO: Author.

American Nurses Association. (1990b). The need for a nursing minimum data set to identify the quality and costs of nursing services. *Summary of Proceedings*. Kansas City, MO: Author.

American Nurses Association. (1991a). *Bylaws*. Kansas City, MO: Author.

American Nurses Association. (1991b). *Standards of Clinical Nursing Practice*. Kansas City, MO: Author.

American Society of Association Executives. (1988). *Principles of Association Management: A Professional Handbook* (2nd ed.). Washington, DC: Author.

American Society of Association Executives. (1990). *Associations Advance America*. Washington, DC: Author.

Bulechek, G., and McCloskey, J. (Eds.). (1992). *Nursing Intervention Classification* (NIC). St. Louis: C. V. Mosby Co.

Caruso, F. C. (1977). *The Challenge of Association Management*. Denver: Association Insight Press.

Council on Computer Applications in Nursing. (1988). *A Computer Nurse Directory*. Kansas City, MO: American Nurses Association.

Grobe, S., Ronald, J.. and Tymchyshyn, P. (1987). *Computers in Nursing Education*. Kansas City, MO: American Nurses Association.

Health Level Seven, Inc. (1991). *Health Level Seven. An Application Protocol for Electronic Data Exchange in Healthcare Environments*. Ann Arbor, MI: Author.

Humphries, B., and Lindberg, D. (1989). Building the unified medical language system. In L. D. Kingsland (Ed.), *Proceedings of the Thirteenth Annual Symposium on Computer Applications in Medical Care*. Washington, DC: IEEE Computer Society Press.

Jencks, S., and Wilensky, G. (1992). The health care quality improvement initiative. A new approach to quality assurance in Medicare. *JAMA, 268*(7), 900-903.

Mack, C. (1991). *The Executive's Handbook of Trade and Business*. New York: Quorum Books.

Martin, K., and Scheet, N. (1992). *The Omaha System Applications for Community Health Nursing*. Philadelphia: W. B. Saunders Co.

Milholland, D. K. (1992). Naming what we do—Nursing vocabularies and databases. *Journal of AHIMA, 63*(10), 58-61.

North American Nursing Diagnosis Association. (1992). *NANDA Nursing Diagnosis: Definition and Classification 1992.* St. Louis: Author.

Saba, V. (1990). *The Classifications of Home Health Nursing Diagnoses and Interventions.* Washington, DC: Author.

Saba, V., Johnson, J., and Simpson, R. (1994). *Computer in Nursing Management.* Washington, DC: American Nurses Publishing.

St. Anthony's ICD-9-CM Book. (1992). Alexandria, VA: St. Anthony Publishing.

Werley, H., and Lang, N. (1988). The consensually derived nursing minimum data set: Elements and definitions. In H. Werley, and N. Lang (Eds.), *Identification of the Nursing Minimum Data Set.* New York: Springer Publishing Co.

Workgroup on Computerization of Patient Records. (1992). *Toward a National Health Information Infrastructure.* Chicago: American Hospital Association.

Workgroup on Computerization of Patient Records. (1993). *Toward a National Health Information Infrastructure.* Chicago: American Hospital Association.

Zielstorff, R., Hudgings, C., and Grobe, S. (1993). *Next-Generation Nursing Information Systems: Essential Characteristics for Professional Practice.* Washington, DC: American Nurses Association.

Zielstorff, R., McHugh, M., and Clinton, J. (1988). *Computer Design Criteria for Systems that Support the Nursing Process.* Kansas City, MO: American Nurses Association.

Standards of Practice and Preparation for Certification

Teresa L. Panniers, PhD, RN, CRNP
Assistant Professor
Department of Education, Administration, Health Policy and Informatics
School of Nursing
University of Maryland at Baltimore

Carole A. Gassert, PhD, RN
Assistant Professor
Department of Education, Administration, Health Policy and Informatics
School of Nursing
University of Maryland at Baltimore

Introduction

In a health care environment where information is crucial to accurate, efficacious, and cost-effective decision making, nursing informatics is emerging as a specialty poised to fulfill these requirements. The area of nursing informatics has developed rapidly during the last decade, and has been recognized formally as a specialty within the nursing profession since 1992 (Simpson, 1992).

To develop as a specialty, nursing informatics must prove its worth to the profession of nursing. The purpose of this chapter is to discuss nursing and nursing specialties, and specifically, to offer recommendations for the development of standards of practice for nursing informatics and the certification of nurses in this specialty.

Background

Nursing specializations were recognized as early as 1938, when nurses were prepared for the first time as clinical specialists (Peplau, 1965). Any expansion in the knowledge upon which a practice is based leads to specialization (Peplau, 1965). Peplau sees the emergence of nursing specialties in the health care field as parallel to the explosive growth of the basic sciences in which new knowledge multiplies the possible relationships among the various sciences. Because only a few entrepreneurs in a particular field may be interested in the relationships between the different sciences, and because curricula in science cannot be revised to include all new knowledge, one result is specialization across sciences (Peplau, 1965). An example of this phenomenon is the rise of nursing informatics, a combination of computer science, information science, and nursing science designed to assist in the management and processing of nursing data, information, and knowledge in order to support the practice of nursing and the delivery of nursing care (Graves and Corcoran, 1989).

Nursing Informatics as a Specialty

Characteristics associated with the maturity of a specialty area are: differentiated practice, educational programs for preparing nurses in a specialty, an established research program, credentialing mechanisms, and representation of the specialty by an organized body (Styles, 1989). Nurse scientists have begun to provide a framework for the specialty of nursing informatics by developing models for organizing the study of nursing informatics (Graves and Corcoran, 1989), for conducting research in nursing informatics (Schwirian, 1986), and for defining nursing information system requirements to support the practice of nursing informatics (Gassert, 1990; Graves and Corcoran, 1988; Staggers and Parker, 1993). As nursing informatics has gained momentum in the practice arena, graduate programs to educate nurses in this field have been developed (Heller, Romano, Moray, and Gassert, 1989). The American Nurses Association Task Force identifies nurses who specialize in nursing informatics as "informatics nurse specialists," with advanced knowledge in both nursing and informatics (American Nurses Association [ANA], 1994). Even though the nursing informatics specialty has been recognized among academicians and practitioners, and most recently by the nursing profession at large (Simpson, 1992), the challenge to define the specialty's standards of practice, scope of practice, and formal methods for recognizing those nurses practicing in the specialty was embraced by the profession.

Scope of Practice

Once a nursing specialty has been defined, standards of practice must be developed. Prior to the development of standards of practice, the specialty of nursing informatics was delineated, i.e., its scope of practice established. Scope of practice refers to the contents of nursing informatics as a distinct segment of nursing practice. It has four defining characteristics: boundary, intersections, core, and dimensions (ANA, 1980).

Boundaries

Nurses practicing in a specialty area experience the boundaries within which their practice occurs. Such boundaries are delineated by: (1) the qualifications of the individual declaring membership in the specialty; (2) the legal and professional regulations related to the practice of the specialty; and (3) the privileges and responsibilities of the practitioner within the specialty. The American Nurses Association (ANA) scope of practice statement for nursing informatics defines the boundaries surrounding nursing informatics by both what the specialty encompasses and what it excludes from the specialty. For example, nursing informatics is viewed as a service specialty within nursing, which includes the development of applications, tools, processes, and structures that can assist nurses to manage data in taking care of patients or in supporting the practice of nursing. Nursing informatics is also viewed as a support function that serves to enable nurses to carry out the work of nursing in an efficient and effective manner. Nursing informatics also exists to support patient care, either directly or indirectly, by supporting nursing education, research and administration. The ANA considers nursing informatics a specialty that overlaps all other areas of nursing practice, yet is distinct in that it focuses on the methods and technology of identifying, naming, organizing and grouping, collecting, processing, analyzing, storing, retrieving, or managing data and information in nursing (ANA, 1994). Informatics nurse specialists promote the practice of nursing by advancing the science of handling nursing information. Finally, the boundaries of nursing informatics practice are distinguished from those of other disciplines by nursing informatics' concern with the application of informatics knowledge to nurses' requirements for information handling.

Intersections

Intersections in a nursing specialty occur when the practice of one specialty intersects with other professions involved in health care. Here, nurses in a particular specialty extend their practice into the domains of other professions. The intersections are not rigid; rather, they are flexible and result from a collaborative effort among professions. All of the health care professions interact, share the same overall mission, have access to the same published scientific knowledge, and in some degree overlap in their professional activities (ANA, 1980). The specialty of nursing informatics intersects with other disciplines concerned with the concepts and structures used to manage data, information, and knowledge. These intersections enhance the delivery of professional nursing care, the generation of nursing knowledge, and the achievement of health outcomes for individuals, families, and communities. (ANA, 1994).

Core

The core of nursing practice in a specialty area are the phenomena that serve as the basis for accepted practice in the specialty (ANA, 1980). In nursing informatics, the core phenomena include all the data, information and knowledge contributed by nursing. Nursing informatics has, as its core operations, the identifying, acquiring, preserving, managing, retrieving, aggregating, analyzing and transmitting of data, information, and knowledge in such a way to make them meaningful and useful to nurses. Because of these requirements, technologies that facilitate the operations performed by nurses practicing in the specialty of nursing informatics are also of concern to nursing informatics (ANA, 1994).

Dimensions

The dimensions of nursing practice are characteristics that fall within and further describe the scope of nursing. A comprehensive statement of these characteristics would include but not be limited to descriptions of what philosophy and ethics guide nurses; what responsibilities, functions, roles, and skills characterize their work; what scientific theories they use and by what methods they apply them; where and when they practice; and with what legal authority they function (ANA, 1980). The ANA states that nursing informatics includes characteristics common to other nursing practice specialties but its dimensions differ from them in that nursing informatics provides nurses with essential information at the point of care, assists nurse managers to develop systems for the effectual use of nursing resources, and facilitates research by aggregating clinical data and making these data available for analyses. Nursing informatics also protects the confidentiality and privacy of personal health information, promotes safe patient care by developing systems that assist with the evaluation of the quality of nursing care, and furthers the science of nursing by making that information on quality of nursing care available to the profession.

Standards of Practice

Standards of practice are principles adhered to by a profession to ensure a level of quality of care accepted by the profession and its clients (ANA, 1991b). Such standards prescribe practices that can be adhered to consistently by members of a profession expressed in language easily understood by the public. Standards of practice can change, however, as a nursing specialty matures.

The ANA first published standards of practice for the profession of nursing in 1973 (ANA, 1991b). In recent years, an increasing number of nursing specialty groups and organizations have begun to develop numerous and disparate sets of standards. Lacking a unifying set of standards, nurses found it difficult to validate their practice patterns. At the same time, the health care environment was shifting its emphasis to the quality of care delivered and to cost-containment issues. Finally, as the profession of nursing has continued to evolve, ANA's former set of generic standards that focused solely on the nursing process seemed outmoded (ANA, 1991b). In response to these issues, the ANA appointed a task force in 1989 to define the nature and purpose of standards of practice for nursing, as well as their interrelationships with quality assurance activities, specialization in nursing practice, credentialing, and the subsequent implications for nursing information systems (ANA, 1991b). Many nursing organizations collaborated in the developmental work (ANA, 1991b). As a result of this effort, the ANA published a revised set of standards for clinical nursing practice in 1991 (ANA, 1991a). This document defines standards of nursing care and standards of professional performance. The intent of these standards of nursing practice is to describe an acceptable level of client care or behavior in the nurse's role (ANA 1991a; 1991b). Philosophical in nature and intended to remain stable over time, these standards apply to all nurses and all clients. Standards are not meant to be operationalized, and criteria have been developed to provide measurable indicators for each of the standards of practice. Criteria are designed to be revised as advancements in science, knowledge, clinical practice, and technology occur (ANA, 1991a).

Nursing informatics has as its core, the data, information, knowledge and the technology needed in the delivery of patient care (ANA, 1994). Therefore, all of the standards of practice in the Standards of Clinical Nursing Practice (ANA, 1991b) pertain to the practice of nursing in the specialty. However, the criteria by which informatics nurse specialists measure adherence to a standard may vary from traditional nursing practice roles, requiring a new criterion to be used to evaluate adherence to the standard. For example, the ANA's *Standards of Clinical Nursing Practice* lists a number of criteria for assessing the standard, "The nurse collects client health data." One such criterion is, "Relevant data are documented in a retrievable form" (ANA, 1991a). Because nursing informatics supports clinical nursing's information needs for patient assessment, new criteria may be required for measuring the practice of informatics nurse specialists. Such a criteria might be, "Appropriate methods and tools of information handling are used to support the collection of atomic-level client health data by the nurse."

As a second example, under the standard for quality of care listed as "The nurse systematically evaluates the quality and effectiveness of nursing practice" is the criteria "The nurse uses the results of quality of care activities to initiate changes in practice" (ANA, 1991a). Again, because nursing informatics supports nurses' handling of information, a new criteria for nurses practicing in the specialty of nursing informatics may be needed. Such a criteria might be, "The informatics nurse specialist manages the analyses of quality of care data to support the initiation of changes in nursing practice." The practice of identifying criterion specific to nursing informatics from the generic standards of practice allows for standardization and less redundancy, while acknowledging the rapid changes in the practice of nursing informatics.

The specialty of nursing informatics also has unique aspects that require the development of a separate set of standards. For example, a standard of practice unique to nursing informatics might be, "Nursing informatics supports the information handling requirements of nurses."

In summary, nurses practicing in the specialty of nursing informatics can use published standards with the addition of specific criterion where appropriate, and can create their own set of standards for areas unique to nursing informatics. This will underscore the unity of the profession of nursing while recognizing the unique qualities of nursing informatics.

Certification

Certification has been described as a voluntary process by which a non-governmental agency or association verifies that an individual licensed to practice a profession has achieved predetermined standards set forth by that profession for practice in the specialty (Carter, 1986). For nearly 50 years, certification of nursing practice has been used as a credentialing mechanism to signify the achievement of predetermined skills and knowledge in a specific field of study (Parker, 1994). The American Nurses Credentialing Center Boards of Certification, as well as numerous other specialty certification boards, provide voluntary certification programs for nurses at the generalist and specialist level in a nursing specialty (American Nurses Credentialing Center [ANCC], 1993a; 1993b; Fickeissen, 1990).

Prior to initiating a certification program, the nursing specialty should have defined its standards of practice and prepared a statement of its scope of practice. Once the specialty has been defined, a certification board can be established. While a certification board may be made up of individuals from the parent or affiliated specialty nursing organization, it is imperative that the board itself be autonomous in matters pertaining to the actual certification of nurses to avoid any potential conflict of interest.

The certification board itself requires a method of determining how to examine potential candidates for certification in the specialty of nursing informatics. One method of determining the content domain to be tested is through use of a group of experts to prepare a test content outline, sometimes called a test blueprint, to determine the domains of practice and the content areas, topics, and subtopics that may be covered on the examination (ANCC, 1993a). Another method of determining the content domain of a specialty area or to validate the content domain as presently depicted is to conduct a job analysis or role delineation study. A job analysis or role delineation study ensures that the content domain tested reflects, and will continue to reflect, the skills and knowledge necessary to competently perform the role of the nurse practicing in a given specialty (Ropka, Norback, Rosenfeld, Miller, and Nielsen, 1992). The results of such a study may be used to guide the content of the certification examinations.

Candidates for certification must meet specific requirements prior to the certification examination. These criterion include requirements for clinical or functional practice in a specialized area of nursing, attainment of a level of education in nursing specified by the certifying body, and the endorsement of one's peers (ANCC, 1993a; 1993b).

Certification as a Generalist

The majority of nursing care to the population is provided by nurse generalists. The nurse generalist brings a comprehensive approach to health care and can meet the health care needs of individuals, families, and communities (ANA, 1980). Certification as a generalist denotes excellence in practice beyond that expected for nursing licensure.

In addition to the general requirements for certification, many certification boards presently (or in the near future will) require a baccalaureate or higher degree in nursing (ANCC, 1993a; 1993b; Parker, 1994). In addition, further requirements for educational preparation inclusive of content in the specified area of the specialty practice are becoming required as the nursing profession seeks to standardize certification across specialties and professional organizations (Pluyter-Wenting and Nieman, 1988).

Integral to the development of an objective examination for nurse generalists in the specialty of nursing informatics is the development of a set of minimum competencies for the specialty of nursing. In the scope of practice document for nursing informatics, a set of minimum competencies required for all graduates of nursing programs has been defined. The fundamental requirements include the ability to identify information requirements for practice, document care and protect the confidentiality and privacy of patient information. In 1987, the International Medical Informatics Association Working Group on Nursing Informatics developed a set of competencies for nurses practicing in the specialty of nursing informatics that were subsequently published by the National League for Nursing (Pluyter-Wenting and Nieman, 1988).

Certification as a Specialist

The specialist in nursing practice is a nurse who, through study and supervised practice at the graduate level (master's or doctorate), has become an expert in a defined area of knowledge and practice in a selected clinical area of nursing (ANA, 1980). The specialist has all the knowledge of the field that a generalist possesses and, in addition, demonstrates an advanced level of expertise in the specialty area. Specialists also conduct research and development, and advance the theory and application of the specialty.

Candidates for certification as nurse specialists are required to have been prepared at the graduate level in the specialty. Further, they are subject to varying requirements regarding the engagement in practice and the endorsement of their peers.

With regard to the competencies required of the informatics nurse specialist that may serve to form the basis for a certification examination, the scope of practice document states that informatics nurse specialists need a specialized set of competencies to advance the practice of the specialty. Required competencies include but are not limited to the design, analysis, and evaluation of nursing informatics science requirements and applications, theory development, research, and collaboration with other health informatics specialists (ANA, 1994).

Standardization Among Certification Programs

One major obstacle to public acceptance of nursing certification has been the profession's inability to standardize its own certification process. As noted earlier, the standards used, the educational background and practice qualifications required vary greatly from organization to organization. Nursing certification programs continue to proliferate, reflecting both the trends in nursing specialty areas and the developing professionalization of the field, as it evolves in substance and complexity.

The American Board of Nursing Specialties (ABNS) (Hartshorn, 1991; Parker, 1994) was established in 1991 as a national peer review program for specialty nursing certification bodies with the purpose of improving nursing practice to meet the increasingly complex demands of the health care system. The ABNS promotes the highest quality of specialty nursing practice through recognition of approved national certification bodies and their programs (Hartshorn, 1991; Parker, 1994). The goals of the ABNS are twofold: (1) to serve as an advocate for consumer protection by establishing and maintaining standards of professional specialty nursing certification, and (2) to increase consumers' awareness of the meaning and value of specialty nursing certification.

ABNS approval requires uniform educational preparation of nurses seeking certification, i.e., a minimum of a baccalaureate degree in nursing and a specified educational program in the area of specialty practice. Advanced specialty nursing practice certification requires a graduate degree in nursing or the appropriate equivalent, including content in the specified area of specialty practice. ABNS requires either that this standard be in effect currently or that a plan be adopted for the standard to be in effect for new certificates no later than the year 2000 (Parker, 1994). Not all certifying bodies have accepted this standard, however (Hartshorn, 1991).

Other standards required of a certifying board include: that the specialty be defined as nursing, be distinct from other nursing specialties, require licensure, be national in scope with an identified need and demand for nurses certified in the specialty, have a substantial number of nurses practicing in the specialty, have a certification body that is autonomous in matters pertaining to certification while maintaining a collaborative relationship with a nursing specialty organization, have educational programs for preparing nurses in the specialty, engage in peer review, and maintain a provision for public consultation or representation (Parker, 1994).

Recommendations

Standards of Practice

Because standards of practice represent the level of quality of care demanded by a profession and the clients that it serves, it is imperative that the nursing profession itself define these standards for the specialty of nursing informatics. Nurses have worked with the ANA, through its Council on Nursing Systems and Administration, to develop separate standards unique to nursing informatics. Communication with members and nonmembers, as well as other nursing organizations, will promote the inclusion of all pertinent data into the ongoing development and revision of the standards document in the future. Incorporation of any research findings into the standards document will enhance the validity of the standards. Because nursing informatics is one element of the broader field of health informatics (ANA, 1994) collaboration with other organizations representing health informatics will enhance the validity of the nursing standards document. Also, because nursing informatics includes clinical nursing practice as an integral part of the specialty, it would be useful to use the ANA Standards of Clinical Nursing Practice (ANA, 1991) to guide the practice of nursing informatics in addition to the document that relates specifically to the areas of practice owned solely by the specialty of nursing informatics.

Certification

Nurses should consider becoming active in their professional organizations, including work towards attaining representation on a certifying board. If this level of involvement is not possible, nurses can consider using their expertise to act as a test-item writer. If all nurses who profess a level of expertise in nursing informatics practice, education, and/or research become involved in the certification process, the validity of the process will be greatly enhanced.

Role delineation studies outlining the practice of both the generalist in nursing informatics and/or the informatics nurse specialist should be undertaken by the nursing profession. In addition to working with the requirements of the certifying body on a certification program in nursing informatics, nurses involved in this process should also use the ABNS standards (Parker, 1994) for approval of certification programs in their planning process to ensure that the certification program will receive ABNS approval.

Nurses should act as advocates for each other in the nursing informatics certification process. Nurse administrators should recognize the standard of excellence demonstrated by nurses certified in nursing informatics. Nurse educators and researchers should strive to continue to move the field of nursing informatics forward through curriculum development, nursing informatics research, and funding appropriation for nursing informatics education and research.

Summary

The specialty of nursing informatics holds much promise for the future as providers strive to manage the data produced from a myriad of information sources to provide high-quality, cost-effective health care to society. Nursing informatics' place as a specialty in nursing can be fostered and validated by defining and reinforcing its standards of practice. Further, the development of a certification program in nursing informatics announces to the public and to the profession the standard of excellence in practice that can be expected of individuals specializing in nursing informatics. Through these efforts nursing informatics will demonstrate its unique contributions to the profession of nursing, to other health informatics disciplines, to the health care profession as a whole and, most importantly, to the well-being of the society it serves.

References

American Nurses Association. (1980). *Nursing: A Social Policy Statement.* Kansas City, MO: Author.

ANA American Nurses Association. (1991a). *Standards of Clinical Nursing Practice.* Washington, DC: American Nurses Association.

American Nurses Association. (1991b). Task force on nursing practice standards and guidelines: Working paper. *Journal of Quality Assurance, 5*(3), 1-17.

American Nurses Association. (1994). *Nursing Informatics Scope of Practice.* Washington, DC: American Nurses Association.

American Nurses Credentialing Center. (1993a). *American Nurses Credentialing Center Certification Catalog.* Washington, DC: Author.

American Nurses Credentialing Center. (1993b). *Study Guide for ANCC Certification Examinations* (1993 ed.). Washington, DC: Author.

Carter, E. W. (1986). *Credentialing in Nursing: Contemporary Developments in Nursing. The 1979 Study of Credentialing in Nursing Recommendations: Where Are We Now?* Kansas City, MO: American Nurses Association.

Fickeissen, J. L. (1990). 56 ways to get certified. *American Journal of Nursing, 90*(3), 50-57.

Gassert, C. A. (1990). Structured Analysis: Methodology for developing a model for defining nursing information requirements. *Advances in Nursing Science, 13*(2), 53-62.

Graves, J., and Corcoran, S. (1988). Design of nursing information systems: Conceptual and practice elements. *Journal of Professional Nursing, 4*(3), 8-177.

Graves, J., and Corcoran, S. (1989). The study of nursing informatics. *Image, 21*(4), 227-231.

Hartshorn, J. C. (1991). A national board for nursing certification. *Nursing Outlook, 39*(5), 226-229.

Heller, B. R., Romano, C. A., Moray, L. R., and Gassert, C. A. (1989). Special follow up report: The implementation of the first graduate program in nursing informatics. *Computers in Nursing, 7*(5), 209-213.

Parker, J. (1994). Development of the American Board of Nursing Specialties (1991-1993). *Nursing Management, 25*(1), 33-35.

Peplau, H. (1965). Specialization in Professional Nursing. *Nursing Science, 3*(4), 268-287.

Pluyter-Wenting, E., and Nieman, H. B. J. (1988). Computer technology and nursing management: The need for education. In H. E. Peterson, and U. Gerdin-Jelger (Eds.), *Preparing Nurses for Using Information Systems: Recommended Information Competencies* (pp. 111-138). New York: National League for Nursing.

Ropka, M. E., Norback, J., Rosenfeld, M., Miller, C., and Nielsen, B. (1992). Evolving a blueprint for certification: The responsibilities and knowledge comprising American professional oncology nursing practice. *Oncology Nursing Forum, 19*(5), 745-759.

Schwirian, P. M. (1986). The NI pyramid—A model for research in nursing informatics. *Computers in Nursing, 4*(3), 134-136.

Simpson, R. (1992). Informatics: Nursing's newest specialty. *Nursing Management, 23*(8), 26-27.

Staggers, N., and Parker, P. L. (1993). Description and initial applications of the Staggers & Parks nurse-computer interaction framework. *Computers in Nursing, 11*(6), 263-268.

Styles, M. M. (1989). *On Specialization in Nursing: Toward a New Empowerment.* Kansas City, MO: American Nurses Foundation, Inc.

Nursing Informatics: Education for a New Specialty and Career

Barbara R. Heller, EdD, RN, FAAN
Dean and Professor
School of Nursing
University of Maryland at Baltimore

Mary Etta C. Mills, ScD, RN, CNAA
Chair and Associate Professor
Department of Education, Administration, Health Policy, and Informatics
School of Nursing
University of Maryland at Baltimore

Carol A. Romano, PhD, RN, FAAN
Director, Clinical Systems and Quality Improvement
Clinical Center Nursing Department
National Institutes of Health

Introduction

In this era of unprecedented change in the health care industry, nursing must be prepared to move into the fast lane on the information superhighway. It is evident that computer technology will be both a driving force and a resource facilitating radical revision of the health care system (Van Cour, 1990). Nurses must become involved in directing the development of computer and information technologies and in managing the information systems that will advance nursing practice, administration, research, and education.

Key to the successful implementation of nursing information systems is their acceptance and integration into professional nursing practice. The designation of nursing informatics as a nursing specialty (American Nurses Association [ANA], 1992) as well as the recent articulation of Standards of Practice for Nursing Informatics (ANA, 1994) has heightened the awareness of the basic competencies required for specialized practice in nursing informatics.

The need for a cadre of knowledgeable nursing professionals able to respond proactively to the increased use of computers and to provide leadership in the design, application, management, and evaluation of information technology in nursing and health care has become abundantly clear. Greater nursing participation in information systems management has been mandated by the Joint Commission on Accreditation of Healthcare Organizations guidelines as well as by the Institute of Medicine's vision for a computer-based patient record.

While automated systems have already begun to revolutionize the management of patient care and other aspects of health care delivery, a significant impediment to the optimal integration of information systems in nursing practice is a knowledge deficit among nurses, ambivalence about the value of information systems in supporting their practice, as well as a dearth of leadership in the field. Many practicing nurses often are unaware of the potential benefit of information technology in decision support and in the organization of patient care including outcomes measurement. Both for these professionals and for students, instructional programs in the application of information technology can improve clinical and management decision-making skills. Greater educational opportunities also are needed to prepare nurses for careers in informatics, including leadership positions, in order to ensure that these information systems provide maximum value to nurses both in clinical practice and in management.

Informatics as an Area of Nursing Specialization

In little less than three decades considerable progress has been made in broadening the range of applications of computers in nursing and in developing a specialization in the field of nursing informatics. Continued evolution and enhanced credibility of nursing informatics as an area of specialization and a scientific discipline will depend on the further development of scholarly inquiry in the field.

In the early 1970's, a study to identify the needs of the health professions for education in medical computing was conducted under the auspices of the International Federation of Information Processing. This survey of Western countries concluded that not only should nurses have a general knowledge of computer and data processing, but also that a large number of nurses be should specially educated to contribute effectively to the development of automated systems for information handling (J. Anderson, Gremy, and Pages, 1974).

In 1985, Hannah defined nursing informatics as the use of information technologies in relation to the functions that are within the purview of nursing and are carried out by the nurse in the care of patients or in the educational preparation of individuals to practice the discipline. Informatics encompasses a wide range of activities related to the use of information management technologies to facilitate the conduct of nursing practice, education, administration and research (Schwirian, 1986).

According to Schwirian (1986, p. 134), the development of nursing informatics as a critical specialized professional focus is appropriate because the field of informatics: (1) contributes to the development of knowledge in the discipline of nursing; (2) enhances the communication of knowledge to present and new generations of nurses; and, finally, (3) enhances the application of knowledge in nursing practice. Schwirian's model for nursing research in the field of nursing informatics defined fertile areas for research in this field. She noted that information, computer technology and nursing form an interactive, interdependent relationship that typifies nursing informatics activity.

Graves and Corcoran (1989) further defined nursing informatics as combining computer science, information science and nursing science to assist in the management and processing or transformation of nursing data, information and knowledge. They viewed nursing informatics as a legitimate area of study in nursing science because it deals with the rules and processes of symbolically representing the phenomena of nursing. This statement supported S. Nelson's (1984) interpretation of informatics as having a focus on the nature of information, its access, the problem requiring information for resolution, and decision making based on the information obtained.

Today, nursing informatics can be characterized as an interdisciplinary field that combines nursing with management technologies and the information and computer sciences. It provides methodologies by which these fields can contribute to better use of the nursing knowledge base and ultimately to improved nursing practice. In this new environment, nurses must acquire a solid foundation in the use of automated systems both for nursing management and for the delivery of patient care. The health care field also requires nursing personnel who can control existing systems and stay abreast of emerging technology.

Need for Education in Nursing Informatics

It has been suggested that one reason for nursing's failure to fully capitalize on the potential of computer technology has been the paucity of specialized education programs (Heller, Romano, Damrosch, and Parks, 1985; Parks, 1986). At this point, only a few schools of nursing, including the University of Maryland, the University of Utah and Case Western Reserve University have programs or tracks in nursing informatics at the graduate level. However, a growing number of programs offer cognates in information science.

According to R. Nelson and Joos (1992), most informatics nurses have educated themselves through networking and a variety of informal learning opportunities including institutes and workshops in informatics sponsored by national and international special interest membership groups. Numerous continuing education conferences address nursing informatics issues, and several book and journal publications support research related to computer applications in nursing. In addition, two of the major national nursing organizations, the American Nurses Association and the National League for Nursing, support councils targeted specifically to nursing informatics members. However, Carty (1994) concludes that there is at present no systematic process for developing competencies in nursing informatics.

Competencies in Nursing Informatics

In 1988, Working Group Eight, Nursing Informatics, of the International Medical Informatics Association, identified three levels of competencies in nursing informatics (Peterson and Gerdin-Jelger, 1988). At the first level, nurses are users of information systems and have an awareness of, understand, use, and interact with those systems in their practice. At the second level, nurses modify and evaluate information systems. At the third level, nurses are system innovators and are responsible for designing and developing new information systems for nursing.

Work by Romano and Heller (1990) identified some key responsibilities of the Nursing Informatics Specialist. These included:

1. The identification of the properties, structure, use, and flow of clinical and management information from the patient, to the health care provider, and subsequently throughout the health care organization.

2. The assessment of real and potential problems related to the communication, accessibility, availability and use of information for clinical and administrative decision-making.

3. The determination of alternative methods of information handling and of system design options that consider subtle differences and the need for a high degree of flexibility. (p. 16)

The ANA (1994) has taken steps to initiate certification of the informatics nurse specialist. Standards of practice include the design, analysis, and evaluation of information systems to support the nursing process, decision-making, outcome identification, and planning.

The Role of the Nursing Informatics Specialist

Nurses are increasingly being employed in the health care environments in such capacities as Nursing Information Systems Specialists, Nursing Informaticians, and Nursing Informatics Specialists. Milholland (1992) estimated that approximately 5,000 nurses have identified nursing informatics as their area of specialty and interest. Advertisements and position descriptions for these jobs confirm the major responsibilities of these positions: planning, designing and implementing clinical and management information systems that facilitate clinical and administrative decision making. Nurses are functioning as project managers for the development and implementation of information technologies, as user training coordinators and as consultants for companies that are developing marketable information systems for nursing and health care. B. Anderson (1992) has outlined a variety of roles for the nursing informatics specialist including team liaison, coordinator of patient care systems, installer of information systems, product manager consultant, system specialist, system analyst and knowledge engineer.

Nurses also will be needed who can conduct research on the concepts underpinning the effective and creative design and use of information systems. These individuals will be instrumental in incorporating research results into new applications and evaluating their effectiveness. This type of informatics research can lead to a more effective interface of humans and computers in a synergistic model that favors and supports patient care.

Organizational Priorities

A national study conducted by Mills (1994) described the relationship of current and future organizational priorities for nursing informatics specialists as identified by Vice Presidents of Nursing in tertiary care hospitals. Responses from 111 individuals indicated that a majority of facilities surveyed (79.3%) had established positions for nursing informatics specialists. The positions had been in place for an average of 5.5 years. The individuals holding the positions had a wide range of educational experiences related to informatics, the most common being continuing education workshops and conferences. Less than half of the respondents (47.1%) had obtained college credits in informatics or computer science. Mills found that nursing information specialists were most heavily engaged in the areas of project management, staff training and implementation of clinical systems, and in advisory and coordinating capacities. Vice Presidents of Nursing also identified several areas of need, specifically communication between the Vice President of Nursing and the Nursing Information Specialist in the areas of systems planning, implementation of clinical nursing systems and strategic planning.

Educational Preparation for Nursing Informatics

Nursing informatics preparation is largely focused on the development of nursing expertise in the use of computer-based information systems in health care organizations and industry. Although it is recognized that all nurses will be using computer applications in their working environment, it was proposed by the International Federation for Information Processing (Anderson, 1974) and by the National League for Nursing Working Group on Nursing Informatics (Peterson, 1988) that education be stratified depending on the degree of involvement of the health professional. A stepped approach is recommended to make this vision a reality (Romano and Heller, 1990).

Baccalaureate Level Education—The Generalist Degree

Baccalaureate programs should produce competent generalists in informatics. While not specialists in informatics, these generalists should have an understanding of the various applications of information technology that support nursing processes (Travis, Root, Hoehn, Brennan, and Fitzpatrick, 1992). Graduates should have not only technical competence to use computers in nursing, but the skills to use information. In a model developed at Case Western Reserve University (Travis, Hoehn, Spees, Hribar, and Youngblut, 1993), undergraduate students complete an integrated informatics curriculum in which informatics courses are designed to articulate with the clinical experience and comprehensive course progression. The framework of the model consists of three basic components: information, technology and clinical care processes. Content areas include information flow in a patient-centered system, technical aspects of nursing informatics applications, and concepts such as the lifetime electronic medical record, nursing minimum data set and clinical decision making.

Master's-Level Education—The Degree of Specialization

Graduates at the master's level are generally known as Nursing Information Systems Specialists or Informatics Nurse Specialists. In practice settings, position titles for persons responsible for nursing information systems vary widely. In addition to Nursing Informatics Specialist, they may include Nursing Systems Analyst; Director of Nursing Systems; Program Director, Nursing Informatics; Nursing Automated Data Processing Coordinator; and Coordinator of Information Systems (Mills, 1994, p. 10).

Specialists at the master's level are prepared as experts to analyze nursing information requirements; design system alternatives; manage information technology; identify and implement user training strategies; and evaluate the effectiveness of clinical and/or management information systems in patient care. Graduate programs combine detailed study of the discipline of nursing with theoretical and practical foundations of management, clinical and information science. Post-master's study also may be a means of obtaining specialized knowledge in the field of nursing informatics.

While the application focus may be primarily based in clinical or administrative support, curricula specific to computer science and information technology may include courses on operations analysis, database systems, data communication and networks, decision support, modeling and simulation, artificial intelligence, and the human-computer interface. The application of computerization and information science in nursing and health care is addressed through the principles and processes of design, implementation and evaluation of computerized systems within the context of management, clinical, information and systems theory with a focus on nursing. Also emphasized is the analysis of information needs related to clinical and management decision making.

Doctoral-Level Education—The Degree of Scholarship

The University of Maryland School of Nursing, in 1991, established the first formal doctoral program with a specialization in nursing. While not organizing informatics as a specialization within the doctoral program, other universities such as the University of Utah, the University of Texas, the State University of New York at Buffalo, and Case Western Reserve University offer computer science cognates in order to build expertise in information technology. Doctoral program objectives in nursing informatics at the University of Maryland School of Nursing include preparing graduates to conceptualize nursing information requirements; to design effective nursing information systems; to create innovative information technology; to conduct research on integrating technology with nursing practice, administration, education and research; and to develop theoretical, practice, and evaluation models for nursing informatics.

The focus of educational preparation is on nursing theory, research, nursing informatics and related disciplines, particularly information science and computer science. Subject matter treated in courses includes nursing, information, ergonomic, cognitive and organizational theories as they apply to computer technology; research design and statistics; research issues in clinical and management information systems, administration, ethics and evaluation as areas of scholarly inquiry; innovation process design; decision analysis; and information needs analysis related to advanced practice in health care.

Nursing Informatics as a Career

Because of the pervasiveness of computer technology and information management systems, career opportunities in information services can be found in every national and international health-care-related industrial, governmental, and service organization. Nurses with preparation in informatics are highly sought to fill jobs in health care agencies, vendor companies, consulting firms, and academia (Gassert, 1991). Positions for Nursing Information Specialists were reported in 79.3% of tertiary care hospitals responding to a national survey (Mills, 1994). Most positions (65.8%) had been in place 5 years or less. Many of these positions were middle managers responsible for coordinating nursing information systems, serving as liaisons between nursing and information systems departments, and systems analysts. Vice Presidents of Nursing enthusiastically endorsed the need for nurses to be prepared at the graduate level (master's and doctoral) in nursing informatics for these positions as well as for upper level management positions responsible for directing information services.

Vendors employ informatics nurse specialists to assist with systems installation, to demonstrate systems and to serve as project managers. Consulting firms utilize nurses in informatics to analyze communications and organizational systems needs and to assist in or manage the process of systems selection, implementation and evaluation. Academic institutions seek qualified informatics faculty with doctoral preparation to engage in student instruction, program development and research.

As health care increasingly automates the process of information management and diversifies the type and location of service delivery, there will be concomitant growth in the need for nurses prepared in informatics. Standardization of data, computerized patient records, integrated information systems and network management will create special opportunities for those nurses prepared to accept them.

Summary

Computers have come into use in virtually every aspect of modern health care. Future-oriented schools of nursing are incorporating nursing informatics into the basic baccalaureate curriculum and offering an opportunity for students to specialize in nursing informatics at the master's and doctoral levels. Careers in nursing informatics extend across such diverse organizations as health care agencies, vendors, consulting firms and education and research institutions.

As the use of information technology in health care continues to surge and as automated systems continue to revolutionize the management of patients and the organization of health care delivery, educational programs must be more widely available to provide the requisite knowledge and skills for the effective management of information systems. The impact of such programs will be to improve the quality of nursing services through the preparation of nursing informatics specialists who are qualified to practice in acute care, long-term care, or community-based settings. To be successful, nurses will require a long-term commitment to formal education in addition to work-related continuing education. As health care organizations come to recognize the nurse's role in information resource management, the nurse will be even more of a key player in planning and decision making. Computer and information technology has only begun to affect nursing practice. Nursing leaders are increasingly realizing the value of clinically driven technology and are actively participating in the development, management and integration of automated nursing information systems. The importance of education in nursing informatics has been acknowledged and several university-level programs have been developed to prepare Nursing Informatics Specialists. The increased availability of informatics specialists who possess the skills and knowledge to direct the use of information technology will help to keep nurses in the driver's seat on the information superhighway.

References

American Nurses Association. (1994). *Nursing Informatics Scope of Practice.* Washington, DC: Author.

Anderson, B. (1992). Nursing Informatics: Career Opportunities inside and out. *Computers in Nursing, 10*(4), 165-170.

Anderson J., Gremy, F., and Pages, J. C. (1974). *Education in Informatics of Health Personnel.* New York: Elsevier.

Carty, B. (1994). The protean nature of the nurse informaticist. *Nursing and Health Care, 15*(4), 174-177.

Gassert, C. A. (1991). Preparing for a career in nursing informatics. In P. B. Marr, R. L. Axford, and S. K. Newbolt (Eds.), *Nursing Informatics '91: Proceedings of the Post Conference on Health Care Information Technology: Implications for Change* (pp. 163-166). New York: Springer-Verlag New York.

Graves, J. R., and Corcoran, S. (1989). The study of nursing informatics. *Image, 21*(4), 227-231.

Hannah, K. J., Guillemin, E. J., and Conklin, D. N. (Eds.). (1985). *Nursing Uses of Computers and Information Sciences.* Amsterdam: Elsevier Science.

Heller, B. R., Romano, C., Damrosch, S., and Parks, P. (1985). Computer applications in nursing: Implications for the curriculum. *Computers in Nursing, 7*(5), 209-213.

Milholland, D. K. (1992, March). Congress says informatics is a specialty. *American Nurse,* p. 2.

Mills, M. E. (1994). Organizational priorities for the nursing informatics specialist. In S. J. Grobe, and E. S. P. Pluyter-Wenting, (Eds.), *Nursing Informatics: An International Overview for Nursing in a Technological Era* (pp. 8-12). Amsterdam: Elsevier Science.

Nelson, R., and Joos, I. (1992). Strategies and resources for self-education in nursing informatics. In J. Arnold, and G. Pearson, (Eds), *Computer Applications in Nursing Education and Practice.* New York: National League for Nursing.

Nelson, S. (1984). Education and research in medical information science. *Medical Informatics, 9*(3/4), 265-267.

Parks, P., Damrosch, S., Heller, B., and Romano, C. (1986). Comparison of nursing faculty and student definitions of computer learning needs. In R. Salamon, B. Blum, and M. Jorgensen, (Eds.), *MEDINFO 86: Proceedings of the 5th World Congress on Medical Informatics* (pp. 950-954). Amsterdam: North Holland.

Peterson, H. E., and Gerdin-Jelger, U. (Eds.). (1988). *Preparing Nurses for Using Information Systems: Recommended Informatics Competencies.* New York: National League for Nursing.

Romano, C., and Heller, B. (1990). Nursing informatics: A model curriculum for an emerging role. *Nurse Educator, 15*(2), 16-19.

Schwirian, P. (1986). The NI pyramid—A model for research in nursing informatics. *Computers in Nursing, 4*(3), 134-136.

Travis, L. L., Hoehn, B., Spees, C., Hribar, K., and Youngblut, J. (1993). Supporting collaboration through a nursing informatics curriculum. In *Proceedings of the Seventeenth Annual Symposium on Computer Applications in Medical Care* (pp. 419-423). New York: McGraw-Hill Book Co.

Travis, L. L., Root, A., Hoehn, B., Brennan, P., and Fitzpatrick, J. J. (1992). An integrated informatics curriculum in a baccalaureate nursing program. In *Proceedings of the Sixteenth Annual Symposium on Computer Applications in Medical Care* (pp. 278-282). New York: McGraw-Hill Book Co.

Van Cour, P. J. (1990). Abating information anxiety: A proactive vision. In M. R. Bleich, and M. J. Bratton, (Eds.), *Information Management and Computers* (pp. 171-179). Baltimore: Williams & Wilkins Co.

Research Focus Areas in Informatics

Carol A. Romano, PhD, RN, FAAN
Director, Clinical Systems and Quality Improvement
National Institutes of Health Clinical Center

Barbara R. Heller, EdD, RN, FAAN
Professor And Dean
School of Nursing
University of Maryland at Baltimore

Mary Etta C. Mills, ScD, RN, CNNA
Associate Professor And Chair
Department of Nursing Education, Administration, Health Policy and
Informatics
School of Nursing
University of Maryland at Baltimore

Introduction

In the last three decades, considerable progress has been made in wide-ranging applications of computers in nursing (Heller and Romano, 1985) and the emergence of specialization in the field of nursing informatics (Heller and Damrosch, 1989). Experts acknowledge, however, that further evolution and enhanced credibility of nursing informatics as a scientific discipline will depend on scholarly inquiry in the field as well as dissemination and application of research results (Jacox and Meyer-Petrucci, 1988; Ozbolt, 1989).

To establish future directions and goals for a research agenda in nursing informatics, an assessment of past achievement is essential. To accomplish this, a study was undertaken to critically examine the published research literature in nursing informatics. The purpose of this paper is : (1) to report the state-of-the-art scholarly research in the field; (2) to identify the foci and scope of the research; (3) to categorize the literature into key areas of study; and (4) to describe trends and issues identified in nursing informatics research over a 30-year span. Based on this review, specific recommendations are proposed regarding potential priorities for a program of research in informatics. In addition, recommendations for establishing national priorities for federal funding in nursing informatics are also set forth.

Review of Existing Studies

For purposes of this study, nursing informatics was defined as the use of information technology by nurses in the care of patients, administration of health care facilities, and education of individuals in the discipline (Peterson and Gerdin-Jegler, 1988). The study consisted of a review of 11 sources of published nursing research literature. Manuscripts selected for this review were those that presented results or conclusions based on reported systematic research in an area of study. Most of the sources of publication were handsearched, rather than computer-searched. No attempt was made to evaluate the quality, rigor, content, or methodology used by the authors. Descriptive and experimental as well as quantitative and qualitative studies were included. All studies were classified by one author at two different points in time several months apart to ensure intrarater reliability. In addition, interrater reliability was established with the help of a research assistant.

The 11 sources consulted were distributed into three primary groups: journals/books, dissertations, and proceedings. The journals/books sources included Nursing Reference (Pocklington and Gutmann, 1984), an annotated bibliography for computer literature; nursing research journals (Nursing Research, Western Journal of Nursing Research, Research in Nursing and Health Care, Advances in Nursing Science, Journal of Professional Nursing); and the specialty journal Computers in Nursing.

In addition, a booklet prepared by the National League for Nursing (NLN) entitled Preparing Nurses for Using Information Systems (Peterson and Gerdin-Jegler, 1988) was reviewed for potential research resources. Two proceeding sources included Proceedings of the Symposium on Computer Applications in Medical Care (SCAMC) (1981-1990), and Proceedings of the 5th World Congress of Medical Informatics (Soloman, Blum, and Johnson, 1986). Dissertation Abstracts was also consulted. A total of 264 citations regarding nursing informatics research were identified and categorized into discrete research areas.

Although citations were found in the nursing literature as early as 1963, the latter half of the 1980s yielded the majority of research publications, with the highest number of 32 (12%) occurring in 1986. A total of 141 citations (53%) were found in the earlier 25-year period (1961-1985), while 123 citations (47%) were found within the last 5 years (1986-1990), alone.

The greatest number of research publications (40%) was found in the Proceedings of the Annual Symposium on Computer Applications in Medical Care (SCAMC), which began formal sessions on nursing content in 1981. Dissertation Abstracts yielded the second highest volume of identified research (26%), followed by both the Nursing Reference (12%), and the refereed journal Computers in Nursing (14%), which began publication in 1984. The remaining three sources consisted of nursing research journals, the NLN booklet, and the Proceedings of the 5th World Congress of Medical Informatics, which comprised 4% of the total research publications found.

Conceptual Framework and Results

The organizing framework used to categorize the 264 identified studies was adapted from a model devised by the National Library of Medicine (NLM), (Graves and Corcoran, 1989). This framework was used to propose a plan for reaching the long-range goals of medical informatics research defined by the NLM as the computer-supported accumulation, structuring, management, and dissemination of biomedical knowledge and expertise. The NLM defined eight areas of study to include the following categories: knowledge representation; knowledge and data acquisition; medical decision making; cognitive aspects of decision support; the human-machine interface; information storage and retrieval; technology transfer and dissemination; and supporting technologies and enabling activities. Each research area is described below.

Knowledge Representation

This first category of research based on the NLM model, knowledge representation, refers to the depiction of medical knowledge through its expression in mathematical and symbolic form. This includes representing numerical values of data, non-numeric forms of information, and methodologies for expressing symbolic knowledge (factual, experiential, judgmental, or problem solving). The study of knowledge representation includes the use of logic, with well-developed semantic theory and rules for inference. It also includes use of semantic networks and systems with well-developed methods for structuring knowledge about the relationships between objects, facts, concepts, and constraints. Twelve nursing studies from this review were grouped into the category of knowledge representation, totaling approximately 5% of the research sample. Three were published in journals, two were cited in Dissertation Abstracts, and seven were published in conference proceedings.

Knowledge and Data Acquisition

The second category used by NLM to classify informatics research is knowledge and data acquisition. This category encompasses concepts and relations in knowledge bases defined by standard terms and language. A uniform system of terms and language creates standardized formats for collecting and reporting clinical data. In this area new tools are used for processing data and information into knowledge bases for intelligent retrieval and decision support, and the knowledge bases are extended by inference from raw data and processing text. Thirteen studies were grouped into this category, representing 5% of the total studies. Nine were cited in Dissertation Abstracts and four were published in conference proceedings.

Medical Decision Making

The third category, medical decision making, refers to any technology that can support a health care provider or administrator in the process of evaluating options and making choices to optimize patient care in terms of risk, outcome, costs, efficiency, and patient satisfaction. This includes deterministic, probabilistic, and heuristic strategies related to predefined outcomes, quantitative estimates of uncertainties, and descriptive decision analysis, respectively. Forty studies were grouped into this category, representing 15% of the total sample. Eight were published in journals, 11 were cited in Dissertation Abstracts, and 21 were published in conference proceedings.

Cognitive Issues

The fourth category, cognitive issues in medical informatics, encompasses research that describes and analyzes the processes of information search, storage, retrieval, utilization, and integration of knowledge that is based in the literature, along with the clinician's individual experience and understanding. Included are evaluation of the impact of biases on decision making; task and user characteristics that affect decision making; the effect of risks, benefits, values, and attitudes on decision making; the knowledge structure and reasoning strategies that characterize experts and novices. A total of 92 studies were grouped into the category of cognitive issues, representing 35% of the total research sample. Thirty were studies published in journals, 42 were cited in Dissertation Abstracts, and 20 were published in conference proceedings. This category of research encompassed the greatest number of citations found. Within this group, 32 manuscripts addressed the effect of computer-assisted instruction, and 28 focused on attitudes toward computerization.

Human-Machine Interface

The fifth category, human-machine interface, refers to the interaction or interface of the machine world of input/output devices and the cognitive world of information/knowledge assimilation, organization, and presentation. Human-machine interaction, such as the mechanics of computer use, graphics, and devices, as well as cognitive issues related to modeling and natural language interaction and explanation are encompassed in this area. Five studies were grouped into this category, representing 2% of the total research sample. One study was published in a nursing journal, two were cited in Dissertation Abstracts, and two were published in conference proceedings.

Storage and Retrieval

The sixth category, information storage and retrieval, involves the organization and structuring of knowledge, and its storage and retrieval as needed. Studies in this area include the application of knowledge in an efficient, efficacious, and cost-effective fashion. Seventeen studies were grouped into this category, representing 6% of the total research sample. Ten were studies published in journals, one was cited in Dissertation Abstracts and six were published in conference proceedings.

Technology Transfer and Dissemination

The seventh category, technology transfer and dissemination, describes the development of consensus for generic standards for operations and interfaces expected of machines, operating system environments, programs, and communication links among sites. This category includes efforts to define evaluation methodologies, standards for informatics applications, and training programs to instruct personnel in the development and dissemination of medical information systems. Sixty-two studies were grouped into the technology transfer and dissemination category, representing 23.5% of the total research sample. Nineteen were studies published in journals, three were studies cited in Dissertation Abstracts and 40 were published in conference proceedings.

Supporting Technologies and Enabling Activities

The eighth category, supporting technologies and enabling activities, identifies the problems surrounding design, implementation, dissemination, interface, integration, and maintenance of large medical information systems. This category explores the development of new hardware and software computing resources to collect, store, manipulate, and display the diverse kinds of information used in biomedicine and nursing, as well as programs that assist clinical care, research, library retrieval, communications, and financial management. Other areas identified for development are communication systems that link health personnel to each other and to information resources, and the training of health professionals to work in this highly specialized area. Twenty-three studies were grouped into the category of supporting technologies and enabling activities, representing 9% of the total research sample. Three were published in journals, five were cited in Dissertation Abstracts, 14 were published in conference proceedings, and one was an NLN publication.

Discussion

There are acknowledged limitations to this research classification process: the probability of nursing informatics research studies being reported in journals, the imprecision and difficulties involved in extracting studies from the literature, and the inaccessibility of proceedings that were not reviewed. The results of this survey, however, do offer a significant indicator of the status of informatics research and the trend of direction of inquiry. While research in all focus areas has increased, the greatest growth occurred in the categories of cognitive aspects of decision support, technology transfer and dissemination, and medical decision making (see Table 1).

Prior to 1986, the focus of research was almost evenly divided between cognitive aspects and technology transfer; in the past five years, however, the majority of research studies (by almost two to one) have focused on cognitive aspects. The key to this trend is the quantity of studies in this category related to computer-assisted instruction, skill training in critical thinking and cognitive monitoring, and perceptions and attitudes related to the implementation and utilization of computer systems. In the category of supporting

Table 1. Informatics Studies by Category and Timeframe

CATEGORIES	1961-1965	1966-1970	1971-1975	1976-1980	1981-1985	1986-1990
Knowledge Representation					5	7
Knowledge and Data Acquisition				2	3	8
Medical Decision-Making			2	2	14	22
Cognitive Aspects	2	2	3	6	37	42
Human-Machine		1			3	1
Information Storage			2	2	8	5
Technology Transfer		1	3	5	30	23
Supporting Technologies					8	15

technologies, the focus is now on the evaluation of system applications, including educational simulations and clinical and administrative data management. The absence of research in the area of clinical nursing practice is critical. The patient/consumer as the focus of study is also absent in all categories. Attention to the patient as the unit of analysis, especially in research related to computer-assisted instruction and learning, is clearly needed.

Several problems with the categorization framework were identified. For example, education and training are currently included within the definition of two existing focus areas (technology transfer and enabling activities) and are implied in the category of cognitive aspects, which addresses the learning processes of novices and experts. Education and training in the field of informatics, versus the use of information technology to educate clinicians, are cited as discrete areas for future study. The NLM categories are not mutually exclusive. For example, the technology transfer category refers to standardization of hardware, software, and communication networks for the purposes of the diffusion of usage, whereas the enabling activities category encompasses implementation strategies directed toward the "peopleware" issues of diffusing usage and acceptance of information technology with the professional communities.

The results of this research review and classification have implications for guiding research in nursing informatics. For example, the focus of informatics interest at the University of Maryland School of Nursing, which offers a graduate specialization program in informatics, has been in the four areas of cognitive aspects of decision support, human-machine interface, technology transfer and dissemination, and enabling activities. Related publications have involved decision making, evaluation, information technology, communication networks, screen design and computer interaction measures, and the diffusion of technology innovations.

Nursing Informatics Research Priorities

This study classified informatics research in nursing using the broad definition of nursing informatics (Peterson and Gerdin-Jegler, 1988). The findings uncovered the dearth of attention given to nursing informatics as it relates to enhancing patient care. In 1988, this concern was echoed by the National Center for Nursing Research's (NCNR—forerunner of the National Institute of Nursing Research) Priority Expert Panel on Nursing Informatics. This Panel was charged with defining national research priorities for funding to address the gaps in knowledge that impair clinical practice and that can be filled by new research. The panel concurred that the study of nursing informatics should address the structuring and processing of nursing information to arrive at clinical decisions and to build systems to support and/or automate that processing (Graves and Corcoran, 1989). With this consideration, the panel proposed the following six program goals for informatics research (National Center for Nursing Research, 1991):

•To establish nursing's language, including lexicons, classification systems, and taxonomies, as well as standards for nursing data.

•To develop methods to build data bases of clinical information (including data, diagnoses, objectives, interventions, and outcomes) and of management information (including staffing, charge capture, turnover, and vacancy rates) and to analyze relationships among them.

—To exploit the data bases to discover new clinical knowledge, including descriptions of diagnoses to which nurses attend and to test relationships among diagnoses, objectives, interventions, and outcomes;

—To exploit the data bases to discover relationships between management variables and patient care, e.g., to determine how nursing care is affected by staffing; and to develop methods of assessing cost-effectiveness, cost-benefits, and productivity that take into account the quality of care (including structure, process and patient outcomes) and institutional outcomes (nurse turnover and vacancy rates).

•To determine how nurses use data, information, and knowledge to give patient care, and how that is affected by differing levels of expertise and by organizational factors and working conditions; and to design information systems accordingly.

•To develop and test patient care decision support systems and knowledge delivery systems that are appropriate for nurses' needs, with consideration for expertise and organizational factors and working conditions.

•To develop prototypes and eventually working models of nurse workstations equipped with tools to provide nurses with all the information needed for patient care, research, and education, at the point of use, and linked to an integrated information system.

•To develop and implement appropriate methods to evaluate nursing information systems and applications, with particular attention to their effects on patient care.

Research Trends in the 1990s

The decade of the nineties witnessed not only defined national priorities for nursing informatics, with federal funding allocated to develop this body of knowledge, but also the nursing professional organizations' recognition of informatics as a specialty (Milholland, 1992). In addition, graduate curriculums in nursing informatics were developed at the University of Maryland and University of Utah School of Nursing. A doctoral program of study in nursing informatics also was initiated at the University of Maryland (Gassert, Mills, and Heller, 1991). Given this fertile environment conducive to research, these authors conducted a follow-up literature analysis in 1994 to determine if current trends in the beginning of this decade were consistent with the prior foci of study. An on-line literature analysis was begun in 1994 to determine if current trends in the beginning of this decade were consistent with the prior foci of study. An on-line literature search of three data bases was conducted by a nurse-librarian. The data bases were Dissertation Abstracts, Medline, and Computer Index in Nursing and Allied Health Literature. The search yielded 346 references. All of the references that reported abstracts were reviewed; of these, 26 reported research studies.

Of these 26 abstracts of research, 11 references focused on medical/nursing decision making, which was the category with the largest number of studies. Six references focused on knowledge representation. Also, these six studies included work on the development of nursing's language and taxonomies, and standards for nursing data. Interestingly, of the five studies cited in Dissertation Abstracts, three focused on decision making, one focused on knowledge acquisition, and one on human-machine interface.

The above data suggest that the prior focus on decision making is continuing and evolving (see Table 1). It is also important to recognize that the need to develop the language used by nursing is being addressed. This is consistent with the defined research priorities of the National Institutes of Nursing Research. Another evolving trend of significance is that the focus of research is beginning to emphasize clinical care. Ozbolt and Graves (1993) report that current research in clinical nursing informatics is proceeding along three important dimensions: (1) identifying and defining nursing language and the structure of its data; (2) understanding clinical judgment and decision making and how it can be facilitated by computer-based systems; and (3) discovering how systems can not only help process information, but also how access to information can change nursing care. The studies reviewed in this second literature analysis validate these three dimensions.

Summary

The ability to identify, evaluate, and use research studies in the field of informatics will contribute to the development of a unique body of knowledge to direct the application of information technology in nursing. Scholarly critique and research rigor will enable new studies to build on strengths of current work and to correct weaknesses. Current research can provide a platform upon which research replication can increase the applicability of research findings. The proposed NLM framework offers an initial step to begin assessing nursing research to date. The informatics program goals of the new National Institute of Nursing Research (formerly NCNR) also offers a focus for designing new studies. We conclude, however, that a framework for research and targeted areas for focus can provide a basis for future research and hence support collaborative efforts across disciplines to enhance patient care.

References

Ackerman, M. J. (Ed.). (1985). Proceedings of the Annual Symposium on Computer Applications in Medical Care (SCAMC). New York: Institute of Electrical Electronics Engineers.

Blum, B. I. (Ed.). (1982). Proceedings of the Annual Symposium on Computer Applications in Medical Care (SCAMC). New York: Institute of Electrical Electronics Engineers.

Cohen, G. S. (Ed.). (1984). Proceedings of the Annual Symposium on Computer Applications in Medical Care (SCAMC). New York: Institute of Electrical Electronics Engineers.

Dayhoff, R. E. (Ed.). (1983). Proceedings of the Annual Symposium on Computer Applications in Medical Care (SCAMC). New York: Institute of Electrical Electronics Engineers.

Gassert, C. A., Mills, M. E., and Heller, B. R. (1991). Doctoral specialization in nursing informatics. In P. D. Clayton (Ed.), Proceedings of the Annual Symposium on Computer Applications in Medical Care (SCAMC) (pp. 263-267). New York: Institute of Electrical Electonics Engineers.

Graves, J. R., and Corcoran, S. (1989). The study of nursing informatics. Image: Journal of Nursing Scholarship, 21, 227-231.

Greenes, R. A. (Ed.). (1988). Proceedings of the Annual Symposium on Computer Applications in Medical Care (SCAMC). New York: Institute of Electrical Electronics Engineers.

Hefferman, H. G. (Ed.). (1981). Proceedings of the Annual Symposium on Computer Applications in Medical Care (SCAMC). New York: Institute of Electrical Electronics Engineers.

Heller, B., Damrosch, S., Romano, C., and McCarthy, M. (1989). Graduate specialization in nursing informatics: A needs assessment. Computers in Nursing, 7(2), 68-77.

Heller, B., Romano, C., Damrosch S., and Parks, P. (1985). Computer application in nursing implications for the curriculum. Computers in Nursing, 3(1), 14-21.

Jacox, A., and Meyer-Petrucci, K. (1988). Support for Research in Computer Applications in Nursing Journal. In M. Ball, K. Hannah, V. G. Jelger, and H. Peterson (Eds.), Nursing Informatics—Where Caring and Technology Meet (pp. 253-259). New York: Springer-Verlag New York.

Kingsland, L. C. (Ed.). (1989). Proceedings of the Annual Symposium on Computer Applications in Medical Care (SCAMC). New York: Institute of Electrical Electronics Engineers.

Milholland, D. K. (1992). Congress says informatics is nursing specialty. American Nurse, 24(7), 10.

Miller, R. A. (Ed.). (1990). Proceedings of the Annual Symposium on Computer Applications in Medical Care (SCAMC). New York: Institute of Electrical Electronics Engineers.

National Center for Nursing Research. (1991). Nursing Informatics: Enhancing Patient Care. Bethesda, MD: U.S. Department of Health and Human Services, USPHS, NIH.

National Library of Medicine. (1986). Medical Informatics Report of Panel for Long Range Plan. Bethesda, MD.

Ozbolt, J. (1989). A Research Program in Nursing Informatics. Unpublished manuscript.

Ozbolt, J. G., and Graves, J. R. (1993). Clinical nursing informatics: Developing tools for knowledge workers. Nursing Clinics of North America, 28(2), 407-425.

Peterson, H. E., and Gerdin-Jegler, U. (Eds.). (1988). Preparing Nurses for Using Information Systems: Recommended Informatics Competencies. New York: NLN Publication N#14-2234.

Pocklington, D., and Guttman, L. (1984). Computer Literature. In Nursing Reference. Philadelphia: J. B. Lippincott Co.

Soloman, R., Blum, B., and Johnson, M. (Eds.). (1986). Proceedings of the 5th World Congress of Medical Informatics. North Holland: Elsevier Science Publishing Company.

Stead, W. W. (Ed.). (1987). Proceedings of the Annual Symposium on Computer Applications in Medical Care (SCAMC). New York: Institute of Electrical Electronics Engineers.

A Global Perspective on the Future of Informatics

Marion J. Ball, Ed.D.
Vice President, Information Services
University of Maryland at Baltimore
President
International Medical Informatics Association

Introduction

The new discipline of informatics is changing the field of health care throughout the world. A total of 39 contributors to this book have documented a wide range of informatics initiatives (see Figure 1). Efforts on the establishment of the computer-based patient record (CPR) within their bailiwick and on minimum data sets promise to establish databases for clinical decision making. Other activities target the development of strategies and support for clinical and administrative information. Despite their diversity, however, all of these efforts are designed to use information technologies to meet the needs of health care.

For the most part, the efforts described in this book are based in the United States. Yet much is occurring throughout the world that could enrich nursing informatics and improve health care. Moreover, an organization exists that is dedicated to international sharing and collaboration within and across the many disciplines and professions that contribute to the delivery of quality health care, whether through research, administration, professional education, or clinical services. This organization, the International Medical Informatics Association (IMIA), supports informatics worldwide with the purpose of advancing global health.

The International Medical Informatics Association

Membership and Governance

In the 1960s, a small band of pioneers, predominantly computer professionals, under the auspices of the International Federation of Information Processing (IFIP) began to explore the application of technology to health care. In 1967, the IFIP formed the TC4 committee under the leadership of Francois Gremy of France, who subsequently recruited the first generations of IMIA officers from the medical and health care communities. The interest of the TC4 members intensified and their numbers grew, until, in 1979, the IMIA was formally established by IFIP. In 1989, IMIA became an IFIP Affiliate Member and is now an apolitical, independent international organization with its Secretariat maintaining an office in Geneva, Switzerland.

IMIA has the status of a Non-Governmental Organization with special relations to the World Health Organization. Regional groups within IMIA include the European Federation for Medical Informatics, IMIA-Europe, and the Federation of Health Informatics Societies in Latin America. IMIA is also exploring the possibility of organizing a Pacific Rim Regional Group. Since its beginnings, IMIA has evolved and matured. Its aims are clearly stated and serve to focus its activities (see Figure 2). As it prepares to enter the

Figure 1.
What Is informatics?

What Is Informatics?

It is a new concept for health care. It can be defined on a number of dimensions. In terms of time, health care informatics is quite simply the next generation after traditional health care information systems. In terms of function, health care informatics is where caring and technology meet. In nursing, the clinical laboratory, radiology and the pharmacy, informatics is the application of information technology to enhance the quality of care, facilitate accountability and assist in cost containment.

Source: Healthcare Informatics. (1990, May). *Healthcare Informatics, 7*(5), 37.

Figure 2.
Aims of IMIA

Aims

To promote informatics in health care and biomedical research

To advance international cooperation

To stimulate research, development, and routine application

To further the dissemination of exchange of information

To encourage education and responsible behavior

To represent the medical and health informatics field within the World Health Organization and any other relevant professional or governmental organization

next century, IMIA is taking on a new role, that of a bridge organization, committed to moving from theory into practice. The IMIA Board has advocated this role in the conviction that collaboration is critical to the future of informatics. From its beginnings, IMIA has fostered international exchanges, with members coming from officially designated national societies and with a triennial international congress known as MedInfo.

Today IMIA comprises 35 member nations (see Figure 3). Each year a representative named by each attends a general assembly meeting and votes on issues. Over the years, IMIA's officers and board have reflected this international makeup, with informaticians from Europe, Asia, and the Americas playing leadership roles (see Figure 4).

In 1993, IMIA created a new membership category and began to actively recruit institutional members. Those joining include professional associations, medical centers, universities, consulting firms, and hardware and software companies (see Figure 5). In September 1993, IMIA offered its first Institutional Member Day in conjunction with the board and general assembly meetings in Japan. These events allow institutional members to learn from IMIA and its member nations about their activities in support of informatics. In turn, IMIA can gain from the expertise of individuals working outside academic medicine, in vendor organizations, professional associations, and elsewhere. Such collaboration is critical to the future of informatics and offers new opportunities for IMIA. Only through such liaisons can IMIA build upon the synergies emerging in the international community. The IMIA Board, comprised of the President, the Vice Presidents, Secretary, and Treasurer, conducts the ongoing business of IMIA. These officers are elected by the general assembly for a three-year term of office.

The extension of IMIA into new sectors replicates and reinforces its earlier efforts. As befits an organization born of two disciplines, medicine and computer science, IMIA has long encouraged crossdisciplinary and interdisciplinary activities. These are fostered by working groups, working conferences, and IMIA's triennial congress, MedInfo.

Figure 3.
IMIA membership

National Members (N=35)

Argentina	China	France	Italy	Nigeria	Spain
Australia	Croatia	Germany	Japan	Norway	Sweden
Austria	Cuba	Hong Kong	Korea	Portugal	Switzerland
Belgium	Czechoslovakia	Hungary	Mexico	Singapore	United Kingdom
Brazil	Denmark	Ireland	The Netherlands	Slovenia	United States of
Canada	Finland	Israel	New Zealand	South Africa	America

Correspondents (N=18)

Algeria	Greece	Indonesia	Malaysia	Romania	Uruguay
Bulgaria	Georgia	Iraq	Morocco	Saudi Arabia	Commonwealth of
Chile	India	Kuwait	Poland	Thailand	Independent
Egypt					States

Figure 4.
IMIA presidents (1968–1998)

Francois Gremy, France, 1968–1975

Jan Roukens, The Netherlands, 1975 –1980

David B. Shires, Canada 1980–1983

Hans Peterson, Sweden, 1983–1986

Shigekoto Kaihara, Japan, 1986–1989

Jos L. Willems, Belgium, 1989–1992

Marion J. Ball, United States, 1992–1995

Otto Rienhoff, Germany, 1995–1998

Figure 5.
Institutional members (effective 9/93)

American Health Information Management Association (AHIMA)

Apple Computer

Bayfront Life Services

Baylor College of Medicine

Bell Atlantic Healthcare

Center for Applied Medical Information Systems

Center for Healthcare Information Management (CHIM)

Digital Equipment Corporation

Emory Clinic

Ernst & Young

First Consulting Group

First Data Health Systems International

HBO & Company

Health Information and Management Systems Society (HIMSS)

Hewlett-Packard

Kaiser Permanente

M. D. Anderson Cancer Center

Monash University

PHAMIS Incorporated

Peat Marwick

Working Groups/Conferences

Of special significance for the readers of this book is the IMIA Working Group (WG) 8 on Nursing Informatics, formally authorized by the IMIA General Assembly meeting in Australia in September 1982, immediately following the first international forum on the impact of computers on nursing held in England earlier that same month. Today WG8 serves as an international focus for activities in nursing informatics and provides valuable global linkages for those working in this evolving discipline.

WG8 is currently headed by Elly S. P. Pluyter-Wenting, who is also Vice President of the BAZIS Foundation in The Netherlands. Today, representatives of 21 countries are members of WG8 (see Figure 6). The group sponsors a triennial international symposium

Figure 6.
Countries represented on WG8

Australia	Denmark	Hong Kong	Italy	Norway	Switzerland
Belgium	Finland	Iceland	Japan	Portugal	United Kingdom
Brazil	France	Ireland	The Netherlands	Spain	United States
Canada	Germany	Israel	New Zealand	Sweden	

Figure 7.
Working groups

WORKING GROUPS

WG1. Information Science and Medical Education

WG4. Data Protection in Health Information Systems

WG5. Primary Health Care Informatics

WG6. Coding and Classification of Health Data

WG7. Biomedical Pattern Recognition

WG8. Nursing Informatics

WG9. Health Informatics for Development

WG10. Hospital Information Systems

WG11. Dental Informatics

WG13. Organizational Impact of Medical Informatics

WG14. Health Professional Workstation

WG15. Technology Assessment and Quality Development in Health Informatics

on nursing informatics. Traditionally, this symposium is scheduled one year prior to the MedInfo Conference and has associated with it a closed invitational working conference which discusses issues critical to the nursing profession and the nursing informatics discipline. Proceedings are published for the symposium; in 1994, the fifth of these well-attended events was held in Texas, USA.

Working groups in IMIA address a range of areas, from data protection and biomedical pattern recognition to hospital information systems (see Figure 7). As nursing informatics has grown, it has made its presence known within these other working groups. For example, in September 1992, the Heidelberg Working Conference sponsored by WG1 on Information Science and Medical Education touched upon two U.S. programs in nursing informatics, at the universities of Maryland and Utah. Two other health disciplines, pharmacy and dentistry, also have established working groups.

Working conferences and working groups enable IMIA to respond to the rapid evolution of informatics in health care. Working conferences can address emerging areas, as did two 1993 working conferences, one on health care professional workstations and another on the organizational impact of informatics.

As invited participants at the workstation conference, nurses helped to address critical issues surrounding the workstation as an enabling technology for the CPR. Subgroups addressed functional requirements, user interfaces, data and knowledge management, processing (hardware/software), and networking/communications.

Such conferences serve to establish the viability of new working groups in their areas. Proposals are now before IMIA to grant working group status to the health professional workstation. Other proposals have been submitted in the areas of technology assessment, health evaluation, and radiology; others will no doubt emerge over time.

Since 1985, fourteen working conferences have published proceedings (see Figure 8). Generally these have been invitational working conferences; however, a few have been open to all interested parties. Plans for certain groups, such as the working conference on hospital information systems held in Atlanta, Georgia, in 1994, reflect the nursing model. The HIS group proposed a closed working conference to be offered in tandem with an

Figure 8.
Selected IMIA publications since 1985

MedInfo Proceedings

MedInfo 86. R. Salamon, B. I. Blum, M. Jorgensen, (Eds.), 1986.

MedInfo 89. B. Barber, D. Cao, D. Qin, G. Wagner, (Eds.), 1989.

MedInfo 92. K. C. Lun, P. Degoulet, T. E. Piemme, O. Rienhoff (Eds.), 1992.

Working Conference Proceedings

Human-Computer Communications in Healthcare. H. E. Peterson and W. Schneider, (Eds.), 1986.

System Analysis of Ambulatory Care in Selected Countries. Reichertz, Engelbrech, and Piccolo. (Eds.), 1986. Springer-Verlag
   GmbH.

Maintaining a Healthy State Within the Individual. E. K. Harris and T. Yasaka. (Eds.), 1987.

Progress in Biological Function Analysis. J. L. Willems, J. H. van Bemmel and J. Michel, 1988.

Nursing and Computers. N. Daly and K. J. Hannah, (Eds.), 1988. C. V. Mosby Company.

Towards New Hospital Information Systems. A. R. Bakker, M. J. Ball, J. R. Scherrer, and J. L. Willems. (Eds.), 1989.

Computerized Natural Medical Language Processing for Knowledge Representation. J. R. Scherrer, R. A. Cote, S. Mandil.
   (Eds.), 1989.

International Primary Care Computing. G. M. Hayes and H. Robinson. (Eds.). 1991.

Knowledge, Information and Medical Information. J. H. van Bemmel and J. Zvarova, (Eds.), 1991.

Software Engineering in Medical Informatics. T. Timmers and B. Blum. (Eds.), 1991.

Telecommunication in Medicine. J. S. Duisterhout, R. Salamon, A. Hasman. (Eds.), 1991.

Trends in Modern Hospital Systems. A. R. Bakker, C. T. Ehlers, J. R. Bryant, and W.E. Hammond, 1992.

Yearbook of Medical Informatics 92. J. H. van Bemmel and A. T. McCray. (Eds.), 1992: Schattauer Verlagsgesellschaft mbH.

Yearbook of Medical Informatics 93. J. H. van Bemmel, A. T. McCray. (Eds.), 1993: Schattauer Verlagsgesellschaft mbH.

The Health Professional Workstation. M. J. Ball, J. S. Silva, J. V. Douglas, P. Degoulet, and S. Kaihara, 1993.

All are published by North-Holland/Elsevier Science Publishers unless otherwise noted, in addition to the IMIA Newsletter.

---

open meeting. This model allows IMIA to further its expertise in highly defined areas while also sharing information with the wider community. Such a strategy is structured to bring theory into practice.

MedInfo

The main event sponsored by IMIA remains the triennial congress on medical informatics. Member nations compete for the opportunity to host this event, which strives to reach the widest audience (see Figure 9.) The next MedInfo—the eighth in the series—is scheduled to be held July 1995 in Vancouver, British Columbia, Canada. Planning and managing the meeting are the responsibilities of the Organizing Committee (OC) and the Scientific Program Committee (SPC); the Editorial Committee is responsible for the proceedings. The specifics of this MedInfo reflect the directions that IMIA is taking: The chair of the OC for MedInfo 95 is a leading nurse informatician, Dr. Kathryn J. Hannah. Her co-chair, Steven Huesing, comes from a vendor association. The site, between Asia and the Western Hemisphere, on the edge of the Pacific Rim, reflects IMIA's commitment to collaboration. With the theme "From Theory into Practice," this will be the first MedInfo to include institutional members among its participants.

Like past congresses, MedInfo 95 will be clearly international and interdisciplinary. Consider MedInfo 92 and its scientific program as illustrative. After 1,166 inquiries from 51 countries, the SPC received 627 submissions from 41 countries. Of those, 414, including 33 workshops, were accepted. Arranged thematically into 17 sections, the proceedings covered a wide range of topics, from computer systems technology to quality assessment and assurance. A section on nursing informatics included a total of 23 contribu-

Figure 9.
MedInfo sites

Stockholm, 1974	Washington, DC, 1986
Toronto, 1977	Beijing and Singapore, 1989
Tokyo, 1980	Geneva, 1992
Amsterdam, 1983	Vancouver, 1995

tions in three sections: concepts, issues and standards; computer approaches to nursing education; and computer systems for nursing management and practice. Contributions to the nursing section came from nine countries, with strong representation from the United States and the United Kingdom.

New Initiatives

As the decade of the 1990s moves toward a mid-point, IMIA continues to launch new initiatives. For IMIA, informatics is the discipline that transforms computing and communications into enabling technologies. These technologies are the building blocks for enterprise systems-_systems that will ultimately comprise global networks. We stand on the threshold of the world informaticians have envisioned, with health care information available when, where, and how it is needed. In the United States, we can build upon federal undertakings like the Unified Medical Language System and High Performance Computing and Communications and use them to bridge the differences and distances which have in the past separated us from the rest of the world. We can benefit from advances in knowledge engineering and the development of interfaces based upon a growing understanding of cognitive processing.

With informatics as our enabler, we can go beyond the limitations of hardware and software. As health professionals, we will be free to focus on the "learnware" and "peopleware" that teach and deliver health care. We will be empowered to collaborate on vital issues, from patient care to research to education. Today the door is open to a new wave of knowledge sharing. As an organization dedicated to furthering informatics, IMIA is pledged to see the health professions into that future. For IMIA, informatics truly is the discipline "where caring and technology meet."

For more information about IMIA, contact:
Marion J. Ball, Ed.D.
President
International Medical Informatics Association
100 North Greene Street
Baltimore, MD 21201-1502 USA

Index

A

Adoption of Innovation Theory, 116-120, 123
Advance directives, 194-195
Alcohol treatment, patient confidentiality and, 266-267
Allergy identification, 195-196
Agency for Health Care Policy and Research (AHCPR), 167
AIDSLINE, 175
AIDSNET, 186
AJN-Net, 178
ALERT, 176
American Board of Nursing Specialties, 285
American Nurses Association, policy development and, 272-278
Americans with Disabilities Act, 269
Ambulatory care, Omaha System and, 39-43
American Organization of Nurse Executives, 28, 31
Automated speech recognition (ASR), 239-244
AVLINE, 175-176

B

Bedside systems
  and restructuring of nursing care, 222-228
  technology assessment and, 74-81
Bench marking, 30
Benefits management, 99-107
BITNET, 174, 180
Blood administration, 195
Bulletin boards, 184
Business systems, 96

C

CANDI, 47
CareMap, 200-215
Case management
  CareMap and, 200-215
  technology and, 144-151
Center for Health Policy Research (CHPR), 155-156
Certification, 283-286
Change, preparation for, 117, 118-120
Cleveland Free-Net, 185
Coding standards, 273
Collaborative Pathways, 210
Communication technologies, nurse executives and, 230-238
Community Health Management Information Systems (CHMIS), 34, 62, 183
Comprehensive Community Health Information Networks (C-CHIN), 5
Comprehensive Health Enhancement Support System (CHESS), 186-187
Computer-Aided Instruction (CAI), 96-97, 216-217
Computer-based Patient Record (CPR), 17, 32, 35, 138-143, 260
Computer-based training (CBT), 129-135, 218
Computerized adaptive testing (CAT), 218
ComputerLink, 85
Confidentiality, patient data and, 257-263, 264-270
Content standards, 274
Continuity of care, 197
Continuous Quality Improvement (CQI), 68-69, 156-158, 193-194
Contracts, in joint-development projects, 110-113
Cost justification model, 103-104

D

Data
  confidentiality of, 257-263, 264-270
  definition of, 2-3
  input of, 34
  nursing practice and, 28-29
  output of, 35
  processing of, 34-35
  storage and retrieval of, 35
Data bases
  for ambulatory and home care, 39-43
  purpose of, 3
Deceased patient, medical records and, 267-268
Decision-support systems (DSS)
  descriptions of, 46-49
  for acute care nurses, 32-37
  for nurse managers, 45-53
  patient care and, 95-96
  purchase of, 52-53
Denver Free-Net, 187-191
Desktop computers, integrated, 236
Documentation systems, 93, 197-198, 239-244
Drug treatment, patient confidentiality and, 266-267

E

Easley-Storfjell Caseload/Workload Analysis, 160
Ecology, organizational, 84-85
Education of staff, 216-221
E-mail, 174, 230-233
Eo, 236
Ethical issues, patient data and, 257-263
E.T. Net, 218

F

Federal Computer Security Act, 269
FidoNet, 174, 178-179
FITNET, 174, 175, 180
Food and Drug Administration, 176
FREENETS, 177

G

GRATEFUL MED, 176

H

Hardware
  installation of, 121-122
  selection of, 217
Health Care Financing Administration (HCFA), 171, 275
Health care networks, 4-5
Health care reform, 29-30, 260-261
Health Care Technology Assessment (HCTA), 74-81
Health Maintenance Organizations (HMOs), 56-57
Home care, Omaha System and, 39-43
Hospital Information Systems (HIS), 93-94, 194-198, 219-220
HSTAR, 176
HSTAT, 176
Human immunodeficiency virus, patient confidentiality and, 265-266

I

Incompetent patient, medical records and, 267
Indicator Measurement System (IMSystem), 65, 70-72
Infection control, 196
Informatics. *See* Nursing informatics
Information management
administrative information and, 4
clinical information and, 4, 97-98
data bases and, 3
definition of, 2-3
environmental context of, 4
ethics and, 257-263
framework for, 3-4
future of, 4-5
information systems and, 3
Information standards, 273-274
Information systems
cost-effectiveness of, 77, 220, 223
cost justification model and, 103-104
culture and, 83-84
definition of, 3
implementation of, 116-127
innovation models and, 88
managed care and, 200-215
managed competition and, 56-57
nurse participation in, 7-8
organizational impact of, 83-90
patient-centered outcomes and, 153-165
requirements for, 7-14
resistance to, 87-88
standards for, 64-73
strategic planning and, 57-62
technology assessment and, 74-81
trends in, 97-98
types of, 92-97
user training for, 101-102, 123-124
Innovation models, 88
International Classification of Diseases (ICD), 274
International Medical Informatics Association, 303-308
Internet, 174-175
Intervention Scheme, 42

J-K

Joint Commission on Accreditation of Healthcare Organizations (JCAHO), and standards for informations systems, 64-73
Joint-development projects
benefits of, 109-110
contract negotiations for, 110-113
health care computing and, 109
nurse executives and, 113-115
schedule for, 112
vendor-client teams in, 108

L

LISTPROCs, 177
LISTSERVs, 180

M

Managed care, 200-215
Managed competition, 56-57
Medication administration, 196-197
Medical records, confidentiality and, 264-270
MedInfo, 307-308
MEDLARS, 175-176
MEDLINE, 175
Message standards, 273
Minor patient, medical records and, 267
Model for Defining Nursing Information System Requirements (MDNISR), 8-14
Multidisciplinary Action Plan (MAP), 211

N

National League for Nursing, 177
Networking, electronic, 174-191
Newsgroups, 177
Newton, 236
Nightingale, Florence, 28, 29
North American Nursing Diagnosis Association (NANDA), 18, 33
Nurse Corner, 184
Nurse executives
communication technologies for, 230-238
joint-development projects and, 113-115
Nurse extenders, 226

NurseLink, 184-185
Nurse managers
decision-support systems for, 45-53
role of in system implementation, 116-127
Nursing documentation, 24-25, 93, 197-198, 239-244
Nursing education, 96-97
Nursing informatics
certification in, 280-287
description of, 3
education and, 288-293
future of, 303-308
patient outcomes and, 171-172
research areas in, 295-301
standards of practice for, 280-287
Nursing Interventions Classification (NIC), 18-21, 33
Nursing language, computerization of, 16-26, 169, 276
Nursing Management Minimum Data Set (NMMDS), 30-31
Nursing Minimum Data Set (NMDS)
acute care and, 32-37
elements of, 33
information standards and, 275-276
nursing interventions and, 17
nursing's future and, 30-31
Nursing process
American Nurses Association and, 274
bedside computers and, 226-228
Nursing research, 97, 295-301

O

Omaha System, 39-43
Oncology Clinical Information System (OCIS), 49
Organization
culture of, 83-84
ecology of, 84-85
psychosocial system of, 86
roles of, 86
resistance within, 87-88
structure of, 85
Outcome Concept Systems (OCS), 162-164
Outcomes management (OM), 156-158
Outcome measurement, 167-172

P

PACE, 46
Pain Management System, 47
Patient acuity/intensity, 159-160
Patient care decision-support systems, 95-96
Patient care departmental systems, 94-95
Patient care documentation systems, 93
Patient Care Information System (PCIS), 131
Patient care stand-alone systems, 95
Patient outcomes, 153-165, 167-172
Peer Review Organizations (PROs), 167
Privacy of patient, 257-263, 264-270
Problem Classification Scheme, 41
Problem Rating Scale for Outcomes, 42-43
Professional associations, policy development and, 272-278
Psychiatric treatment, patient confidentiality and, 266

Q

Quality assurance programs, 156-158
Quality improvement (QI), 156-158, 193-198
Quality management systems, 96

R

Rehabilitation Potential Patient Classification System (RPPCS), 160
Research, 97, 295-301
Resistance, theories of, 87-88
Resource allocation, 50-51, 245-255
Restructuring of nursing care, 222-228
Rogers, Everett, 116, 117, 118-120, 123

S

Scheduling, computerized, 245-255
Software
availability of, 216-217
installation of, 121-122
pitfalls of, 218
quality of, 218
workflow, 233-235
workgroup, 233, 235
SON-NET, 184
Speech-recognition devices, 239-244
Staff
scheduling of, 245-255
training of, 101-102, 123-124, 216-221, 253-254
Standards of practice, 282-283, 286
Strategic planning, 57-62
Structured analysis (SA), 11
System testing, 122-123

T

Technology assessment, 74-81
Telnet sessions, 175
Total Quality Management (TQM), 50, 68-69, 156-158, 193
Training
computer-based, 129-135
group sessions and, 128-129
tutorials and, 132-134
of staff, 101-102, 123-124, 216-221

U

Uniform Clinical Data Set (UCDS), 171, 275
Uniform Nursing Language System (UNLS), 276
Unit staffing, 50, 245-255
Universal precautions, 196

V

Variance analysis, 207-208
Vendors, joint-development projects and, 108-115
Videoconferencing, 236
Virginia Henderson International Nursing Library, 176, 221
Voice-activated computers, 239-244

W-Z

White House Task Force on Healthcare Reform, 183
Workflow software, 233-235
Workgroup software, 233, 235